Cellular and Molecular Targets
in Allergy and Clinical Immunology

Cellular and Molecular Targets in Allergy and Clinical Immunology

Proceedings of the 26th Symposium of the
Collegium Internationale Allergologicum

**Edited by Stephen Holgate, Gianni Marone,
and Johannes Ring**

*Allergy & Clinical Immunology International –
Journal of the World Allergy Organization,* Supplement 2, 2007

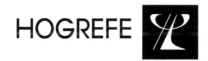

Library of Congress Cataloguing-in-Publication Data

is available via the Library of Congress Marc Database
under the LC Control Number 2007934920

Library and Archives Canada Cataloguing-in-Publication Data

Collegium Internationale Allergologicum. Symposium (26th : 2006 : St. Julian's, Malta)
Cellular and molecular targets in allergy and clinical immunology: proceedings of the 26th Sympo-
sium of the Collegium Internationale Allergologicum / edited by Stephen T. Holgate, Gianni Marone,
Johannes Ring.

Symposium held May 5–10, 2006.
Includes bibliographical references.
ISBN 978-0-88937-358-7

1. Allergy—Congresses.   I. Holgate, S.T.   II. Marone, G. (Gianni)   III. Ring, Johannes, 1945–
IV. Title.
RC583.2.C64 2007   616.97   C2007-905273-8

PUBLISHING OFFICES
USA: Hogrefe & Huber Publishers, 875 Massachusetts Avenue, 7th Floor,
                Cambridge, MA 02139
                Tel. (866) 823-4726, Fax (617) 354-6875, E-mail info@hhpub.com
Europe: Hogrefe & Huber Publishers, Rohnsweg 25, 37085 Göttingen, Germany
                Tel. +49 551 99950-0, Fax +49 551 99950-425, E-mail hhpub@hogrefe.de

SALES AND DISTRIBUTION
USA: Hogrefe & Huber Publishers, Customer Service Department, 30 Amberwood
                Parkway, Ashland, OH 44805, Tel. (800) 228-3749, Fax (419) 281-6883
                E-mail custserv@hhpub.com
Europe: Hogrefe & Huber Publishers, Rohnsweg 25, 37085 Göttingen, Germany
                Tel. +49 551 99950-0, Fax +49 551 99950-425, E-mail hhpub@hogrefe.de

OTHER OFFICES
Canada: Hogrefe & Huber Publishers, 1543 Bayview Avenue, Toronto, Ontario, M4G 3B5
Switzerland: Hogrefe & Huber Publishers, Länggass-Strasse 76, CH-3000 Bern 9

Hogrefe & Huber Publishers
Incorporated and registered in the State of Washington, USA, and in Göttingen, Lower Saxony,
Germany

Printed and bound in Germany
ISBN 978-0-88937-358-7

Table of Contents

Immune Effector Cells

Preface
Cellular and Molecular Targets in Allergy and Clinical Immunology

The prevalence of allergies, asthma, and related allergic diseases has dramatically increased in recent decades. It is no longer true that only developed countries are affected – these diseases are now placing an enormous strain on the health resources in many developing countries around the world.

At the same time, there has been rapid progress in translating molecular science into diagnostic and therapeutic applications. Even with these tremendous developments, large gaps still remain in the way that allergists practice medicine in the office.

One of the aims of the *Collegium Internationale Allergologicum's* biennial symposium and of this book is to bridge this ever-widening gap.

The *Collegium* is a unique organization of the world's most prominent physicians and scientists in the field of allergy and immunology. Membership to the society is by invitation only, and the selection of members is based on scientific accomplishment. As a result of these membership guidelines, the science presented at the biennial symposia of the *Collegium* is considered by many to be the most late-breaking information available.

This volume stands in a long tradition of monographs featuring the highlights of allergy research over the decades. It reflects the most important discussions and summarizes the state of the art across the wide spectrum of experimental and applied, clinical research, as presented at the latest *Collegium* symposium.

Finally, we would like to extend our gratitude to Professor Stephen Holgate and Professor A Barry Kay for their wonderful organization of the 26th Symposium of the *Collegium* on the beautiful and historical island of Malta. Also, to Christina Sarembe and Robert Dimbleby of Hogrefe & Huber for their help in preparing this book and to Stanley Mandarich and Katie Vande Zande at the CIA Secretariat for planning such a wonderful meeting in Malta.

Stephen Holgate
26th Symposium Organizer

Gianni Marone
President

Johannes Ring
Past President

Carl Prausnitz Lecture

From Wheals and Wheeze to Tolerance: Allergy quo vadis?

Johannes Ring

Division Environmental Dermatology and Allergology GSF/TUM, Department of Dermatology and Allergology Biederstein, Technische Universität München, Munich, Germany

Introduction

A little over 100 years ago, in July 1906, the term "allergy" was born in the *Münchner Medizinische Wochenschrift*, vol. 30, page 1457, in an one-and-a-half-page essay by the Viennese pediatrician Clemens von Pirquet (see Figure 1) [46]. It seems adequate on an occasion like this, when we are celebrating this centennial, to reflect briefly on the history and the development of allergy and allergy research over the past century [1, 13, 15, 26, 31, 34, 35, 39, 40, 54, 56, 61, 64, 65, 68, 70] – especially with respect to the work and discoveries contributed by members of the Collegium Internationale Allergologicum (CIA) (see Table 1; the list is, of course, not complete).

Von Pirquet's contribution was to introduce some clarity into a confusion between noxious and protective immunity: While the protective effects of immunization had become apparent and widely used through the work of Jenner,

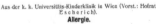

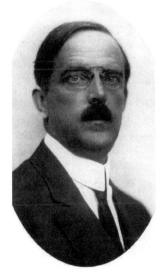

Figure 1. Clemens von Pirquet and the original publication on "Allergie" in the *Münchener Medizinische Wochenschrift* [46].

Pasteur, and Behring, it was the observation of a dramatic adverse reaction after repeated im-

Table 1. Allergy progress in the past century and CIA members.

- Antibodies in serum – IgE: Prausnitz, Ovary, Ishizaka T + K, Johansson, Metzger . . .
- Histamine, mast cells and basophils: Dale, Riley, Uvnas, Selye, Brocklehurst, Feldberg, West, Hahn, Giertz, Schmutzler, Lichtenstein, Austen . . .
- Complement: Kabat, Mayer, Vogt, Rother K + U . . .
- Antigens – allergens – immunochemistry: Ouchterlony, Waldenstroem, Westphal, Inderbitzin, Kraft . . .
- Basic immunology: Coombs, Gell, Roitt, Sela, Milgrom, Macher, Turk, Tada, Ricci, DeWeck, Capron . . .
- Clinical allergy: Hansen, Löffler, Miescher, Kallos P + L, Hjorth, Serafini, Pepys, Salvaggio, Pauwels, Hoigné . . .
- Therapy: Bovet, Loveless, Dukor, Heusser . . .

munization, named "anaphylaxis," which showed that immunization may also be harmful [47]. While von Pirquet's definition comprised all kinds of specifically altered immune reactivity, including decreased immune responses [34], we define allergy today as "specific immunological hypersensitivity leading to disease."

One of the major breakthroughs in the young history of allergy research in the 20th century was the observation of Carl Prausnitz and his fish-allergic colleague Küstner that allergy was transferable with serum: Carl Prausnitz injected serum of Küstner into his own forearm, waited 24 h and then scratched fish allergen onto this area inducing a strong wheal and flare reaction [51]. It is interesting to note that in his original and very exacting publication, Prausnitz mentioned that some days later after a fish meal he felt an itch and a localized flare reaction at the skin test site.

In the following I would like to illustrate through a subjective selection some present-day hotspots in allergy research, with an outlook to future perspectives.

Table 2. Atopy and eczema: Associated candidate genes.

Region	Candidate gene	Additionally associated phenotypes
1q21	EDF, Filaggrin	Ichthyosis vulgaris, eczema
1q31–32	?	Psoriasis
3p24	Chemokine RANTES	–
3q21	CD80, CD86, ?	Eczema
4q35.1	IRF2	–
5q31	SPINK5	Netherton
(Common loci with IBD)	IL-4 cluster	Asthma, Rhinitis, SPT, Total IgE
	IL-13	Asthma, BHR, SPT, Total IgE
	CD14	Asthma, Rhinitis, SPT, Total IgE, Specific IgE
11q13	FCER1B	Atopy, asthma, total and specific IgE
13q12–14	?	–
14q11.2	Mast-cell chymase	–
16p11.2 ± 12.1	IL-4-receptor alpha	Asthma, BHR, Rhinitis, Total IgE
17qcen-q11	NOD2A	Asthma, SPT
17q11-q12	RANTES	Asthma, Eosinophil level
	MCP1	Asthma, Eosinophil level
17q21	Eotaxin	Asthma, BHR
19p13.3	TXA2	Total IgE
19q13.1	TGFB1	Asthma, SPT, Total IgE, Specific IgE

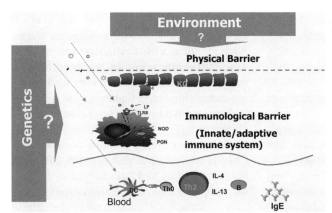

Figure 2. Aspects of disturbed barrier function in atopy (see Weidinger [73]).

The Genetics of Allergy

The fact that certain allergies occur in families was already described for the Julian-Claudian imperial family in Rome [quoted at 53] and gave rise to the creation of the term of "atopy" by Coca and Cooke [15, 61]. Advances in molecular genetics allowed the definition of certain gene loci for clinical phenotypes using different methods like association studies, coupling analyses, or candidate gene analyses. Measuring mutations of DNA sequences within candidate genes and their promoters (single nucleotide polymorphisms – SNPs) yielded exciting new data with regard to many different genes on a high number of chromosomes [16, 70, 73, 75] (see Table 2).

Recently, it was shown that mutations on the filaggrin molecule, coded in the epidermal differentiation complex on chromosome 1, probably cause the barrier defect observed in *ichthyosis vulgaris* (McLean) and are also responsible for the dry skin in atopic eczema [75]. This fits the abnormalities observed in epidermal proteases (like SPINK5 found in Netherton's syndrome), which also act at the pro-filaggrin–filaggrin maturation steps of epidermal keratinization and stratum corneum formation.

These findings have made clear that in the analysis of the pathophysiological events in atopic diseases not only the immunological barrier, be it of the adaptive or the innate immune system, but also the physico-chemical barrier in the epithelial layer [27, 70, 73] play a clear role (see Figure 2).

Future perspectives should include new strategies for the prevention and therapy of this disturbed epithelial barrier in atopic diseases.

Environmental Influences in Allergy

Allergies have shown a dramatic increase in prevalence worldwide over the last decades. The causes for this increase are not yet clear; there are many hypothetical concepts (see Table 3) including several aspects both from allergen exposure, altered immune reactivity, but also regarding environmental influences, both protective and enhancing in nature [24, 36, 37, 40, 42, 51, 53, 57, 71, 73, 74]. The so-called "jungle" [53] or "hygiene" [62] hy-

Table 3. Hypothetical concepts to explain increase in prevalence of atopic diseases [53].

- Increased awareness and improved diagnostics
- Genetic susceptibility
- Psycho-social influences
- Acceleration of daily life
- Allergen exposure
- Decreased stimulation of the immune system ("jungle" or "hygiene" hypothesis)
- Underlying disease
- Iatrogenic (pharmacotherapy)
- Environmental pollution (modern type smog)
- Climate change

pothesis describes decreased immune stimulation through less "immune system training" – triggered by improved hygiene, fewer infections, fewer parasite infestations, and leading to a predominant Th2 response compared to the natural protective Th1 immune response. While this hygiene hypothesis has been valuable in contributing to research, it holds especially true for allergic airway disease, but probably not so for atopic skin disease [57–58]. It is too early to draw practical recommendations for primary prevention. It is, however, clear that vaccination programs are not harmful with regard to allergy development; on the contrary, we were able to show that pertussis vaccination was a major contributor to the decreased asthma prevalence in East German children observed after German reunification in 1990 [53a].

Based on the example of pollinosis, the problem of allergen exposure seems to be a major contributor to increased prevalence [8]. During the last decades we have been exposed to

- more pollen,
- new pollen, and
- altered pollen.

Because of the temperature increase from climate change observed in the northern hemisphere, the average length of the pollen period in Central Europe has increased between 10–14 days for many pollinating plants [72]. This means that pollen are in the air for a longer time and are being emitted in higher quantities.

New pollen species such as *Ambrosia artemisiifolia* have been observed in many regions of Central Europe, where it was unknown 20 years ago, having followed highway motor roads or traveled in bird-food mixtures containing sunflower seed contaminated by ragweed seeds [23a]. It may be estimated that in modern-day Bavaria 10–15% of all patients are skin-prick test positive to ambrosia [unpublished data].

Pollen grains are altered by air pollutants in a polluted atmosphere. Pollen agglomerations have been found over West German cities together with air pollutant particles leading to surface structure changes and to altered aller-

gen liberation [8]. Recently, Behrendt et al. [7] showed that pollen grains themselves release not only allergens but proinflammatory, eicosanoid-like substances as bioactive lipids – pollen-associated lipid mediators (PALMs) – which are either proinflammatory in nature, as leukotriene-like PALMS (octadecaenoic acids attracting and activating neutrophil and eosinophil granulocytes), or immunomodulatory PALMs like prostaglandins (phytoprostanes), thus contributing to the development of a Th2-favoring milieu in the epithelium [63].

Psychosomatic Aspects of Allergy

There is a remarkable analogy between the immune system and the nervous system with regard to the specificity of discrimination, the diversity of signals recognized, and the memory of this specific information over decades [2].

The new field of "psycho-neuro-allergology" has rapidly developed in recent years and proved that factors of the central nervous system such as neurotrophins and neurotransmitters can influence the pathways and cellular reactions of the allergic cascade. On the other hand, cytokines and other important mediators of the allergic reaction also act on nervous cells [2, 10, 29, 33, 53, 65].

Some time ago, John Bienenstock and co-workers [10] showed that anaphylaxis in egg-allergic rats can be conditioned by using an audiovisual stimulus (flashlight and Rolling Stones music); after a few weeks the animals would shock already to the audiovisual stimulus alone, without the presence of ovalbumin. Classic psychological stimuli conditioning allergic symptoms (asthma or itch) include the simple mentioning of allergens (sometimes only anecdotic in character) and the mentioning of the disease, the presence of physicians, being at a hospital, anxiety, or even negative experiences such as personal criticism or lack of acceptance.

The itch sensation is a central feature of many allergic skin diseases and as such an ideal phenomenon to study with regard to psycho-

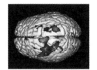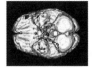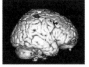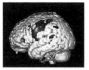

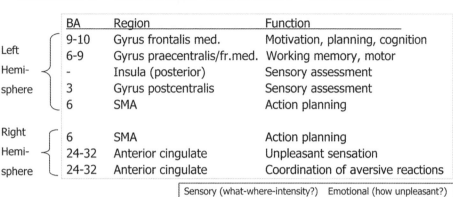

	BA	Region	Function
Left Hemi-sphere	9-10	Gyrus frontalis med.	Motivation, planning, cognition
	6-9	Gyrus praecentralis/fr.med.	Working memory, motor
	-	Insula (posterior)	Sensory assessment
	3	Gyrus postcentralis	Sensory assessment
	6	SMA	Action planning
Right Hemi-sphere	6	SMA	Action planning
	24-32	Anterior cingulate	Unpleasant sensation
	24-32	Anterior cingulate	Coordination of aversive reactions

Sensory (what-where-intensity?)	Emotional (how unpleasant?)
Cognitive (circumstances?)	Countermeasures

Figure 3. Projection of itch sensation on cerebral cortex (Brodmann areas and function) (see [18]).

neuro-allergological mechanisms. It was amazing to become able to visualize itch in the brain using positron emission tomography (PET) (see Figure 3) [18]. One problem of itch research was that there are no on- and off-switches in the itch studies: Once the itch sensation has started, it usually continues for 10–20 minutes. Recently, we were able to develop a methodology using an alternate temperature module to switch histamine-induced itch sensations in humans on and off within 20 s [48]. This will allow future studies using functional MRI associating cerebral activation patterns with distinct characteristics of the itch sensation.

It has also become clear that itch has different qualities that can be differentiated using specialized questionnaires like the Eppendorf Itch Questionnaire (EIQ) (also available in English [19]). Using this EIQ, we found different patterns in descriptive items with regard to suffering and pruritofensive actions between itch induced in atopic eczema, itch in prurigo simplex, or itch in chronic urticaria [19]. These studies found in a cluster component analysis that itch in atopic eczema has parts and components that do not correlate with the intensity or extent of eczematous skin lesions, but rather describe a compulsory component in the CNS associated with atopic itch.

Allergy Diagnostics

While there has been little progress in the last decades with regard to skin and provocation tests, new aspects have emerged from *in vitro* allergy diagnostics [45], with chip array techniques measuring a multitude of allergen specific IgE on one chip [Baron et al., pers. comm], cellular tests like basophil activation [55], as well as measurement of free and bound IgE, a problem that ensues during anti-IgE treatment.

In patients undergoing treatment with a monoclonal antibody against IgE (e.g., omalizumab), IgE measurement is difficult. The classic techniques do not discriminate between free and bound IgE in immune complexes. Therefore, we were interested in developing a tool for overcoming this problem by binding the anti-IgE part of the variable region to a heavy chain of avian origin while not interfering with human antibodies. With this tool we were able to measure reproducibly and reliably free IgE under omalizumab therapy [Ollert, Ariquant, in preparation]. This technique may become more important in the future when several anti-IgE preparations of different sources are available for treatment.

Progress in Therapy

Progress in therapy has usually gone slowly. Almost 20 years have passed from the discovery of leukotrienes in 1979 by Samuelson and coworkers [61] to the first commercially available leukotriene antagonist for clinical practice! Therefore, it helps to look back over longer stretches and compare the progress in allergy therapy today with the procedures and modalities recommended in textbooks before 1950 [15, 25, 32, 56, 61, 66, 69] (see Table 4). Some of it seems still topical, some things have gained new attention through recent hypotheses, and of course some things are just obsolete.

What was already practiced and well-known back then as it is today is allergen-specific immunotherapy (ASIT), soon to celebrate its 100th birthday in 2011 [43]. A short history of this type of essential therapy in allergy, namely, the only causal therapy except allergen avoidance strategies, may help to elucidate the progress. It is beyond question that this type of therapy works for some allergens and for some allergic diseases, as shown in many placebo-controlled randomized clinical trials [22, 41, 44]. The mechanism is still not exactly understood. The increase in IgG antibodies as blocking antibodies was a favored explanation some time ago, while more recently it has been regarded as a marker of a shift from Th2 to Th1 response or of regulatory T cells in the presently favored mechanism [4, 5, 9, 60].

While suppressor cells were in fashion in the 1980s, they have since disappeared and returned as regulatory T-cells through the work of Sakaguchi and coworkers [54]. Recently, several groups found that this concept of the regulatory cells does in fact explain many things that occur during allergen-specific immunotherapy, such as secretion of interleukin 10, TGFβ, and induction of actual tolerance [5, 9, 64].

A major progress in ASIT seems to be the use of recombinant allergens [12, 13, 14, 35, 67], as shown in a number of studies [31, 41]. With this procedure it will in the future be pos-

Table 4. Allergy treatment before 1950 [15, 25, 32, 61, 66, 69].

- Abstinence (avoidance)
- Peptone
- Vaccines (bacterial, tuberculin, etc.)
- Desensitization
- Nonspecific desensitization (histamine, histaminase, etc.)
- Sympathomimetics (ephedrine, amphetamine, adrenaline, etc.)
- Parasympathicolytics (Belladonna, atropine, hyscyamus, stramonium powders, etc.)
- Opiates (opium, codeine, cocaine, etc.)
- Antihistamines
- Expectorants (iodide, etc.)
- Hormones (insulin, pituitary and adrenal extracts)
- Vitamins and calcium
- Hypnotics (urethane, ether, tribromethanol)
- X-ray (thorax, spleen)
- Surgery (cervical sympathectomy, ganglion, etc.)
- Miscellaneous (aspirin, whisky, etc.)

sible to treat individual allergic responses with individually tailored recombinant allergen mixtures, thus avoiding unwanted possible sensitizations via allergen-specific immunotherapy against innocent bystander proteins contained in the extract.

Further progress is to be expected through the use of new adjuvants. For decades, aluminium hydroxide was the only adjuvant, though later tyrosine was used. New adjuvants are emerging based on the above-mentioned hypothetical concepts, trying to shift the deviated immune response from Th2 toward normal. Monophosphoryl lipid as an analogon to lipids from endotoxin is already in clinical use with good results [21]. Certain motives from the bacterial DNA (CpG) of mycobacterial origin have been shown to act very effectively, shifting Th2 responses toward normal both in animal experiments as well as in first clinical trials [17, 38]. Other similar strategies using mycobacterium vaccae or other immunostimulants are in progress.

New progress in allergy therapy also has

been achieved (and further progress is expected) through the use of biologicals, be it soluble receptor antagonists, recombinant cytokines [50], or immunologically active substances. The major breakthrough was achieved through use of antibodies against human IgE [26], which are already employed in the treatment of moderate to severe asthma. Anti-IgE also has been tried in atopic eczema, but with unclear effects. We were able to demonstrate a marked improvement of clinical symptoms in some patients with severe atopic eczema and dramatically increased serum IgE levels (over 10,000 kU/l); also, by studying IgE-secreting plasma cells in the peripheral blood with an immunoscope technique, there was a switch from IgE production toward IgG under omalizumab treatment [Lim, Mempel et al., JACI, in press].

Allergy Prevention

Allergy prevention may be seen on three levels:

- *primary prevention* comprises measures to prevent the occurrence of disease and to eliminate causal factors in disease development in allergy, meaning preventing sensitization;
- *secondary prevention* denotes the earliest recognition of a disease prior to clinical manifestation and prophylaxis in susceptible individuals;
- *tertiary prevention* comprises procedures to prevent sequelae of disease after manifestation as well as the treatment of acute disease including rehabilitation and prevention of a renewed exacerbation.

Primary prevention should start during pregnancy (for instance, smoking avoidance) and includes practical recommendations like breastfeeding, late and then only stepwise addition of solid food in infants, etc.) [11, 30, 33, 71]. The question of pet keeping in the household is still controversial. Platts-Mills [49] showed that increasing concentrations of cat allergen in the air first lead to an increase of IgE antibodies and sensitization, but in higher concentrations, tolerance and IgG4 production may occur with decreased IgE responses. However, to date, most preventive recommendations still advise to avoid pet-keeping as a preventive treatment [11].

In *secondary prevention*, pharmaco-therapeutic intervention strategies have been successfully used, such as cetirizine in the Early Treatment of the Atopic Child (ETAC) study, where it was possible to reduce the incidence of asthma in children with atopic eczema, sensitized to grass pollen and housedust mite [23]. Similar results were obtained using the mast cell blocker and H1 antagonist ketotifen in allergic rhinoconjunctivitis and consequent inhibition of asthma development.

Tertiary prevention strategies include educational programs (asthma and eczema "schools"), climate therapeutic approaches at high altitude or at sea-level as well as long-term pharmaco-therapeutic treatment in a complex patient management approach [53].

Future strategies should strive to implement active allergy prevention programs using "true" vaccination for infants at risk with a mixture of the most common allergen epitopes used as vaccine early in life [28, 71]; however, the ethical implications of these strategies – which have been proven effective in animal experiments – have to be thoroughly considered.

What Makes an Allergist an Allergist?

A look at the diversity of clinical symptoms of allergic diseases, the multitude of trigger factors and elicitors from the environment, and the complex pathophysiological reaction patterns makes it obvious that allergology is nothing but interdisciplinary in character. It is a clinical discipline that gains knowledge from several theoretical specialties, which it then uses in different clinical fields.

The most common bonds keeping allergy specialists together and defining them are

- an expertise and understanding of the relevant clinical diseases,
- a basic understanding of the physiology and

pathophysiology of the human immune response, and

- a profound knowledge on the many and ever more numerous factors contributing to allergy – be they causal (allergens) or modulating (adjuvant factors) – from the environment.

Conclusion

A look at the life of Carl Prausnitz, who after his breathtaking discoveries in basic allergy research became a modest general practitioner on the isle of Wight, shows us that work with patients and the well-being of patients should always be our major aim. Carl Prausnitz-Giles, as he then called himself was such a charismatic doctor that people spoke only of him as "Father Giles." Still, he kept up his interest in scientific progress as a founder of the Collegium Internationale Allergologicum in 1954 together with a group of excellent and dedicated allergists and immunologists from all over the world. Therefore, the CIA has dedicated its main honorary lecture to Carl Prausnitz – and it is with a great feeling of admiration for our predecessors in allergy research and in the humble spirit of scientific inquiry and friendship among colleagues that I want to conclude this lecture.

References

1. Aalberse RC: Structural features of allergenic molecules. Chem Immunol Allergy 2006; 91:134–146
2. Ader R, Felton DL, Cohen N (Eds.): Psychoneuroimmunology (3rd ed.). Academic Press, London, 2001
3. Akdis CA, Akdis M, Trautmann A, Blaser K: Immune regulation in atopic dermatitis. Curr Opin Immunol 2000; 12:641–646
4. Akdis CA, Blaser K: Mechanisms of allergen-specific immunotherapy. Allergy 2000; 55:522–530
5. Akdis M, Blaser K, Akdis CA: T regulatory cells in allergy. Chem Immunol Allergy 2006; 91:159–173
6. Behrendt H, Traidl-Hoffmann C, Plötz S, Mariani V, Kasche A, Thiel M, Jakob T, Ring J: Pollen-associated lipid mediators in the elicitation of allergic reactions. Allergy Clin Immunol Int: J World Allergy Org 2004; Suppl. 1:5–10
7. Behrendt H, Kasche A, Ebner von Eschenbach C, Risse U, Huss-Marp J: Secretion of proinflammatory eicosanoid-like substances precedes allergens release from pollen grains in the initiation of allergic sensitization. Int Arch Allergy Immunol 2001; 124:121–125
8. Behrendt H, Becker W-M: Localization, release and bioavailability of pollen allergens: the influence of environmental factors. Curr Opin Immunol 2001; 13:709–715
9. Bellinghausen I, Brand U, Steinbrink K, Enk AH, Knop J, Saloga J: Inhibition of human allergic T-cell responses by IL-10-treated dendritic cells: differences from hydrocortisone-treated dendritic cells. J Allergy Clin Immunol 2001; 108:242–249
10. Bienenstock J, Befus AD: Mucosal immunology. Immunology 41 1980; 249–270
11. Borowski, C, Schäfer T, Aktionsbündnis (abap): "Allergieprävention – Evidenzbasierte und konsentierte Leitlinie," München: Urban & Vogel, 2005
12. Breiteneder H, Ferreira F, Reikerstorfer A et al.: Complementary DNA cloning and expression in *Escherichia coli* of Aln g I, the major allergen in pollen of alder (*Alnus glutinosa*). J Allergy Clin Immunol 1992; 90: 909–917
13. Breiteneder H, Pettenburger K, Bito A, Valenta R, Kraft D, Rumpold H, Scheiner O, and Breitenbach M: The gene coding for the major birch pollen allergen Betv1, is highly homologous to a pea disease resistance response gene. EMBOJ 1989; 7:1935–1938
14. Chapman MD, Smith AM, Vailes LD, Arruda LK: Recombinant mite allergens. Allergy 1997; 52:374–379
15. Cooke RA: Allergy in theory and practice. Philadelphia: Saunders, 1947
16. Cookson WO, Ubhi B, Lawrence R, Abecasis GR, Whalley AJ, Cox HE et al.: Genetic linkage of childhood atopic dermatitis to psoriasis susceptibility loci. Nat Genet 2001; 27:372–373
17. Creticos PS, Schroeder JT, Hamilton RG, Balcer-Whaley SL, Khattignavong AP, Lindblad R, Li H, Coffman R, Seyfert V, Eiden JJ, Broide D; Immune Tolerance Network Group: Immunotherapy with a ragweed-toll-like receptor 9 agonist vaccine for allergic rhinitis. N Engl J Med 2006; 355:1445–1455
18. Darsow U, Drzezga A, Frisch M, Munz F, Weilke F, Bartenstein P, Schwaiger M, Ring J: Processing of histamine-induced itch in the human cerebral cortex: a correlation analysis with dermal reactions. J Invest Dermatol 2000; 115:1029–1033
19. Darsow U, Scharein E, Simon D, Walter G, Bromm B, Ring J: New aspects of itch patho-

physiology: component analysis of atopic itch using the Eppendorf Itch Questionnaire. Int Arch Allergy Immunol 2001; 124:326–331

20. Denburg JA: Allergy is in the blood at birth. ACII-JWAO 2005; 1–3

21. Drachenberg KJ, Wheeler AW, Stuebner P, Horak F: A well-tolerated grass pollen-specific allergy vaccine containing a novel adjuvant, monophosphoryl lipid A, reduces allergic symptoms after only four preseasonal injections. Allergy 2001; 56:498–505

22. Durham SR, Walker SM, Varga EM et al.: Long-term clinical efficacy of grass-pollen immunotherapy. N Engl J Med 1999; 341:468–475

23. ETAC Study Group. Allergic factors associated with the development of asthma and the influence of cetirizine in a double-blind, randomized placebo-controlled trial: first results of ETAC. Pediatr Allergy Immunol 1998; 9:116–124

23a Gabrio T, Behrendt H, Eitle C et al.: Verbreitung von Ambrosia-Pflanzen in Deutschland. Derm 2006; 12:293–303

24. Gassner-Bachmann B, Wüthrich B: Bauernkinder leiden selten an Heuschnupfen und Asthma. Dtsch med Wschr 2000; 125:924–931

25. Hansen K, Werner M (Eds.): Lehrbuch der klinischen Allergie. Stuttgart: Thieme, 1960.

26. Heusser C, Jardieu P: Therapeutic potential of anti-IgE antibodies. Curr Opin Immunol 1997; 9:805–813

27. Holgate ST, Davies DE, Lackie PM, Wilson SJ, Puddicombe SM, Lordan JL: Epithelial-mesenchymal interactions in the pathogenesis of asthma. Eur Respir J 2000; 105:193–204

28. Holt PG, Macaubas C: Development of long term tolerance versus sensitization to environmental allergens during the perinatal period. Curr Opin Immunol 1997; 9:782–787

29. Iamandescu IB: Psychoneuroallergology. Bucharest: Romcartexim, 1998.

30. Johansson SGO, Haahtela T (Eds.): Prevention of allergy and allergic asthma. World Allergy Organization project report and guidelines. Chemical Immunol Allergy, Vol. 84. Karger: Basel, 2006

31. Jutel M, Jaeger L, Suck R, Meyer H, Fiebig H, Cromwell O: Allergen-specific immunotherapy with recombinant grass pollen allergens. J Allergy Clin Immunol 2005; 116:608–613

32. Kämmerer H: Allergische Diathese. Munich: Bergmann, 1928

33. Kay B (Ed.): Allergy and allergic diseases. Oxford: Blackwell, 1997

34. Kay B: 100 years of "Allergy": can von Pirquet's word be rescued? Clinical and Experimental Allergy 2006; 36:555–559

35. Kraft D, Sehon A (Eds.): Molecular biology and immunology of allergens. Boca Raton: CRC Press, 1993

36. Krämer U, Lemmen CH, Behrendt H, Link E, Schäfer T, Gostomzyk J, Scherer G, Ring J: The effect of environmental tobacco smoke on eczema and allergic sensitization in children. Br J Dermatol 2004; 150:111–118

37. Krämer, U, Koch, T, Ranft, U, Ring, J, Behrendt, H: Traffic-related air pollution is associated with atopy in children living in urban areas. Epidemiology 2000; 11:64–70

38. Krieg AM, Hartmann G, Yi AK: Mechanism of action of CpG DNA (review). Curr Top Microbiol Immunol 2000; 247:1–21

39. Lanzavecchia A: Mechanisms of antigen uptake for presentation. Curr Opin Immunol 1996; 8:348–354

40. Marone G (Ed.): Superantigens and superallergens. Chem Immunol Allergy, Vol 93, pp. I–XIV. Basel, Karger, 2007

41. Müller UR: Recent developments and future strategies for immunotherapy of insect venom allergy. Curr Opin Allergy Clin Immunol 2003; 3:299–303

42. Mutius E von, Weiland SK, Fritzsch C: Increasing prevalence of hay fever and atopy among children in Leipzig, East Germany. Lancet 1998; 351:862–866

43. Noon L: Prophylactic inoculation against hayfever. Lancet 1911; 1572

44. Norman P S: An overview of immunotherapy. J Allergy clin Immunol 1980; 65:87

45. Ollert M, Weissenbacher St, Rakoski J, Ring J: Allergen-specific IgE measured by a continuous random-access immunoanalyzer: Interassay comparison and agreement with skin testing. Clinical Chemistry 2005; 51:1241–1249

46. Pirquet C von: Allergie. Münch Med Wochenschr 1906 30:1457

47. Portier P, Richet C: L'action anaphylactique de certains venins. C R Soc Biol 1902; 54:170–172.

48. Pfab F, Valet M, Sprenger T, Toelle TR, Athanasiadis GI, Behrendt H, Ring J, Darsow U: Short-term alternating temperature enhances histamine-induced itch: A biphasic stimulus model. J Invest Dermatol 2006; 126:2673–2678

49. Platts-Mills T, Vaughan J, Squillace S, Woodfolk J, Sporik R: Sensitization, asthma, and a modified Th2 response in children exposed to cat allergen: a population-based cross-sectional study. Lancet 2001; 357:752–756

50. Plötz S, Simon HU, Darsow U, Simon D, Vassina E, Yousefi S, Hein R, Smith T, Behrendt H, Ring J: Use of an anti-interleukin-5 antibody in the

hypereosinophilic syndrome with eosinophilic dermatitis. N Engl J Med 2003; 349:2334–2339

51. Prausnitz C, Küstner H: Studien über die Überempfindlichkeit. Zentralbl Bakteriol Parasitenkol Infektionkr Abt I Originale 1921; 86:160–169

51a Riedler J, Edler W, Oberfeld G, Schreuer M: Austrian children living on a farm have less hay fever, asthma and allergic sensitization. Clin Exp Allergy 2000; 30:194–200

52. Ring J, Krämer U, Schäfer T, Behrendt H: Why are allergies increasing? Current Opinion Immunology 2001; 13:701–708

53. Ring J: Allergy in practice. Berlin, New York: Springer, 2005

53a Ring J, Krämer U, Oppermann H, Ranft U, Behrendt H: Influence of pertussis/pertussis vaccination on asthma and allergy prevalence in East and West Germany. ACII-JWAO 2004; Suppl. 1, 16:17–24

54. Sakaguchi S: Regulatory T-cells: key controllers of immunologic self-tolerance. Cell 2000; 101:455–458

55. Sanz ML, Maselli JP, Gamboa PM, Oeling A, Dieguez I, de Weck AL: Flow cytometric basophil activation test: a review. J Invest Allergol Clin Immunol 2002; 12:143–154

56. Schadewaldt H.: Geschichte der Allergie (4 volumes). München-Deisenhofen: Dustri, 1980–1984

57. Schäfer T, Merkl J, Klemm E, Wichmann HE, Ring J (KORA Study Group): Does my partner cause my allergy? Allergy 2004; 59:781–785

58. Schäfer T, Krämer U Vieluf D, Abeck D, Behrendt H, Ring J: The excess of atopic eczema in East Germany is related to the intrinsic type. Br J Dermatol 2000; 143:992–998

59. Schäfer T., Meyer T, Ring J, Wichmann HE, Heinrich J: Worm infestation and the negative association with eczema (atopic/nonatopic) and allergic sensitization. Allergy 2005; 60:1014–1020

60. Schmidt-Weber CB, Blaser K: Immunological mechanisms in specific immunotherapy. Springer Semin Immunopathol 2004; 25:377–390

61. Simons, E (Ed.): Ancestors in allergy. New York: Global Med. Com, 1994

62. Strachan DP: Hay fever, hygiene and household size. BMJ 1989; 299:1259–1262

63. Traidl-Hoffmann C, Mariani V, Hochrein H, Karg K, Wagner H, Ring J, Müller MJ, Jakob T, Behrendt H: Pollen-associated phytoprostanes inhibit dendritic cell interleukin-12 production and augment helper type 2 cell polarization. J Exp Med 2005; 201:627–635

64. Umetsu DT, Akbari O, DeKruyff RH: Regulatory T-cells control the development of allergic disease and asthma. J Allergy Clin Immunol 2003; 112:480–487

65. Undem BJ, Kajekar R, Hunter DD, Myers AC: Neural integration and allergic disease. J Allergy Clin Immunol 2000; 106:213–220

66. Urbach E: Klinik und Therapie der allergischen Krankheiten. Wien: Maudrich, 1935

67. Valenta R, Kraft D: From allergen structure to new forms of allergen-specific immunotherapy. Curr Opin Immunol 2002; 14:718–727

68. Valenta R, Seiberler S, Natter S, Mahler V, Mossabeb R, Ring J, Stingl, G: Autoallergy: A pathogenetic factor in atopic dermatitis? J Allergy Clin Immunol 2000; 105:432–437

69. Vaughan WT, Black JH: Practice of allergy. St. Louis: Mosby, 1948

70. Vom Eerdewegh, P, Little, RD, Dapuis, J et al.: Association of the ADAM33 gene with asthma and bronchial hyperresponsiveness. Nature 2002; 418:426–430

71. Wahn U, von Mutius E: Childhood risk factors for atopy and the importance of early intervention. J Allergy Clin Immunol 2001; 107:567–574

72. Walther GR, Post E, Convey P, Menzel A, Parmesan C, Beebee TJC, Fromentin JM, Hoegh-Guldberg O, Bairlein F: Ecological responses to recent climate change. Nature 2002; 416: 389–395

73. Weidinger S, Rodriquez E, Stahl C, Wagenpfeil S, Klopp N, Illig T, Novak N: Filaggrin mutations strongly predispose to early-onset and extrinsic atopic dermatitis. Journal of Investigative Dermatology 2007; 127:724–726

74. Wichmann HE: Environment, life-style and allergy: the German answer. Allergo J 1995; 6:315–316

75. Smith F, Irvine A, Terron-Kwiatkowski A, Sandilands A, Campbell L, Zhao Y, KLiao H, Evans A, Goudie D, Lewis-Jones S, Arseculeratne G, Munro C, Sergeant A, O'Regan G, Bale S, Compton J, DiGiovanna J, Presland R, Fleckman P, McLean WH I: Loss-of-function mutations in the gene encoding filaggrin cause ichthyosis vulgaris. Nature Genetics 2006; 38: 337–342

Johannes Ring

Director, Klinik und Poliklinik für Dermatologie und Allergologie am Biederstein, Technische Universität München, Biedersteiner Str. 29, D-80802 München, Germany, Tel. +49 89 4140-3271, Fax +49 89 4140-3171, E-mail johannes.ring@lrz.tum.de

Regulation of c-Kit Expression in Human Mast Cells

Inhibition of SCF-Induced c-Kit Downregulation by STI 571 (Gleevec) in LAD 2 and HMC-1 Cells

M. Babina, C. Rex, S. Guhl, F. Thienemann, M. Artuc, B.M. Henz, and T. Zuberbier

Department of Dermatology and Allergy, Charité Campus Mitte, Berlin, Germany

Summary. *Background:* c-Kit is of fundamental relevance to mast cell (MC) development and maintenance. However, little is known about the regulation of Kit cell surface levels in normal tissue-derived human MC. *Methods:* Terminally differentiated MC were isolated from human skin and compared with the less mature MC lines LAD2 and HMC-1. Cells were exposed to stem cell factor (±STI571), cycloheximide, actinomycin D, and combinations thereof for 20 min to 16 h, before determination of Kit and other cell surface receptors. *Results:* Ligand-induced Kit internalization was a universal mechanism and detectable in HMC-1, LAD2, and skin MC. STI571, (Gleevec, Novartis, Basel, Switzerland) an inhibitor of the intrinsic Kit kinase, was able to significantly delay Kit internalization in LAD2 and also in HMC-1 cells that carry the D816V mutation and had been considered unresponsive to STI571. Investigations into the natural turnover of Kit expression in the three types of MC revealed that Kit is rapidly affected by the inhibition of fundamental cellular processes, even in nonproliferating skin MC. Only a minor decrease of other cell surface receptors (ICAM-1, ICAM-3, β1 integrin chain) was noticed in the same time frame. On combined treatment, cycloheximide, actinomycin D, and stem cell factor (SCF) displayed additive effects, resulting in an almost complete disappearance of Kit from the cell surface. *Conclusions:* Kit represents a rapidly cycling cell surface receptor. Not only is it rapidly internalized upon binding of its ligand, but it is also greatly affected by inhibition of de-novo-protein synthesis or transcription when viewed against the background of other receptors.

Keywords: mast cells, differentiation, c-Kit, protein turnover, mastocytosis

The receptor tyrosine kinase c-Kit is of fundamental relevance to MC development and maintenance [1–4]. c-Kit expression seems tightly regulated at various levels, including transcription, translation, activation-induced shedding, and internalization upon ligand binding [1, 5]. It is unknown whether posttranscriptional mechanisms contribute to c-Kit expression levels in fully differentiated human mast cells, such as those of the skin. Likewise, the cycling velocity of c-Kit at baseline conditions has not yet been addressed.

Therefore, we studied whether the well-documented pathway of c-Kit internalization induced by the binding of its ligand SCF would also apply to skin MC, and compared the response pattern of the latter with two human mast cell lines (LAD2 and HMC-1). As shown in Figure 1A, SCF-driven downregulation was a universal mechanism and detectable in the three MC subsets alike, suggesting that it was an intrinsic property of c-Kit itself. Among MC subsets, only the kinetics differed slightly with mature skin MC internalizing li-

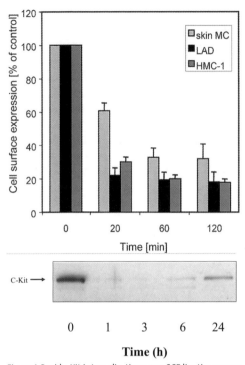

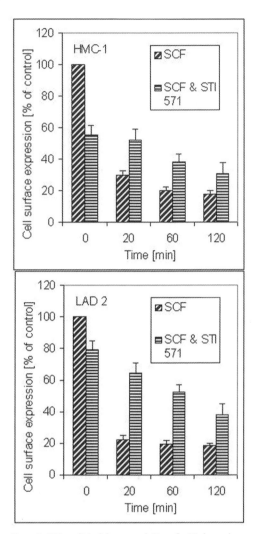

Figure 1. Rapid c-Kit internalization upon SCF ligation occurs independently of the MC subtype and is followed by degradation. (A) MC were purified from human foreskin as described [8]. LAD2 cells were kindly provided by Dr. Metcalfe, and HMC-1 5C6 cells (the parental cell line) by Dr. Butterfield. Skin MC, LAD2 cells (SCF deprived for 24 h) and HMC-1 5C6 cells were treated with SCF (at 100 ng/ml) for the times indicated and cell surface c-Kit expression was evaluated by flow-cytometry (using PE coupled anti-c-Kit mAb 95C3, which recognizes an epitope within the extracellular domain of c-Kit that does not compete with SCF binding). The results are expressed in percent of the mean fluorescence intensity obtained with untreated control cells and are the mean ± SEM of five independent tests: $p < .01$ for LAD2 vs. skin MC and HMC-1 5C6 vs. skin MC at 20 min. All other values were statistically nonsignificant. (B) LAD2 cells (SCF deprived for 24 h) were treated with SCF for 1 h, recovered in fresh media, and then lysed and processed for Western blot analysis after the indicated times, essentially as described [9]. The rabbit anti-c-Kit antibody sc-168 (C-19; Santa Cruz, Heidelberg, Germany) was used at 100 ng/ml at 4° C overnight, followed by goat-anti-rabbit secondary peroxidase conjugate.

Figure 2. SCF-mediated downregulation of c-Kit depends on its intrinsic kinase activity. Both LAD2 and HMC-1 5C6 cells were pretreated with STI 571 (kindly provided by Novartis Pharma, Basel, Switzerland) for 30 min (at 1 μM) and then stimulated with SCF for the times indicated (time 0 = no SCF), as in Figure 1A. The data are the mean ± SEM of four independent experiments.

ganded c-Kit slowly (Figure 1A). Figure 1B demonstrates that SCF-driven downregulation of cell surface c-Kit is accompanied by a rapid degradation that is followed by a relatively slow recovery process.

STI 571 (Gleevec), an inhibitor of the intrinsic c-Kit kinase activity, was then tested for its ability to interfere with SCF-induced loss of c-Kit from the cell surface. As shown in Figure 2, STI 571 was, indeed, able to substantially inhibit and delay the process of c-Kit disappearance in LAD2, but interestingly also in HMC-1 cells that carry the D816V mutation and are considered unresponsive to STI 571 in

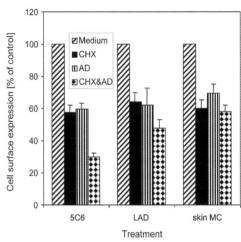

Figure 3. c-Kit dependence on *de novo* protein synthesis is independent of the MC subtype. The three MC subsets were treated with cycloheximide (CHX, 5 μg/ml), actinomycin D (AD, 10 μg/ml) or a combination of both for 16 h analyzed for c-Kit surface expression by means of flow-cytometry. The data are the mean ± SEM of 8 (skin MC), 11 (HMC-1 5C6), and 6 (LAD 2) independent tests. The only statistically significant differences were found in the presence of AD (either alone or when combined with cycloheximide): $p < .05$ for LAD2 vs. HMC-1 5C6 and $p < .001$ for skin MC vs. HMC-1 5C6.

terms of their growth characteristics [6,7]. Our result suggests that SCF-mediated mitogenic promotion is largely uncoupled from SCF-mediated c-Kit internalization and that both may rely on a different array of signaling intermediates activated through the c-Kit receptor. In addition, STI 571 alone, though suppressing SCF-driven internalization, unexpectedly induced some downregulation of Kit on its own, and this was more pronounced in HMC-1 than in LAD2 cells (Figure 2).

To investigate the baseline turnover of c-Kit, the effects of cycloheximide and actinomycin D (either alone or combined) were determined for c-Kit and compared with other cell surface receptors (ICAM-1, ICAM-3, β1 integrin chain). In HMC-1 5C6 cells, only c-Kit was significantly and strongly affected (maximum inhibition > 50% of controls), while only a minor impact on the other cell surface receptors was noted under the same conditions [data not shown].

A comparison among the three MC types revealed that c-Kit levels are rapidly affected by discontinued *de novo* protein translation in all MC subsets, while a suppression of gene transcription had a weaker effect in the two more mature MC subsets as compared to HMC-1 5C6 cells (Figure 3). On combined treatment, cycloheximide, actinomycin D, and SCF displayed additive effects, resulting in an almost complete disappearance of Kit from the cell surface ($p < .01$, data not shown).

In summary, c-Kit represents a rapidly cycling cell surface receptor. The relatively short half-life of Kit, even in the absence of ligand, suggests that carefully balanced Kit levels are of fundamental importance to MC. In addition, it was shown that STI 571 can display some effects in cells expressing one gene copy of Kit that carries the D816V substitution.

References

1. Ashman LK: The biology of stem cell factor and its receptor c-Kit. Int J Biochem Cell Biol 1999; 31:1037–1051.
2. Rönnstrand L: Signal transduction via the stem cell factor receptor/c-Kit. Cell Mol Life Sci 2004; 61:2535–2548.
3. Roskoski R Jr: Signaling by Kit protein-tyrosine kinase – the stem cell factor receptor. Biochem Biophys Res Commun 2005; 337:1–13.
4. Lyman SD, Jacobsen SE: c-kit ligand and Flt3 ligand: stem/progenitor cell factors with overlapping yet distinct activities. Blood 1998; 91:1101–1134.
5. Felli N, Fontana L, Pelosi E, Botta R, Bonci D, Facchiano F, Liuzzi F, Lulli V, Morsilli O, Santoro S, Valtieri M, Calin GA, Liu CG, Sorrentino A, Croce CM, Peschle C: MicroRNAs 221 and 222 inhibit normal erythropoiesis and erythroleukemic cell growth via kit receptor down-modulation. Proc Natl Acad Sci USA 2005; 102:18081–18086
6. Akin C, Brockow K, D'Ambrosio C, Kirshenbaum AS, Ma Y, Longley BJ, Metcalfe DD: Effects of tyrosine kinase inhibitor STI571 on human mast cells bearing wild-type or mutated c-kit. Exp Hematol 2003; 31:686–692.
7. Frost MJ, Ferrao PT, Hughes TP, Ashman LK: Juxtamembrane mutant V560GKit is more sensitive to Imatinib (STI571) compared with wild-type c-kit whereas the kinase domain mutant D816VKit is resistant. Mol Cancer Ther 2002; 1:1115–1124.
8. Babina M, Guhl S, Stärke A, Kirchhof L, Zuberbier T, Henz BM: Comparative cytokine profile

of human skin mast cells from two compartments – strong resemblance with monocytes at baseline, but induction of IL-5 by IL-4 priming. J Leukoc Biol 2004; 75:244–252.

9. Babina M, Schülke Y, Kirchhof L, Guhl S, Franke R, Böhm S, Zuberbier T, Henz BM, Gombart AF: The transcription factor profile of human mast cells in comparison with monocytes and granulocytes. Cell Mol Life Sci 2005; 62:214–226.

Torsten Zuberbier

Department of Dermatology and Allergy, Charité – Universitätsmedizin Berlin, Charitéplatz 1, D-10117 Berlin, Germany, Tel. +49 30 450518135, Fax +49 30 450518919, E-mail torsten.zuberbier@charite.de

Costimulation of Mast Cells via FcεRI and Toll-Like Receptors Markedly Augments Production of Inflammatory Cytokines

H. Qiao, M.V. Andrade, T. Hiragun, Z. Peng, F.A. Lisboa, and M.A. Beaven

Laboratory of Molecular Immunology, National Heart, Lung, and Blood Institute, National Institutes of Health, Bethesda, MD, USA

Summary. *Background:* Mast cells mediate IgE-dependent allergic reactions and protective responses to acute infections through the activation of the pathogen-recognizing Toll-like receptors (TLRs). Clinical reports indicate that allergies are exacerbated by viral/bacterial infections. We investigated whether or not TLRs act in synergy with the IgE receptor, FcεRI, to enhance release of inflammatory mediators from mast cells. *Methods:* Degranulation as well as production of arachidonic acid and cytokines were measured in IgE-primed MC/9 and primary bone marrow-derived mast (BMMC) cells. Signaling events were monitored by immunoblotting and immunoprecipitation techniques, assay of kinase activities, and binding of transcription factors to oligonucleotide arrays. *Results:* Antigen interacted synergistically with TLR2 and TLR4 ligands to enhance the production of TNFα, interleukin (IL)-6, IL-12, and IL-13 by as much as 20-fold. However, the TLR ligands neither stimulated degranulation or release of arachidonic acid nor influenced such responses to antigen probably because these ligands failed to generate a calcium signal. The enhanced cytokine production resulted from synergistic activation of mitogen-activated protein (MAP) kinases in addition to engagement of a broader and more effective repertoire of transcription factors for cytokine gene transcription. Of note, low concentrations of the glucocorticoid, dexamethasone, effectively suppressed responses to antigen and TLR ligands through induction of inhibitory regulators of signaling. *Conclusions:* The synergistic interactions of TLR ligands and antigen may have relevance to the exacerbation of IgE-mediated allergic diseases by infectious agents and to the treatment of these diseases.

Keywords: mast cells, FcεRI, Toll-like receptors, antigen, pathogens, synergy, signaling mechanisms, dexamethasone, cytokines.

Introduction

The underlying feature of IgE-dependent (atopic) diseases such as allergic rhinitis, asthma, atopic dermatitis, food allergies, and systemic anaphylaxis is the activation of mast cells by allergens via the IgE receptor, FcεRI. This results in release of inflammatory and chemotactic mediators and recruitment of leukocytes [1, 2]. The evolutionary benefit of these reactions to the host is unclear. However, recent studies indicate that mast cells express the pathogen-recognizing Toll-like receptors (TLRs) and in doing so provide effective protection against infection through production of inflammatory cytokines [3].

Atopic diseases may be exacerbated by pathogenic agents. Lipopolysaccharide (LPS), a ubiquitous environmental contaminant from Gram-negative bacteria, and respiratory infections caused by viruses, *Mycoplasma pneumoniae*, or *Chlamydiia pneumoniae* may increase the severity of the respiratory manifestations of atopic disease in humans [4] and experimentally induced asthma in mouse [5, 6]. The mechanisms are unclear but circumstantial evidence points to the involvement of TLRs [7, 8]. Of the 13 known TLRs, TLR2 and TLR4 appear to play essential roles in the immune response to pathogens in human lung. Moreover, ligands for TLR2 and TLR4 augment inflammatory responses to inhaled antigen in mouse lung [9, 10]. Each TLR subtype recognizes a particular molecular pattern that is characteristic of pathogen molecules. On binding to the pathogen, the TLRs dimerize and in this manner interact with TLR-associated intracellular signaling molecules [11].

We have suggested that the exacerbation of allergic disease by infection may be fueled by synergistic interactions between FcεRI and TLRs because co-activation of mast cells via FcεRI and TLR2 or TLR4 markedly enhances production of inflammatory cytokines [12]. Here, we review these studies and describe how glucocorticoids suppress responses to both antigen and TLR ligands.

Material and Methods

All procedures were performed as described elsewhere [12]. MC/9, RBL-2H3, and mouse bone marrow-derived mast cells (BMMC) were primed with antigen-specific IgE. Cells were stimulated with TLR ligands, either individually or in combination with the antigen, dinitrophenylated horse serum albumin (DNP–HSA). TLR stimulants included: the synthetic analog of bacterial lipoprotein, tripalmitoyl Cys-Ser-(Lys)$_4$, (P3C) which has preference for TLR2/TLR1 heterodimers; bacterial peptidoglycan (PGN) and macrophage-activating lipopeptide from *Mycoplasma fermentans* (MALP2) which have preference for TLR2/TLR6 heterodimers;

and the TLR4 ligand, *E. coli* lipopolysaccharide (LPS).

Degranulation and release of [^{14}C]arachidonic acid were measured by release of the granule marker, β-hexosaminidase, and of [^{14}C]arachidonate in labeled cultures. Cultures were stimulated for 20 min in a PIPES-buffered saline medium with the indicated stimulants. Commercially available kits were used to analyze production of individual or multiple cytokines by ELISA or antibody arrays. For these determinations, cultures were incubated for 3 h in the presence of stimulants in complete growth medium. Signaling events were evaluated by measurement of cytosolic Ca^{2+} in Fura2-loaded cells, by immunoblotting for detection of activating phosphorylations of protein kinases and transcription factors, by assay of immunoprecipitated kinases *in vitro*, and by use of commercial oligonucleotide binding arrays to determine DNA-binding activity of transcription factors.

Results and Discussion

TLRs and FcεRI Act in Synergy in Stimulating Production of Cytokines

MC/9 and RBL-2H3 cells express TLR2, 3, 4, 5, and 6 and components of TLR-related signaling pathways such as myeloid differentiation protein (MyD88) and the IL-1 receptor-associated kinase, IRAK1 (Figure 1). We found that antigen interacted synergistically with the TLR2 ligands, P3C, PGN, and MALP2, as well as the TLR4 ligand, LPS, to markedly enhance production of TNFα, IL-6, and IL-13 in MC/9 cells and BMMC by up to 20-fold [12]. TNFα production was similarly enhanced in RBL-2H3 cells. This enhancement was most evident at concentrations of antigen or TLR ligand that by themselves elicited minimal production of cytokine. However, the TLR ligands neither stimulated degranulation and release of arachidonic acid nor influenced such responses to antigen probably because these ligands failed to generate a necessary calcium signal. The enhanced cytokine production resulted from synergistic activation of

A. Pathways

B. cDNA Array (MC/9 cells)

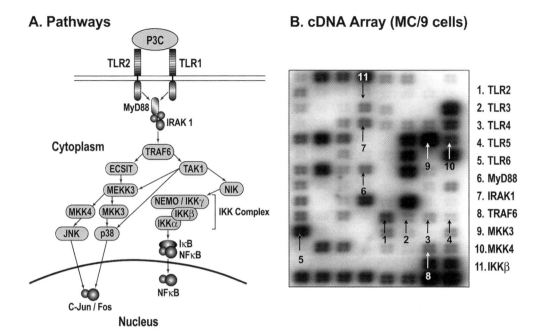

Figure 1. TLRs and related signaling molecules are expressed in mast cells. (A) Pathways activated through the TLR2/TLR1 heterodimer by P3C. (B) Expression of mRNA for the components of these pathways and the individual TLRs as determined by use of a cDNA binding array (Superarray, Frederick MD) in MC/9 cells. Similar results were obtained with RBL-2H3 cells.

JNK and p38 MAP kinase and downstream activation of transcription factors such as AP1 and ATF-2 in addition to the engagement of a more effective repertoire of transcription factors for cytokine gene transcription. For example, some transcription factors were activated more robustly by TLR ligands while others were activated more robustly or even exclusively by antigen.

Inhibitory Actions of Glucocorticoids

Glucocorticoids act through the glucocorticoid receptor to either negatively or positively regulate gene transcription by mechanisms that are referred to as transrepression and transactivation, respectively. The anti-inflammatory actions of glucocorticoids have been attributed to repression of the transcriptional activity of factors that regulate cytokine gene transcription [13]. However, glucocorticoids may act also by transactivation to induce synthesis of inhibitory regulators such as downstream of tyrosine kinase-1 (Dok-1), MAP kinase phosphatase-1 (MKP-1), and Src-like

adaptor protein (SLAP). Dok-1 negatively regulates Ras by activating the Ras GTPase activating protein and as a consequence, the entire Ras/Raf1/Erk pathway as well as release of arachidonic acid in antigen-stimulated mast cells are inhibited [14]. MKP-1 is one of a family of dual-specificity protein phosphatases (also known as DUSPs) that dephosphorylate and inactivate Erk and p38 MAP kinase in mast cells and other types of cells [14–16]. SLAP, first described as an inhibitor of the tyrosine kinase ZAP70 in T-cells, was found to similarly inhibit antigen-stimulated phosphorylation of Syk (a cognate of ZAP70) and downstream signals in RBL-2H3 cells [17]. The induction of these regulators likely accounts for the inhibitory effects of dexamethasone on signaling events in mast cells which are of slow onset, are apparent with as little as 5 nM to 10 nM dexamethasone, and are mediated via the glucocorticoid receptor [18–20].

In addition to suppression of antigen-induced responses, the glucocorticoids effectively suppress TLR-mediated cytokine pro-

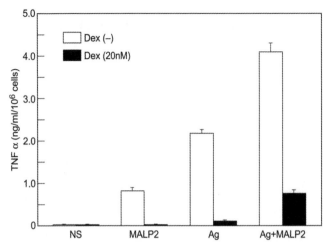

Figure 2. Suppression of TNFα production by dexamethasone. MC/9 cells were incubated for 18 h with 20 ng/ml dexamethasone before stimulation with 100 ng/ml MALP2 for 3 h. TNFα was assayed by ELISA [15]. Values are the mean ± SEM of values from three experiments.

duction. Production of TNFα, for example, is abrogated in dexamethasone-treated cells (Figure 2). As will be reported elsewhere, dexamethasone suppresses key TLR-related signaling pathways. These actions of dexamethasone are shared by other glucocorticoids and are inhibited by the glucocorticoid-receptor antagonist RU486.

Concluding Comments

We suggest that synergy between TLR ligands and allergens might contribute to the exacerbation of atopic diseases by infection. If so, glucocorticoids would be especially effective because of their ability to prevent responses to both types of stimulants.

Acknowledgment

This work is supported by the Intramural Research Program of the National Institutes of Health.

References

1. Wedemeyer J, Tsai M, Galli SJ: Roles of mast cells and basophils in innate and acquired immunity. Curr Opin Immunol 2000; 12:624–631.
2. Prussin C, Metcalfe DD: IgE, mast cells, basophils, and eosinophils. J Allergy Clin Immunol 2003; 111:S486–S494.
3. Marshall JS: Mast-cell responses to pathogens. Nat Rev Immunol 2004; 4:787–799.
4. MacDowell AL, Bacharier LB: Infectious triggers of asthma. Immunol Allergy Clin North Am 2005; 25:45–66.
5. Marsland BJ, Scanga CB, Kopf M, Le GG: Allergic airway inflammation is exacerbated during acute influenza infection and correlates with increased allergen presentation and recruitment of allergen-specific T-helper type 2 cells. Clin Exp Allergy 2004; 34:1299–1306.
6 Kondo Y, Matsuse H, Machida I, Kawano T, SaekiS, Tomari S, Obase Y, Fukushima C, Kohno S: Effects of primary and secondary low-grade respiratory syncytial virus infections in a murine model of asthma. Clin Exp Allergy 2004; 34:1307–1313.
7. Basu S, Fenton MJ: Toll-like receptors: function and roles in lung disease. Am J Physiol Lung Cell Mol Physiol 2004; 286:L887–L892.
8. Cook DN, Pisetsky DS, Schwartz DA: Toll-like receptors in the pathogenesis of human disease. Nat Immunol 2004; 5:975–979.
9. Eisenbarth SC, Piggott DA, Huleatt JW, Visintin I, Herrick CA, Bottomly K: Lipopolysaccharide-enhanced, toll-like receptor 4-dependent T helper cell type 2 responses to inhaled antigen. J Exp Med 2002; 196:1645–1651.
10. Redecke V, Hacker H, Datta SK, Fermin A, Pitha PM, Broide DH, Raz E: Cutting edge: Activation of Toll-like receptor 2 induces a Th2 immune response and promotes experimental asthma. J Immunol 2004; 172:2739–2743.
11. Takeda K, Akira S: Toll-like receptors in innate immunity. Int Immunol 2005; 17:1–14.
12. Qiao H, Andrade MV, Lisboa FA, Morgan K, Beaven MA: FcεRI and Toll-like receptors mediate synergistic signals to markedly augment production of inflammatory cytokines in murine mast cells. Blood 2006; 107:610–618.

13. Hayashi R, Wada H, Ito K, Adcock IM: Effects of glucocorticoids on gene transcription. Eur J Pharmacol 2004; 500:51–62.

14. Hiragun T, Peng Z, Beaven MA: Dexamethasone up-regulates the inhibitory adaptor protein Dok-1 and suppresses downstream activation of the mitogen-activated protein kinase pathway in antigen-stimulated RBL-2H3 mast cells. Mol Pharmacol 2005; 67:598–603.

15. Kassel O, Sancono A, Kratzschmar J, Kreft B, Stassen M, Cato AC: Glucocorticoids inhibit MAP kinase via increased expression and decreased degradation of MKP-1. EMBO J 2001; 20:7108–7116.

16. Jeong HJ, Na HJ, Hong SH, Kim HM: Inhibition of the stem cell factor-induced migration of mast cells by dexamethasone. Endocrinology 2003; 144:4080–4086.

17. Hiragun T, Peng Z, Beaven MA: Cutting Edge: Dexamethasone negatively regulates Syk in mast cells by up-regulating Src-like adaptor protein (SLAP). J Immunol 2006; 177:2047–2050.

18. Rider LG, Hirasawa N, Santini F, Beaven MA: Activation of the mitogen-activated protein kinase cascade is suppressed by low concentrations of dexamethasone in mast cells. J Immunol 1996; 157:2374–2380.

19. Cissel DS, Beaven MA: Disruption of Raf-1/heat shock protein 90 complex and Raf signaling by dexamethasone in mast cells. J Biol Chem 2000; 275:7066–7070.

20. Andrade MV, Hiragun T, Beaven MA: Dexamethasone suppresses antigen-induced activation of phosphatidylinositol 3-kinase and downstream responses in mast cells. J Immunol 2004; 172:7254–7262.

Michael A. Beaven

Bldg. 10 / Rm 8N109, National Institutes of Health, Bethesda, MD 20892-1760, USA, Tel. +1 301 496-6188, Fax +1 301 402-0171, E-mail beavenm@nhlbi.nih.gov

Escherichia coli Hemolysin Provokes Mast Cell Activation

S. Krämer[1,4], G. Sellge[1,3], F. Gunzer[2], and S.C. Bischoff[1,4]

[1]*Department of Gastroenterology, Hepatology and Endocrinology and* [2]*Department of Microbiology and Hospital Hygiene, Medical School of Hannover, Hannover, Germany,* [3]*Pathogénie microbienne moléculaire – INSERM U389, Institut Pasteur, Paris, France,* [4]*Department of Nutritional Medicine and Immunology, University of Hohenheim, Stuttgart, Germany*

Summary. *Background:* Mast cells (MC) are known to play an important role in innate immunity in the murine system. Here we studied the interaction of human intestinal MCs with different *Escherichia (E.) coli* strains. *Methods:* MC, isolated from the human intestine and purified to homogeneity, were infected with different *E. coli* strains. Histamine, sulfidoleukotriens (sLT), TNF-α, and IL-8 were measured by immunoassay. Isogenic *E. coli* mutants were constructed using the suicide vector mutagenesis. *Results: E. coli* hemolysin provoke the expression of mRNA for TNF-α, IL-3, IL-5, IL-6 and IL-8, and the release of histamine, sulfidoleukotrienes, and TNF-α in human intestinal MC. *Conclusion:* Human intestinal MC are sensitive target cells for *E. coli* hemolysin causing degranulation, eicosanoid and cytokine production.

Keywords: human, mast cells, *E. coli*, hemolysin, inflammation

Mast cells (MC) are widely distributed throughout the body. They are preferentially located around blood vessels and nerves and at sites of the host-environment interface such as the skin and the mucosa of the respiratory, gastrointestinal, and urogenital tract. MC are a heterogeneous cell population and those found in different tissues have distinct characteristics. They exert their effector functions by releasing preformed granule-associated and de-novo synthesized mediators such as histamine, proteases, eicosanoids, cytokines, and chemokines. It has been presumed that MC play a relevant role in the defence against bacterial infections [1, 2].

We have established methods for the isolation, purification, and culture of human intestinal MC, providing a unique source of tissue-derived human MC. We investigated the sensibility of human intestinal MC for *E. coli* bacteria and bacterial components. Cytokine mRNA expression was quantified by real-time RT-PCR. Histamine, sulfidoleukotriens (sLT), TNF-α, and IL-8 were measured by immunoassay.

We could show that human intestinal MC were almost unresponsive to apathogenic *E. coli* strains. Noteworthy, also the type 1 fimbriated *E. coli* strain ORN103(pSH2) recognized to stimulate murine and human cord blood-derived MC [3–5] did not affect cytokine gene transcription or the release of proinflammatory mediators despite the fact that the FimH receptor CD48 was expressed [unpublished data]. However, two hemolytic *E. coli* strains provoked the expression of mRNA for TNF-α, IL-3, IL-5, IL-6, and IL-8, and the release of histamine, sulfidoleukotrienes, and TNF-α. Hemolysin (hly) is a member of the RTX (repeats in toxin) family

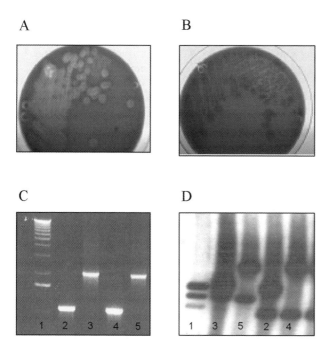

Figure 1. Phenotypical and genotypical characterization of the isogenic hemolysin mutant strains. Phenotypical illustration on blood agar plate from (A) the wildtyp strain *E. coli* ATCC 25922 and (B) the isogenic mutant. Genotypical illustration of the hemolysin gene with (C) PCR and (D) Southern blot. [1] DNA-ladder, [2] isogenic mutant of *E. coli* ATCC 25922, [3] Wildtyp *E. coli* ATCC 25922, [4] isogenic mutant of *E. coli* ATCC 35218, and [5] Wildtyp *E. coli* ATCC 35218.

and has long been described as a cytolytic toxin. However, it is known that sublytic hly concentration mediates degranulation, eicosanoid and nitric oxide production in different cells [6–8]. The hly determinant comprises four genes, hlyC, hlyA, hlyB, and hlyD in transcriptional order. Gene hlyA encodes the inactive prohemolysin which requires posttranslational modification by hlyB. The gene products of hlyC and hlyD are required for the secretion of the 110 kD protein. To test the role of hly we created mutants of the hemolytic *E. coli* strains. PCR fragment, generated from *E. coli* ATCC 25922 and ATCC 35218 by using the primer pair SK1 (5'-GCTCTAGACCACGAGT-TAATAACTGAAGT-3') and SK-2 (5'-CCGAGCTCCAACTGAAACCTCCTGCT-3'), were digested with HpaI, harboring a 1043-bp internal deletion in hlyA. To construct hemolysin-negative mutants of *E. coli* ATCC 25922 and ATCC 35218 we used a suicide vector, as described previously [9]. The phenotypical illustration of the isogenic mutants on blood agar containing erythrocytes shows the lack of large clear zones of hemolysis (Figure 1 A + B). Genotypical illustration of the hemolysin gene were verified with PCR

and Southern blot (Figure 1 C + D). The 1043-bp difference reflects the deletion within the hlyA gene. All tests showed that the presence of an active hly gene was absent.

In contrast to the hemolytic wildtyp strains the isogenic hemolysin-deficient mutant strains failed to induce the release of histamine, sLT, and cytokines in human intestinal MC (unpublished data). In summary, this analysis shows that sublytic hemolysin concentrations of Hly is crucial for bacteria-induced human intestinal MC activation, which enhanced the release of classical MC mediators known to attract and activate granulocytes and other immune cells.

References

1. Echtenacher B, Mannel DN, Hultner L: Critical protective role of mast cells in a model of acute septic peritonitis. Nature 1996; 381:75–77.
2. Malaviya R, Ikeda T, Ross E, Abraham SN: Mast cell modulation of neutrophil influx and bacterial clearance at sites of infection through TNF-α. Nature 1996; 381:77–80.
3. Malaviya R, Ross EA, MacGregor JI, Ikeda T, Little JR, Jakschik BA, Abraham SN: Mast cell

phagocytosis of FimH-expressing enterobacteria. J Immunol 1994; 152:1907–14.

4. Malaviya R, Gao Z, Thankavel K, van der Merwe PA, Abraham SN: The mast cell tumor necrosis factor α response to FimH-expressing *Escherichia coli* is mediated by the glycosylphosphatidylinositol-anchored molecule CD48. Proc Natl Acad Sci USA 1999; 96:8110–8115.

5. Arock M, Ross E, Lai-Kuen R, Averlant G, Gao Z, Abraham SN: Phagocytic and tumor necrosis factor α response of human mast cells following exposure to gram-negative and gram-positive bacteria. Infect Immun 1998; 66:6030–6034.

6. Gunzer F, Bohn U, Fuchs S, Muhldorfer I, Hacker J, Tzipori S, Donohue-Rolfe A: Construction and characterization of an isogenic slt-ii deletion mutant of enterohemorrhagic *Escherichia coli*. Infect Immun 1998; 66:2337–2341.

7. Grimminger F, Scholz C, Bhakdi S, Seeger W: Subhemolytic doses of *Escherichia coli* hemolysin evoke large quantities of lipoxygenase products in human neutrophils. J Biol Chem 1991; 266:14262–14269.

8. Grimminger F, Rose F, Sibelius U, Meinhardt M, Potzsch B, Spriestersbach R, Bhakdi S, Suttorp N, Seeger W: Human endothelial cell activation and mediator release in response to the bacterial exotoxins *Escherichia coli* hemolysin and staphylococcal α-toxin. J Immunol 1997; 159:1909–1916.

9. Rose F, Kiss L, Grimminger F, Mayer K, Grandel U, Seeger W, Bieniek E, Sibelius U: *E. coli* hemolysin-induced lipid mediator metabolism in alveolar macrophages: impact of eicosapentaenoic acid. Am J Physiol Lung Cell Mol Physiol 2000; 279:L100–L109.

Stephan C. Bischoff

Department of Nutritional Medicine and Immunology, University of Hohenheim, Fruwirthstr. 12, D-70593 Stuttgart, Germany, Tel. +49 711 4592-4101, Fax +49 711 4592-4343, E-mail bischoff.stephan@uni-hohenheim.de

Surface Expression, Inhibitory Function and Candidate Ligand for Siglec-8 on Human Mast Cells

H. Yokoi[1], S.A. Hudson[1], N. Bovin[2], R.L. Schnaar[3], and B.S. Bochner[1]

[1]Division of Allergy and Clinical Immunology, Department of Medicine, The Johns Hopkins University School of Medicine, Baltimore, MD, USA, [2]Shemyakin & Ovchinnikov Institute of Bioorganic Chemistry, Russian Academy of Sciences, Moscow, Russia, [3]Department of Pharmacology and Molecular Sciences, The Johns Hopkins University School of Medicine, Baltimore, MD, USA

Summary. Siglec-8 is an inhibitory receptor expressed on eosinophils, basophils and mast cells. While its engagement on eosinophils is known to promote rapid and profound apoptosis, its function on mast cells has not been explored. Using culture-derived human mast cells and an antibody to Siglec-8, no effect of Siglec-8 engagement was seen on cell survival. In contrast, marked inhibition of FcεRI-dependent release of histamine and prostaglandin D2 (PGD2) was observed. Separate studies done in collaboration with the Consortium for Functional Glycomics (www.functionalglycomics.org) identified 6' sulfated sialyl Lewis X as a unique candidate ligand for Siglec-8 and its murine paralog, Siglec-F. These observations suggest that ligand-based future therapies targeting Siglec-8 could have the capacity to reduce both eosinophil survival and mast cell activation.

Keywords: Siglec, mast cell, immunoreceptor tyrosine-based inhibitory motif, mediator release, glycan, ligand

Introduction

Siglecs (sialic acid-binding immunoglobulin-like lectins) are a family of innate immune receptors that are transmembrane I-type lectins characterized by the presence of an N-terminal V-set immunoglobulin domain that binds sialic acid [1]. A unique characteristic of many Siglecs is the presence of conserved cytoplasmic sequences containing tyrosine motifs, suggesting that these molecules possess inhibitory functions (e.g., immunoreceptor tyrosine-based inhibitory motifs or ITIMs). Our previous work has focused on characterizing Siglec-8 expression and function on human eosinophils, where activation by antibody crosslinking induces apoptosis via a process dependent on caspases, generation of reactive oxygen species, and mitochondrial injury [2, 3]. We therefore hypothesized that Siglec-8 crosslinking on mast cells would inhibit their function.

Materials and Methods

Human mast cells were generated from peripheral blood CD34 + precursors using standard culture methods [4, 5]. Stable Siglec-8 transfectants in human embryonic kidney (HEK) cells were generated as described [6]. Mouse IgG1 monoclonal antibody (mAb) 2C4 was generated as described [6]. CD51 mAb was purchased (clone AMF7, IgG1 from Im-

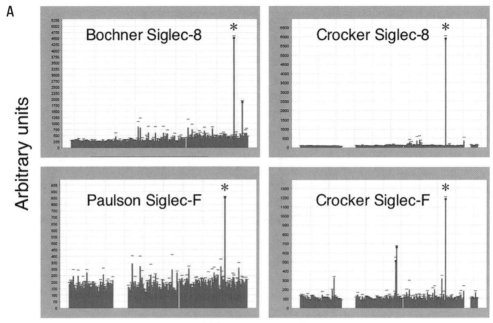

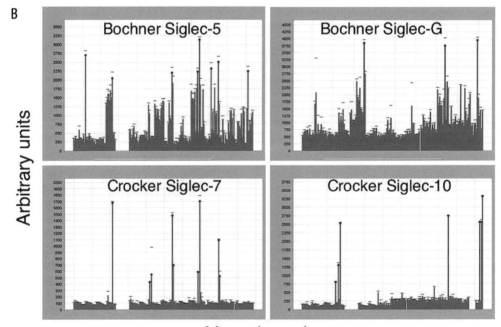

Figure 1. Comparison of results generated by the Consortium for Functional Glycomics Protein-Glycan Interaction Core H using their glycan array and Siglec-8- or Siglec-F-Ig fusion proteins (Panel A) or other CD33-related Siglec-Igs (Panel B) submitted by the investigators indicated. The * in Panel A indicates the location on each array of binding to the glycan 6'-sulfo-sialyl Lewis X, which was not recognized by any of the Siglecs shown in Panel B. Results are reproduced from: www.functionalgly-comics.org/glycomics/publicdata/primaryscreen.jsp

munotech, Miami, FL) as was an antibody recognizing FcεRIα (CRA-1, IgG1 from eBioscience, San Diego, CA). Apoptosis was assayed as previously outlined for eosinophils [2]. Indirect immunofluorescence and flow cytometry were done as described [5]. Release of histamine and prostaglandin D2 were measured by standard assays [7, 8]. Details regarding the development and use of glycan arrays to screen for ligands by the Consortium for Functional Glycomics Protein-Glycan Interaction Core H can be found at www.functionalglycomics.org/static/consortium/resources/resourcecoreh.shtml. Methods specific to screening for Siglec-8 ligand are described in a previous publication [9]. Polyacrylamide polymers were generated as detailed elsewhere [10] (and see www.lectinity.com/catalogonline.php?XX = BP).

Results

As expected, CD34+ blood precursors did not express FcεRI or Siglec-8, but by 4 weeks of culture, cells began to express both FcεRI and Siglec-8 (as detected by immunofluorescence and flow cytometry) in parallel with histamine and tryptase [5]. Siglec-8 surface expression plateaued by 8 weeks. Unlike for eosinophils, antibody crosslinking did not induce mast cell apoptosis, but instead significantly inhibited FcεRI-dependent release of histamine and PGD2 [11].

One of the shortcomings of these studies is that an antibody must be used to engage and crosslink Siglec-8 because its ligand was unknown. However, through the efforts of the Consortium for Functional Glycomics (www.functionalglycomics.org), ligand screening for Siglec-8, along with its mouse paralog, Siglec-F [12] and other CD33-related Siglecs was performed and among about 180 carbohydrate ligands, only one consistent ligand, 6'-sulfo-sialyl Lewis X, was identified, with a relative affinity for Siglec-8 of about 2 μM [9] (Figure 1A). Closely related glycans, including 6-sulfo-sialyl Lewis X (an L-selectin ligand) and sialyl Lewis X (a common selectin ligand) did not bind Siglec-8, and 6'-sulfo-sialyl Lewis X was not found to be a ligand for other CD33-related

Siglecs (Figure 1B). Subsequently, using biotinylated multivalent polyacrylamide polymers, selective binding of 6'-sulfo-sialyl Lewis X, but not structurally related glycan polymers, was confirmed in Siglec-8 transfectants using flow cytometry.

Discussion

Despite the profound proapoptotic effect of Siglec-8 engagement on human eosinophils, and a similar effect of Siglec-9 engagement on human neutrophils [13] as well as preliminary studies showing reduced viability after Siglec-F ligation on mouse eosinophils [14], the Siglec-8 apoptosis pathway does not appear to function in human mast cells. The reason for this is not known but most likely is related to different survival pathways in play for mast cells, as well as their poor ability to generate reactive oxygen species. Instead, the profound inhibitory effect on FcεRI-dependent (and therefore immunoreceptor-based activation motif (ITAM)-dependent) mediator release fits with the present understanding of the importance of the ITIM cytoplasmic domain in CD33-related Siglec signaling including for Siglec-8 [15]. It is also intriguing to note that despite significant genetic and sequence differences, both Siglec-8 and Siglec-F have evolved to preferentially recognize identical glycans. Taken together, these data suggest that aggregation of Siglec-8, either via a monoclonal antibody or perhaps with an appropriate multivalent form of 6'-sulfo-sialyl Lewis X or glycomimetic, could potentially be used therapeutically to reduce eosinophil numbers and mast cell activation in vivo.

Acknowledgments

The authors thank Dr. Walter Hubbard for performing the PGD2 measurements. This work was supported by grant AI41472 from the National Institutes of Health (to BSB), the Consortium for Functional Glycomics grant GM62116 (from NIGMS), and the Russian Academy of Sciences Physicochemical Biology Program (to NB). Dr. Bochner also received support as a Cosner Scholar in Translational Research from Johns Hopkins University. The authors thank Dr. Shelly Heimfeld and David Yadock from the Fred Hutchinson Cancer Research Center and The Program of Excellence in Gene Therapy (PEGT, National Institutes of Health grant HL66947) for providing CD34 + cells. Under a licensing agreement between GlaxoSmithKline and the Johns Hopkins University, Dr. Bochner may be entitled to a share of royalties received by the University on the potential sales of Siglec-8 related products. Dr. Bochner is a paid consultant to GlaxoSmithKline. The terms of this arrangement are being managed by the Johns Hopkins University in accordance with its conflict of interest policies.

References

1. Varki A, Angata T: Siglecs – the major sub-family of I-type lectins. Glycobiology 2006; 16:1R–27R.
2. Nutku E, Aizawa H, Hudson SA, Bochner BS: Ligation of Siglec-8: a selective mechanism for induction of human eosinophil apoptosis. Blood 2003; 101:5014–5020.
3. Nutku E, Hudson SA, Bochner BS: Mechanism of Siglec-8-induced human eosinophil apoptosis: role of caspases and mitochondrial injury. Biochem Biophys Res Commun 2005; 336:918–924.
4. Kulka M, Metcalfe DD: High-resolution tracking of cell division demonstrates differential effects of TH1 and TH2 cytokines on SCF-dependent human mast cell production in vitro: correlation with apoptosis and Kit expression. Blood 2005; 105:592–599.
5. Yokoi H, Myers A, Matsumoto K, Crocker PR, Saito H, Bochner BS: Alteration and acquisition of Siglecs during in vitro maturation of CD34+ progenitors into human mast cells. Allergy 2006; 61:769–776.
6. Kikly KK, Bochner BS, Freeman S, Tan KB, Gallagher KT, D'Alessio K et al.: Identification of SAF-2, a novel siglec expressed on eosinophils, mast cells and basophils. J. Allergy Clin Immunol 2000; 105:1093–1100.
7. Siraganian RP: Refinements in the automated fluorometric histamine analysis system. J Immunol Methods 1975; 7:283–290.
8. Liu MC, Hubbard WC, Proud D, Stealey B, Galli S, Kagey-Sobotka A et al.: Immediate and late inflammatory responses to ragweed antigen challenge of the peripheral airways in asthmatics: cellular, mediator, and permeability changes. Am Rev Respir Dis 1991; 144:51–58.
9. Bochner BS, Alvarez RA, Mehta P, Bovin NV, Blixt O, White JR et al.: Glycan array screening reveals a candidate ligand for Siglec-8. J Biol Chem 2005; 280:4307–4312.
10. Bovin NV: Neoglycoconjugates: trade and art. Biochem Soc Symp 2002:143–160.
11. Yokoi H, Choi OH, Hubbard W, Lee HS, Canning BJ, Lee HH, Ryu SD, Bickel CA, Hudson SA, MacGlashan Jr DW, Bochner BS: Inhibition of Fc(ε)RI-dependent mediator release and calcium flux from human mast cells by Siglec-8 engagement. J Allergy Clin Immunol (in press).
12. Tateno H, Crocker PR, Paulson JC: Mouse Siglec-F and human Siglec-8 are functionally convergent paralogs that are selectively expressed on eosinophils and recognize 6'-sulfo-sialyl Lewis X as a preferred glycan ligand. Glycobiology 2005; 15:1125–1135.
13. von Gunten S, Yousefi S, Seitz M, Jakob SM, Schaffner T, Seger R et al.: Siglec-9 transduces apoptotic and nonapoptotic death signals into neutrophils depending on the proinflammatory cytokine environment. Blood 2005; 106:1423–1431.
14. Zimmermann N, McBride M, Yamada Y, Raper A, Crocker PR, Rothenberg ME et al.: In vivo depletion of murine eosinophils by antibodies to Siglec-F. J Allergy Clin Immunol 2006; 117:S329 (abstr).
15. Guo JP, Nutku E, Yokoi H, Schnaar RL, Zimmermann N, Bochner BS: Siglec-8 and Siglec-F: inhibitory receptors on eosinophils and mast cells. Allergy Clin Immunol Inter – J World Allergy 2007; 19:54–59.

Bruce S. Bochner

Professor of Medicine and Director, Division of Allergy & Clinical Immunology, Johns Hopkins Asthma & Allergy Center, 5501 Hopkins Bayview Circle, Rm. 2B.71, Baltimore, MD 21224-6821, USA, Tel. +1 410 550-2101, Fax +1 410 550-1733, E-mail bbochner@jhmi.edu

Pharmacologic Regulation of Eosinophil Activation: New Therapeutic Targets

M. Capron, D. Staumont, F. Trottein, and D. Dombrowicz

Inserm U547, Institut Pasteur de Lille, Université Lille 2. France

Summary. Eosinophils are associated to various allergic diseases, in particular asthma and atopic dermatitis [1]. In order to investigate new potential therapeutic targets, which would suppress eosinophilia and/or eosinophil function, we examined the role of prostaglandin (PG) D2 and peroxisome proliferator-activated receptors (PPAR) in the regulation of eosinophilia in mouse models of allergen-induced asthma and atopic dermatitis (AD). Mast cells also indirectly participate in asthmatic reactions and potentiate AD [2, 3]. Indeed, upon activation by IgE and multivalent Ag, mast cells release several inflammatory mediators such as histamine, proteases, cytokines, and eicosanoids, including leukotrienes and PGs [4]. Among the latter, PGD_2 is the most abundantly produced. During acute asthmatic episodes, PGD_2 is released by mast cells into the lungs and causes bronchoconstriction. PGD_2, as well as histamine, directly activates eosinophils, promotes their recruitment and affects other key parameters of lung inflammation, in particular vascular permeability.

Keywords: eosinophils, PPAR, PGD_2, allergy, inflammation

PGD_2 acts directly through the D prostanoid receptor (DP)1 ($G_{\alpha s}$-coupled) and DP2 ($G_{\alpha i}$-coupled), two membrane-bound receptors that exert broadly antagonistic effects [5, 6]. Within the immune system, DP1 activation affects the maturation process and the migratory ability of human and mouse dendritic cells (DC), a key cell population involved in the initiation and the regulation of the immune response [7]. On the other hand, DP2 was identified in humans on type 2-polarized lymphocytes (Th2 and Tc2), basophils, eosinophils, and monocytes. Previous studies have revealed that DP2 mediates eosinophil chemotaxis induced by mast cell products and was later identified as a PGD_2 receptor. DP2 activation, thus, accounts for the PGD_2-induced eosinophil chemotaxis and degranulation, while DP1 activation delays their apoptosis onset.

We have demonstrated that mouse eosinophils express DP2 mRNA and provided evidence that DP2 activation induces their migra-tion *in vitro* [8]. We also show that DP2 activation *in vivo* promotes eosinophilia, IgE synthesis, and exacerbates pathology (epithelial thickening in the skin and airway hyperresponsiveness) in two models of Th2-related inflammation: allergic asthma and AD, while DP1 activation exerts opposite effects on these parameters [8]. The mechanisms accounting for DK-PGD_2 action *in vivo* remain unclear, although they likely involve a direct chemotactic effect on eosinophils, while DP1 activation by BW245C rather directly affects DC function and, thus, only indirectly eosinophils. A direct effect of DP2 on eosinophils is of particular relevance in asthma since it has recently been demonstrated, using two strains of eosinophil-deficient mice, that this cell type was crucial to the development of airway remodeling and, according to one report, to airway hyperreactivity.

Taken together, our data reveal an important role of DP2 in promoting Th2-associated skin and lung inflammatory responses in mice, while DP1 activation leads to the opposite outcomes and counter-regulates Th2 inflammation. This suggests that DP2 antagonists might be of therapeutic interest in diseases where eosinophilia could be prevented.

PPARs are members of the nuclear receptor superfamily of ligand-activated transcription factors and key regulators for lipid and glucose metabolism. PPARs are ligand-activated transcription factors existing under 3 isoforms: -α, -β/-δ and -γ and forming dimers with the retinoic acid X receptor (RXR) [9]. Their anti-inflammatory properties, their implication in the mechanism of skin repair after injury, and their expression by several cells types recruited in skin and during inflammatory response suggest a potential regulatory role in allergic pathologies such as asthma and AD. Using PPAR agonists as well as PPAR-α-deficient animals, we found that both PPAR-α and -γ efficiently inhibited allergic asthma, lung eosinophilia, IgE production, and airway remodeling (fibrosis, mucus accumulation) [10] but that PPAR-γ was without effect in AD. By contrast, PPAR-β/-δ most efficiently decreased skin pathology, IgE production, and dermal recruitment of inflammatory cells. Finally, PPAR-α agonists and PPAR-α-deficient animals provided mirror-images in both pathologies, where agonists inhibited disease development and deficient animals displayed a worsening of the symptoms. Taken together, our results suggest that according to the tissue localization of the disease, PPAR isoforms might exert differential effects.

In conclusion, both PGD2 receptors and PPAR could be considered as interesting new therapeutic targets for eosinophil-associated diseases.

References

1. Rothenberg ME, Hogan SP. The eosinophil. Annu Rev Immunol 2006; 24:147–174.

2. Bradding P, Walls AF, Holgate ST. The role of the mast cell in the pathophysiology of asthma. J Allergy Clin Immunol 2006; 117:1277–1284.

3. Bischoff SC. Role of mast cells in allergic and non-allergic immune responses: comparison of human and murine data. Nat Rev Immunol 2007; 7:93–104.

4. Kraft S, Kinet JP. New developments in FcepsilonRI regulation, function and inhibition. Nat Rev Immunol 2007; 7:365–378.

5. Kostenis E, Ulven T. Emerging roles of DP and CRTH2 in allergic inflammation. Trends Mol Med 2006; 12:148–158.

6. Pettipher R, Hansel TT, Armer R. Antagonism of the prostaglandin D2 receptors DP1 and CRTH2 as an approach to treat allergic diseases. Nat Rev Drug Discov 2007; 6:313–325.

7. Angeli V, Faveeuw C, Roye O, Fontaine J, Teissier E, Capron A, Wolowczuk I, Capron M, Trottein F. Role of the parasite-derived prostaglandin D2 in the inhibition of epidermal Langerhans cell migration during schistosomiasis infection. J Exp Med 2001; 193:1135–1147.

8. Spik I, Brénuchon C, Angéli V, Staumont D, Fleury S, Capron M, Trottein F, Dombrowicz D. Activation of the prostaglandin D2 receptor DP2/CRTH2 increases allergic inflammation in mouse. J Immunol 2005; 174:3703–3708.

9. Michalik L, Auwerx J, Berger JP, Chatterjee VK, Glass CK, Gonzalez FJ, Grimaldi PA, Kadowaki T, Lazar MA, O'Rahilly S, Palmer CN, Plutzky J, Reddy JK, Spiegelman BM, Staels B, Wahli W. International Union of Pharmacology. LXI. Peroxisome proliferator-activated receptors. Pharmacol Rev 2006; 58:726–741.

10. Woerly G, Honda K, Loyens M, Papin JP, Auwerx J, Staels B, Capron M, Dombrowicz D. Peroxisome proliferator-activated receptors alpha and gamma down-regulate allergic inflammation and eosinophil activation. J Exp Med 2003; 198:411–421.

David Dombrowicz

Inserm U547, Institut Pasteur de Lille, Calmette BP245, 59019 Lille Cedex, France, Phone +33 320 87 79 67, Fax +33 320 87 78 88, E-mail david.dombrowicz@pasteur-lille.fr

Eosinophil Progenitors at Birth: Intimations of Future Atopy and Inflammation

J.A. Denburg[1], R. Fernandes[1], A.K. Ellis[1], M. Cyr[1], L. Crawford[1], M. Kusel[2], K. Holt[2], B. Holt[2], T. Kebadze[3], S.L Johnston[3], P. Sly[2], S. Prescott[2], and P.G. Holt[2]

[1]Division of Allergy & Clinical Immunology, McMaster University, Hamilton, ON, Canada, [2]Telethon Institute for Child Health Research, Centre for Child Health Research, University of Western Australia, West Perth, Australia, [3]Imperial College London, London, UK

Summary. *Background:* Dysfunctional *adaptive* (T-cell) immunity in the genesis of atopy and asthma is paralleled by abnormalities in *innate* immunity, including the contribution of bone marrow and tissue hemopoietic progenitors, particularly of the eosinophil/basophil (Eo/B) lineage. *Methods:* We examined the relationship between CB progenitor function and phenotype and atopic or respiratory clinical outcomes in the first year of life. *Results:* A consistent relationship was observed between increased numbers of GM-CSF- and IL-3-responsive Eo/B-colony-forming units (CFU) and CB IL-3+ and GM-CSFR+ CD34+ cell numbers, with a reciprocal decrease in the proportion of CB IL-5R+ cells, at birth, and the frequency and severity of respiratory symptoms during early infancy. Kinetic patterns of expression of Eo/B-lineage specific genes, GATA-1, MBP and IL-5Rα were also assessed in random CB samples, in relation to functional Eo/B-CFU present. *Conclusions:* These studies point to potential mechanisms underlying the generation of early life airway inflammatory responses.

Keywords: progenitors; eosinophils; cytokine receptors

Introduction

Allergic diseases are increasing worldwide, including allergic rhinitis and asthma, two important allergic airways diseases with high morbidity [1–3]. It has become apparent that there is an inflammatory basis for these conditions [4]. Efforts to understand the development of these inflammatory responses, their basis in immunity, and factors underlying their increased prevalence have increased in intensity over the last decade, and indeed are critical to the goal of slowing the progression of the allergy epidemic. Being able to identify a biomarker in cord blood (CB) or early life that is strongly predictive of later allergy could allow for early intervention with appropriate treatment, and/or avoidance strategies that could potentially slow or halt the "atopic march."

A number of studies at our institution (with international collaboration) of infants at high risk for developing atopy have shown that the number and functional phenotype of CB stem cells (hemopoietic progenitors) that possess the cell marker CD34 are altered in high-risk infants when compared to low-risk infants [5–7], particularly the eosinophil/basophil (Eo/B) lineage-committed progenitor cell. The collective results of these studies demonstrate that in infants at risk for atopy (based upon maternal skin tests and/or family history), these CD34-positive and Eo/B progenitors are reduced in number, and have a more immature phenotype than those of low risk of atopy (for example, reduced expression of hemopoietic cytokine receptors such as IL-5R or GM-CSFR). Furthermore, we have observed altered clinical outcomes in infants

Allergy Clin Immunol Int: J World Allergy Org, Supplement 2 (2007)

with these dysregulated and immature pheno-types, which are both partially reversible by maternal dietary supplementation with n-3 omega polyunsaturated fatty acids during pregnancy; these results suggest that the CB progenitor phenotype can be *predictive* of future atopic outcomes [7].

It has previously been suggested that the increased severity of respiratory symptoms in infants at high risk for atopy may be due in large part to a developmental delay in postnatal maturation of their adaptive immune functions [8], in particular their diminished capacity to secrete both Th2 and (especially) Th1 cytokines which are central to host defence. However, it is equally feasible that noncognate inflammatory effector cells such as mast cells, basophils, eosinophils (Eo/B) or their progenitors may also play a critical role in determining the degree of inflammation and hence frequency/severity of symptoms accompanying ARI during infancy, thus contributing to asthma development.

Consequently, we have further examined the phenotype and function of CB hemopoietic Eo/B progenitors as potential predictors of the development of inflammation-associated clinical responses.

Results and Discussion

In examining the relationship between CB progenitor function and phenotype and the clinical outcomes in the first year of life, a consistent relationship was observed between increased numbers of GM-CSF- and IL-3-responsive Eo/B-colony-forming units (CFU) and CB IL-3+ and GM-CSFR+ CD34+ cell numbers, with a reciprocal decrease in the proportion of CB IL-5R+ cells, at birth, and the frequency and severity of respiratory symptoms during infancy. Kinetic patterns of expression of Eo/B-lineage specific genes, GATA-1, MBP and IL-5Rα in random CB samples were related to functional Eo/B-CFU present.

The *inverse* correlation between the numbers of *undifferentiated* progenitors (CD34+/45+ cells overall) and respiratory outcomes at one year is in agreement with our previous ob-servation of 'restoration' of a normal, high ambient level of undifferentiated progenitors after PUFA treatment of the mother, which correlates with improved first year atopic outcomes [7,9]. We have also observed that CB CD34+ progenitors of infants at high risk for atopy and asthma (as evidenced by maternal skin prick tests) have an *increased* expression of IL-3R, and *decreased* IL-5R expression. Similarly, in the current study, the absence of IL-5 responsiveness, as well as both IL-3R and GM-CSFR expression on CD34+ CB cells, as well as corresponding functional (CFU) responses to these cytokines, correlated positively and significantly with respiratory symptoms (fever and/or wheeze in response to documented, acute respiratory infection with virus predominantly) from three months through the first year of life. This was also reflected as an apparent *skewing* toward IL-3 and GM-CSF responsive myeloid progenitor phenotypes and functions.

Kinetic patterns of expression of Eo/B-lineage specific genes, GATA-1, MBP and IL-5Rα revealed: expression of MBP mRNA at 48 h and 72 h, correlating positively with the number of Eo/B CFUs, and GATA-1 mRNA expression showing inverse correlations. One interpretation of these findings is that the intensity of acute inflammatory responses in infancy may be directly related to the numbers or phenotype of available hemopoietic progenitors, especially in atopic high-risk infants, in whom an eosinophilic skewing may predominate.

These studies point to potential mechanisms underlying the generation of early life airway inflammatory responses, and indicate that current concepts of the immunological basis for risk of asthma/ atopy must be extended to include *altered progenitor cell differentiation profiles*.

Acknowledgments

This research was supported by grants from the Canadian Institutes for Health Research and AllerGen-NCE Inc. The assistance of Lynne Larocque is gratefully acknowledged.

References

1. Juniper EF: Quality of life in adults and children with asthma and rhinitis. Allergy 1997; 52:971–977.

2. Nathan RA, Meltzer EO, Selner JC, Storms W: Prevalence of allergic rhinitis in the United States. J Allergy Clin Immunol 1997; 99:S808–S814.

3. Executive summary: The impact of allergic rhinitis on quality of life and other airway diseases. Allergy 1998; 53 (Suppl 41):7–31.

4. O'Byrne PM: Pathogenesis of asthma. In: Denburg JA (Ed.), Allergy and allergic diseases: The new mechanisms and therapeutics. Totowa, NJ, Humana Press, 1998, pp. 493–508.

5. Fernandes R, Kusel M, Cyr M, Sehmi R, Holt K, Holt B, Kebadze T, Johnston SL, Sly P, Denburg JA, Holt P. Cord blood hemopoietic progenitor profiles predict acute respiratory symptoms in infancy. Pediatr Allergy Immunol 2007; in press.

6. Cyr MM, Hatfield H, Dunstan JA, Prescott SL, Holt PG, Denburg JA: Relationship of maternal skin test responses to infant cord-blood progenitor cytokine receptor expression [abst]. J Allergy Clin Immunol 2004; 113:S162.

7. Denburg JA, Hatfield HM, Cyr MM, Hayes L, Holt PG, Sehmi R, Dunstan JA, Prescott SL: Fish oil supplementation in pregnancy modifies neonatal progenitors at birth in infants at risk of atopy. Pediatr Res 2005; 57:276–281.

8. Holt PG, Clough JB, Holt BJ, Baron-Hay MJ, Rose AH, Robinson BWS, Thomas WR: Genetic 'risk' for atopy is associated with delayed postnatal maturation of T-cell competence. Clin Exp Allergy 1992; 22:1093–1099.

9. Dunstan JA, Mori TA, Barden A, Beilin LJ, Taylor AL, Holt PG, Prescott SL: Fish oil supplementation in pregnancy modifies neonatal allergen-specific immune responses and clinical outcomes in infants at high risk of atopy: a randomized control trial. J Allergy Clin Immunol 2004; 112:1178–1184.

Judah A Denburg

Department of Medicine, HSC-3V46, McMaster University, 1200 Main Street West, Hamilton, ON L8N 3Z5, Canada, Tel. +1 905 521-2100 ext 76714, Fax +1 905 521-4971, E-mail denburg@mcmaster.ca

CXCR3 Ligand Production by Human Mast Cells in Response to Infection-Associated Stimuli

S.P. Zinn, S.M. Burke, and J.S. Marshall

*Departments of Microbiology & Immunology and Pathology,
Dalhousie University, Halifax, Nova Scotia, Canada*

Summary. *Background:* Mast cells are immune effector cells with a critical role in allergy and host defence. The activation of mast cells by pathogen products or cytokines may contribute to the exacerbations of allergic disease associated with certain infections. *Methods:* Using human umbilical cord blood-derived human mast cells (CBMC) and the human mast cell line HMC-1 5C6 as a model, the selective production of the CCR5 ligand CCL5, and the CXCR3 ligands CXCL10, CXCL9 and CXCL11, was investigated. Following 24 h incubation with IFN-γ, the double stranded RNA analog poly(I:C), synthetic bacterial lipopeptide Pam_3CSK_4 (LP), or Gram positive peptidoglycan, chemokines production was observed. *Results:* Activation with either bacterial lipopeptide or peptidoglycan induced significant production of CCL5 by CBMC. IFN-γ induced high levels of CXCL9 and CXCL10 production while lipopeptide, and poly(I:C) were weaker inducers of CXCL10. Dengue virus infection but not poly(I:C) activation also induced production of other chemokines from CBMC. *Conclusions:* These findings have important implications for the role of resident mast cells in the selective recruitment of effector cells during infection.

Keywords: mast cell, toll-like receptor, IFN-γ, CXCL9, CXCL10, CCL5

Introduction

Mast cells are recognized as immune effector cells important in many physiologic processes. They are considered sentinel cells in host defence and are known to contribute critically to bacterial clearance [1, 2] and parasite expulsion [3, 4]. The ability of mast cells to selectively release a repertoire of both preformed and newly-synthesized cytokines, chemokines and lipid mediators is essential to this defensive dexterity. Their long-term residence in various tissues that interface with the external environment proximal to blood vessels is also critical to this role. Pathogen products, such as bacterial lipopolysaccharide (LPS) and viral dsRNA, have been shown to initiate mast cell mediator release via signaling through Toll-like receptors (TLR) [5–7]. However, during infection mast cells can also be activated via a number of other pathways directly by pathogen products or indirectly by complement components and cytokines [8].

The CXCR3 ligands CXCL9, CXCL10, and CXCL11 are type 1-associated chemokines known to have chemoattractant properties and potent angiostatic ability by virtue of their binding to the chemokine receptor, CXCR3. CXCR3 is expressed on activated T-cells, NK cells, macrophages, dendritic cells and endothelial cells [9–11]. Although CXCR3 ligands are often characterized by their IFN-inducibility, in some cell types they are upregulated following TLR signaling via IFN-regulatory factor (IRF) or NF-κB [12–14].

In the current study, the ability of human mast cells to produce the CXCR3-binding chemokines CXCL9, CXCL10 and CXCL11 was examined following exposure to IFN-γ or a number of pathogen-associated stimuli.

Materials and Methods

Mast Cells

Highly pure human cord-blood-derived mast cells (CBMC) were obtained by long-term culture of umbilical cord blood progenitor cells, as previously described [15], using a modification of the method described by Saito et al. [16]. Briefly, cord blood mononuclear cells were cultured in RPMI 1640 medium (Hyclone, Logan, Utah) supplemented with 20% heat-inactivated FBS (Medicorp), 1% HEPES buffer solution, 1% penicillin-streptomycin (Life Technologies, Burlington, Ontario), 75–100 ng/ml human recombinant stem cell factor (hSCF, Peprotech), 20% CCL-204 conditioned supernatant (source of IL-6) and 10^{-6} M prostaglandin E2 (PGE₂). Following 6–8 weeks of culture, the percentage of mast cells was assessed following toluidine blue staining of cytocentrifuge preparations. Only preparations confirmed to contain 95% pure mast cells based on metachromatic staining were employed.

The human mast cell line HMC-1 5C6 was grown in Iscove's modified Dulbecco's medium (Hyclone) supplemented with 10% FBS and 1% penicillin-streptomycin. Cells were cultured in fresh medium every 3–4 days.

Cell Activation and Cytokine Analysis

CBMC were activated for 24 h with research grade human recombinant IFN-γ (Meloy Laboratories, Inc., Springfield, VA), synthetic lipopeptide (Pam₃CysSerLys₄ from EMC Microcollections, Tübingen, Germany), poly(I:C) (Calbiochem, San Diego, CA), *Staphylococcus aureus* derived peptidoglycan (PGN; Fluka Bio-

Chemika, distributed by Sigma, St. Louis, MO), or yeast zymosan from *Saccharomyces cereviseae* (Sigma). Activation supernatants were examined for CXCL9, CXCL10, CXCL11, CCL5 and IL-12 production by ELISA. Sensitivity for the IL-12 ELISA was 30 pg/ml. Sensitivity for all chemokine assays was 20 pg/ml.

Results and Discussion

Mast Cell CXCR3 Ligand Production in Response to Bacterial and Fungal Products

CBMC and HMC-1 5C6 were activated at a concentration of 1×10^6 cells/ml for 24 h with increasing doses of zymosan or LP. Significant CXCL10 production was observed in HMC-1 5C6 cultures in response to LP at a concentration of 100 μg/ml ($n = 4$; $p < .05$). Although the extent of responses varied between subjects, when evaluated as a group, CBMC stimulation with LP induced significant production of CXCL10 ($n = 7$; $p < .05$, see Figure 1). LP also had a significant detrimental effect on CBMC cell viability over 24 h at this dose. Significant CXCL9 production was not detected following stimulation with LP and no significant production of any CXCR3 ligand was consistently observed in response to zymosan (data not shown). Although both LP and zymosan are known to activate cells via a TLR2 dependent pathway, they differed sub-

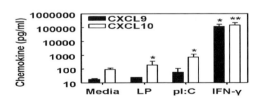

Figure 1. Infection-associated stimuli induce selective production of chemokines by CBMC. CBMC were stimulated with bacterial lipopeptide (LP; 100 mg/ml), peptidoglycan (PGN; 100 μg/ml), poly(I:C) (pI:C; 100 mg/ml), or interferon-γ (IFN; 100 U/ml) (B) for 24 h. Chemokine production was measured in cell-free supernatants by ELISA. Graph is representative of 4–8 separate experiments, where mean ± SEM are displayed. *represents $p < .05$, **represents $p < .01$, compared with media control.

stantially in their ability to induce CXCR3 ligands.

Mast cells have been shown previously to produce the chemokine CCL5 in response to some pathogens [6]. PGN and LP activated CBMC were examined for their production of CCL5 over 24 h. Significant CCL5 production was observed in response to 100 µg/ml PGN (127.8 ± 50.8 pg/ml; $p < 0.05$) and 1 and 100 µg/ml LP (145.2 ± 73.8 pg/ml; $p < 0.05$; 277.2 ± 79.3 pg/ml; $p < .01$; respectively) as compared to 20.4 ± 13.8 pg/ml observed in resting CBMC ($n = 4$, Figure 1). The presence of significant levels of CCL5 production following TLR2 activator stimulation of human mast cells may be complementary to CXCR3 ligand production with respect to effector cell recruitment during early infection.

CXCR3 Ligand Production Following Stimuli Associated with Viral Infection

Poly(I:C) is frequently used to mimic virus-induced double stranded RNA. This can activate cells via TLR3 or by utilizing a number of other mechanisms including interactions with PKR. When CBMC were activated with poly(I:C) we observed a significant CXCL10 response (720.5 ± 465.6 pg/ml; $p < .05$) but no significant induction of production of other CXCR3 ligands (Figure 1). Similarly, active infection of HMC-1 cells with dengue virus strongly induced CXCL10 (data not shown). This demonstrates the ability of viral associated stimuli to directly activate human mast cells to produce this chemokine.

IFN-γ is known to be produced in the context of viral infection, predominately by T-cells. In other cell types, IFN-γ is a potent inducer of CXCR3 ligand [17]. CBMC treatment for 24 h with IFN-γ led to a highly significant CXCL9 and CXCL10 response. The CXCR3 ligand response to IFN-γ was much greater than that observed using LP or poly(I:C). In the context of infection, IFN-γ responses arising later in primary infection or as a result of secondary infection could dramatically enhance the chemokine production

by local resident mast cells and subsequent effector cell recruitment.

Overall, these findings demonstrate that human mast cells are able to produce significant levels of CXCR3 ligands when stimulated with pathogen products. During early infection, resident mast cells can respond to a variety of pathogen products by producing CXCR3 ligands, particularly CXCL10 and CXCL11, with concurrent production of CCL5 observed in many cases. As the specificities of mast cell stimulation and mediator release during infection are explored, opportunities to control these responses therapeutically can be exploited.

Acknowledgments

This work was supported by the Atlantic Chapter of the Canadian Breast Cancer Research Foundation and the Canadian Institutes of Health Research.

References

1. Echtenacher B, Mannel DN, Hultner L: Critical protective role of mast cells in a model of acute septic peritonitis. Nature (1996; 381:75–77.

2. Malaviya R, Ikeda T, Ross E, Abraham SN: Mast cell modulation of neutrophil influx and bacterial clearance at sites of infection through TNF-α. Nature 1996; 381:77–80.

3. Knight PA, Wright SH, Lawrence CE, Paterson YY, Miller HR: Delayed expulsion of the nematode *Trichinella spiralis* in mice lacking the mucosal mast cell-specific granule chymase, mouse mast cell protease-1. J Exp Med 2000; 192:1849–1856.

4. Maruyama H, Yabu Y, Yoshida A, Nawa Y, Ohta N: A role of mast cell glycosaminoglycans for the immunological expulsion of intestinal nematode, Strongyloides venezuelensis. J Immunol 2000; 164:3749–3754.

5. McCurdy JD, Olynych TJ, Maher LH, Marshall JS: Cutting edge: distinct Toll-like receptor 2 activators selectively induce different classes of mediator production from human mast cells. J Immunol 2003; 170:1625–1629.

6. Marshall JS, King CA, McCurdy JD: Mast cell cytokine and chemokine responses to bacterial

and viral infection. Curr Pharm Des 2003; 9:11–24.

7. Kulka M, Alexopoulou L, Flavell RA, Metcalfe DD: Activation of mast cells by double-stranded RNA: evidence for activation through Toll-like receptor 3. J Allergy Clin Immunol 2004; 114:174–182.

8. Prodeus AP, Zhou X, Maurer M, Galli SJ, Carroll MC: Impaired mast cell-dependent natural immunity in complement C3-deficient mice. Nature 1997; 390:172–175.

9. Janatpour MJ, Hudak S, Sathe M, Sedgwick JD, McEvoy LM: Tumor necrosis factor-dependent segmental control of MIG expression by high endothelial venules in inflamed lymph nodes regulates monocyte recruitment. J Exp Med 2001; 194:1375–1384.

10. Loetscher M, Gerber B, Loetscher P, Jones SA, Piali L, Clark-Lewis I, Baggiolini M, Moser B: Chemokine receptor specific for IP10 and mig: structure, function, and expression in activated T-lymphocytes. J Exp Med 1996; 184:963–969.

11. Penna G, Sozzani S, Adorini L: Cutting edge: selective usage of chemokine receptors by plasmacytoid dendritic cells. J Immunol 2001; 167:1862–1866.

12. Jaruga B, Hong F, Kim WH, Gao B: IFN-γ/STAT1 acts as a proinflammatory signal in T-cell-mediated hepatitis via induction of multiple chemokines and adhesion molecules: a critical role of IRF-1. Am J Physiol Gastrointest Liver Physiol 2004; 287:G1044–G1052.

13. Majumder S, Zhou LZ, Chaturvedi P, Babcock G, Aras S, Ransohoff RM: Regulation of human IP-10 gene expression in astrocytoma cells by inflammatory cytokines. J Neurosci Res 1998; 54:169–180.

14. Borgland SL, Bowen GP, Wong NC, Libermann TA, Muruve DA: Adenovirus vector-induced expression of the C-X-C chemokine IP-10 is mediated through capsid-dependent activation of NF-κB. J Virol 2000; 74:3941–3947.

15. Lin TJ, Issekutz TB, Marshall JS: Human mast cells transmigrate through human umbilical vein endothelial monolayers and selectively produce IL-8 in response to stromal cell-derived factor-1 α. J Immunol 2000; 165:211–220.

16. Saito H, Ebisawa M, Tachimoto H, Shichijo M, Fukagawa K, Matsumoto K, Iikura Y, Awaji T, Tsujimoto G, Yanagida M, Uzumaki H, Takahashi G, Tsuji K, Nakahata T: Selective growth of human mast cells induced by Steel factor, IL-6, and prostaglandin E2 from cord blood mononuclear cells. J Immunol 1996; 157:343–350.

17. Proost P, Vynckier AK, Mahieu F, Put W, Grillet B, Struyf S, Wuyts A, Opdenakker G, Van Damme J: Microbial Toll-like receptor ligands differentially regulate CXCL10/IP-10 expression in fibroblasts and mononuclear leukocytes in synergy with IFN-γ and provide a mechanism for enhanced synovial chemokine levels in septic arthritis. Eur J Immunol 2003; 33:3146–3153.

Jean S. Marshall

Department of Microbiology & Immunology, Sir Charles Tupper Medical Building, Dalhousie University, Halifax, Nova Scotia B3H 1X5, Canada, Tel. +1 902 494-5118, Fax +1 902 494-5125, E-mail jean.marshall@dal.ca

Molecular Mechanisms of Hygiene Hypothesis

N. Kondo, Z. Kato, H. Kaneko, T. Fukao, E. Matsui, and M. Aoki

Department of Pediatrics, Graduate School of Medicine, Gifu University, Japan

Summary. The occurrence of autoimmune diseases (Th1 diseases) and allergic diseases (Th2 diseases) has increased in more affluent, Western, industrialized countries. One theory proposed to explain the increase in the prevalence of autoimmune and allergic diseases is that it results from a decrease in the prevalence of childhood infections. This theory dates back to the mid-1960s in relation to Th1-mediated diseases. In 1989, Strachan first proposed that this theory might also explain the increase in Th2-mediated diseases, and it has subsequently come to be called the hygiene hypothesis. Here, we explore the molecular mechanisms of the hygiene hypothesis.

Keywords: hygiene hypothesis, Th1, Th2, IL-10

Imbalance in the Th1 and Th2 System

Atopy is characterized by enhanced IgE responses to environmental antigens. The production of IgE is upregulated by Th2 cytokines, in particular, IL-4, and is downregulated by Th1 cytokines, in particular, IFN-γ. IL-12 and IL-18, which produce IFN-γ, are the important cytokines that downregulate IgE production. Imbalance in the Th1 and Th2 system induces the allergic diseases.

Molecular Mechanism of Hygiene Hypothesis

Several molecular mechanisms concerning the hygiene hypothesis have been suggested. The stimulation of the innate immune system by endotoxin (lipopolysaccharide, LPS) may be important in the ontogeny of the normal immune system and a decreased frequency of allergic diseases. CD25-positive T-cells and other regulatory T-cells produce IL-10 and TGF-β, and act to downregulate both Th1-mediated responses and Th2-mediated responses. The decrease in antigenic or endotoxin (LPS) stimulation related to the decrease in the frequency of childhood infections has resulted in a decrease in the levels of regulatory cytokines such as IL-10.

We investigated the effects of IL-10 on Th1 and Th2 cytokine production, and IL-10 and TGF-β production of LPS or Der f-1-stimulated peripheral blood mononuclear cells (PBMCs).

First, we investigated the effects of IL-10 on IL-12, IFN-γ and IL-4 production of PHA-stimulated PBMCs (data not shown). We demonstrated that exogenous IL-10 suppressed dose-dependently the production of IL-12 and IFN-γ, which are Th1 cytokines. In contrast, IL-10 did not suppress the production of IL-4, which is a Th2 cytokine. However, in this case IL-4 levels were very low. Therefore, we used antigen-specific T-cell clones to further investigate the effects of IL-10. In this case, IL-4 levels were detectable and IL-10 was shown to suppress the production of IL-4 from the T-cell clone. TGF-β did not effect the IL-4 production. Therefore, we conclude that IL-10 suppresses accelerated production of both Th1 and Th2 cytokines and in doing so serves as an immunomodulator and preserves the Th1 and Th2 balance.

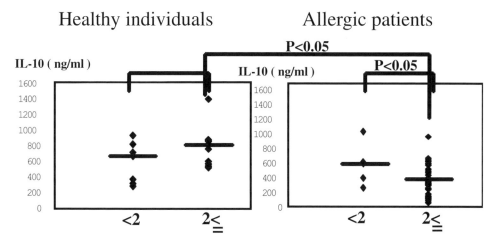

Figure 1. Comparison of IL-10 production from LPS-stimulated PBMCs, in children less than 2 years old and more than 2 years old.

We then investigated IL-10 and TGF-β production by LPS- or Der f/1-stimulated PBMCs; IL-10 production from PBMCs from stimulated with LPS allergic patients was significantly lower than that of the healthy controls. Moreover, we compared IL-10 production of LPS-stimulated PBMCs from children who were less than 2-years old and more than 2-years old. In allergic children, IL-10 production in those less than 2-years old was the same as the healthy controls, but in those older than 2 years it was significantly lower than that of the healthy controls (Figure 1): In the case of Derf-1 stimulated PBMCs, IL-10 production by the allergic patients was significantly lower than that of the healthy controls.

These data suggest that in allergic patients, IL-10 production by PBMCs, by LPS or Derf-1 stimulation, is impaired when compared with healthy controls. This may result from poor development of regulatory T-cells since these are the principle sources of IL-10.

Conclusion

In innate immunity, in childhood infections such as bacterial endotoxin, LPS stimulation through toll-like receptors (TLRs) may induce regulatory T-cells and IL-10 production, and these may regulate the level of Th2 balance. As a result we suggest this can prevent the development of allergic disorders. If the level of stimulation is insufficient then it fails to regulate Th1 and Th2 balance and as a consequence will reduce the protection from developing allergic diseases.

Reference

1. Weiss ST: Eat dirt – the hygiene hypothesis and allergic diseases. N Engl J Med 2002; 347:930–931.

Naomi Kondo

Department of Pediatrics, Graduate School of Medicine, Gifu University, Yanagito 1-1, Gifu 501-1193, Japan, Tel. +81 58-230-6380, Fax +81 58 230-6387, E-mail nkondo@gifu-u.ac.jp

Vascular Endothelial Growth Factor-A Is Stored in and Immunologically Released from Human Basophils

G. Marone[1], N. Prevete[1], I. Fiorentino[1], S. Staibano[2], F.W. Rossi[1], C.A. Leone[3], A. Genovese[1], A.F. Walls[4], and A. de Paulis[1]

[1]Divisione di Immunologia Clinica ed Allergologia e Centro Interdipartimentale di Ricerca di Scienze Immunologiche di Base e Cliniche (CISI), Università di Napoli Federico II, Naples, Italy, [2]Dipartimento di Scienze Biomorfologiche e Funzionali – Sezione di Anatomia Patologica, Università di Napoli Federico II, Naples, Italy, [3]Divisione di Otorinolaringoiatria e Chirurgia Cervico-facciale, Azienda Ospedaliera Monaldi, Naples, Italy, [4]Immunopharmacology Group, Southampton General Hospital, Southampton, UK

Summary. Angiogenesis is a multistep complex phenomenon critical for several inflammatory and neoplastic disorders. Basophils, normally confined to peripheral blood, can infiltrate the sites of chronic inflammation. We have characterized the expression and localization of vascular endothelial growth factor-A (VEGF-A) in these cells. Basophils express mRNA for three isoforms of VEGF-A (121, 165, and 189). Peripheral blood basophils contain VEGF-A localized in secretory granules. Immunologic activation of basophils induced the release of VEGF-A. Our data suggest that basophils play a role in angiogenesis and inflammation through the expression and release of several isoforms of VEGF-A.

Keywords: angiogenesis, mast cells/basophils, chemotaxis, vascular endothelial growth factor

Angiogenesis is a complex multistep process that culminates in the growth of new blood vessels from the microcirculation [1]. It is critical for such chronic inflammatory disorders as bronchial asthma [2, 3], rheumatoid arthritis [4] and tumor growth [1]. Vascular endothelial growth factor (VEGF) is the most potent pro-angiogenic mediator known so far. Originally identified from its ability to induce vascular permeability [5], VEGF is a potent inducer of endothelial proliferation, migration, and survival. It also acts as a proinflammatory cytokine [1]. The VEGF family includes VEGF-A, VEGF-B, VEGF-C, VEGF-D, and placental growth factor (PlGF) [6]. Some components of the VEGF family have differentially spliced forms that differ in their ability to enhance angiogenesis. For example, human VEGF-A has at least six isoforms: 121, 145, 165, 183, 189, and 204. Of these, VEGF-A$_{165}$ and VEGF-A$_{121}$ are the most potent proangiogenic isoforms [7].

Human basophils express the high affinity receptor for IgE (FcεRI) and synthesize several proinflammatory mediators and a restricted Th2-like profile (IL-4 and IL-13) (8–10).

Basophils are normally present only in peripheral blood; however, they can infiltrate the sites of chronic inflammation [11, 12].

In this study we found that peripheral blood basophils express mRNA for various members of the VEGF-A family. VEGF-A was detected in secretory granules of basophils, and immunologically activated basophils released VEGF-A.

Materials and Methods

Purification of Peripheral Blood Basophils

Basophils were purified from the peripheral blood of healthy volunteers, aged from 20 to 39 years, negative for HIV-1, HIV-2, HCV and HBV antibodies [10].

Reverse Transcriptase-Polymerase Chain Reaction

Total cellular RNA was isolated by TRIzol Reagent (Invitrogen, Ltd., Paisley, UK). Reversely-transcribed DNA were then amplified, using VEGF-A$_{121-165}$ specific 5' sense (GTGAATGCAGACCAAAGAAAG) and 3' antisense (AAACCCTGAGGGAGGCTC) primers, VEGF-A$_{189}$ specific 5' sense (GTA-TAAGTCCTGGAGCGT) and 3' antisense (AAACCCTGAGGGAGGCTC) primers. The reaction products were analyzed by electrophoresis in 1% agarose gel containing ethidium bromide, followed by photography under ultraviolet illumination [13].

VEGF-A ELISA

VEGF-A was measured in duplicate determinations with a commercially available ELISA (R & D System, Minneapolis, MN).

Double-Immunofluorescence Staining on Cytospin

Basophils left to adhere on glass precoated with 1% poly-L-lysine (Menzel-Glaser, Germany) (1 hour at 22°C) were fixed in 4% paraformaldehyde. Nonspecific bonds were blocked by preincubating fixed basophils with nonimmune normal horse serum (30 min at 22°C) [14]. Double-immunofluorescence staining was carried out by incubation overnight at 4°C with the primary antibodies BB1 (1:100) [15] and rabbit polyclonal anti-VEGF-A (Santa Cruz Biotechnology, Inc.) (1:300). Cells were then incubated with FITC-conjugated rabbit anti-mouse secondary antibody (Dako, Glostrup, Denmark) (1:50) (1 h at 22°C) and with TRITC-conjugated swine anti-rabbit secondary antibody (Dako, Glostrup, Denmark) (1:50) (1 h at 22°C). Nuclear counterstaining was carried out with DAPI (4',6-diamidine-2'-phenylindole dihydrochloride; Roche, Basel, Switzerland) (15 min at 22°C). Finally, the glasses were mounted with coverslips using a synthetic mounting medium. Basophils were observed under a Zeiss Axiovert 100 M microscope fitted with an LSM 510 confocal system. Images were recorded with LSM 510 software (Zeiss, Oberkochen, Germany).

Results

The human VEGF-A gene encodes three major peptides constituted by 121, 165, and 189 amino acids as a result of alternative splicing. VEGF-A$_{165}$, the predominant isoform in several normal and tumor cells, lacks the residues encoded by exon 6, whereas VEGF-A$_{121}$ lacks the residues encoded by exons 6 and 7 [1]. We investigated the expression of VEGF mRNA in basophils purified (> 99%) from peripheral blood of normal donors. The analysis of PCR products by electrophoresis in agarose gel revealed three VEGF-A isoforms (VEGF-A$_{121}$, VEGF-A$_{165}$, and VEGF-A$_{189}$) and two VEGF-B isoforms (VEGF-B$_{167}$, and VEGF-B$_{186}$). By contrast, VEGF-C and VEGF-D mRNA were not detected in human basophils [data not shown].

We next investigated VEGF-A expression in basophils at protein level. Basophils were lysed in 1% Triton X-100/PBS in the presence of protease inhibitors, and the total content of immunoreactive VEGF-A was measured by specific ELISA. In eight experiments, the mean ± SEM concentration of VEGF-A in basophils was 144.4 ± 10.8 pg/10^6 cells.

To verify the intracellular localization of VEGF-A, we analyzed cytospins of enriched preparations of peripheral blood basophils by confocal microscopy. BB1 is a monoclonal antibody that specifically recognizes basogranulin in secretory granules of human basophils, but not in neutrophils, lymphocytes or monocytes (11, 15). We also used a rabbit polyclonal antibody raised against amino acids 1–140 of human VEGF-A. In addition to VEGF-A reactivity in BB1$^+$ basophils, the presence of VEGF-A in BB1$^-$ cells was also shown. This indicates that in peripheral blood there are other cells, in addition to basophils, that constitutively express VEGF-A. An interesting feature was the colocalization of BB1$^+$ secretory granules with VEGF-A immunoreactivity. These results are compatible with the hypothesis that VEGF-A is stored in secretory granules of peripheral blood basophils.

In five experiments we evaluated the release of VEGF-A and of histamine in basophils immunologically activated with anti-IgE. Basophils challenged with anti-IgE rapidly released histamine, which peaked at 15 min. Stimulation of basophils with anti-IgE caused a small increase in VEGF-A secretion that was detectable after 30 min. The release of VEGF-A induced by anti-IgE reached a plateau after 2–4 h of incubation [data not shown].

Discussion

In this study we have found that basophils purified from healthy donors express mRNA for three major isoforms of VEGF-A (121, 165, and 189) and two isoforms of VEGF-B (167 and 186). Interestingly, VEGF-C and -D mRNA, two mediators of lymphatic development [1], were not detected in basophils. Therefore, basophils display a selective expression of certain members of the VEGF family.

We also demonstrate that VEGF-A is stored in secretory granules and that the immunologic release of this cytokine from basophils follows a biphasic pattern: rapid release (30 min)

after the anti-IgE challenge and a second wave, 2–4 h after challenge. The first wave of release is probably due to the secretion of preformed VEGF-A, whereas the second wave presumably represents *de novo* synthesis.

It is possible that VEGF-A synthesized and released from basophils plays a dual role in inflammatory angiogenesis. First, VEGF-A released from circulating basophils might activate VEGF receptors present on circulating endothelial cell precursors and immune cells; second, VEGF-A released from basophils infiltrating the sites of chronic inflammation might represent a local source of an important angiogenic factor.

Mast cells, basophils and eosinophils are considered primary effector cells in allergic disorders [8]. It has been shown that human mast cells synthesize and release several isoforms of VEGF-A [16–19]. Also human eosinophils exert direct proangiogenic effects [20]. Here we demonstrate that human basophils express and release VEGF-A. Taken together, these findings support the hypothesis that the release of angiogenic factors from primary effector cells of allergic inflammation could represent a relevant aspect of tissue remodeling in chronic allergic disorders.

The results of this study might have practical implications in several inflammatory disorders in which basophils that infiltrate sites of inflammation play a prominent role [8, 11, 12]. In fact, we found that basophils are a source of VEGF-A, which is the most potent angiogenic factor known so far. This finding raises the possibility that basophils might modulate angiogenesis. Pharmacological manipulation of the VEGF network, which is already showing promise in relation to neoplastic angiogenesis [21], might also be effective in disorders associated with basophil recruitment and activation.

Acknowledgments

This work was supported in part by grants from the Ministero dell'Istruzione, dell'Università e della Ricerca, the Istituto Superiore di Sanità (AIDS Project 40D.57), Ministero della Salute "Alzheimer Project" and Regione Campania.

We would like to dedicate this paper to Rita Levi Montalcini on the occasion of the 20th anniversary of the Nobel Prize. We thank Graziella Persico for her inspiring comments and encouragement during these studies.

References

1. Carmeliet P: Angiogenesis in life, disease and medicine. Nature 2005; 438:932–936.
2. Hoshino M, Nakamura Y, Hamid QA: Gene expression of vascular endothelial growth factor and its receptors and angiogenesis in bronchial asthma. J Allergy Clin Immunol 2001; 107:1034–1038.
3. Chetta A, Zanini A, Foresi A, Del Donno M, Castagnaro A, D'Ippolito R, Baraldo S, Tesi R, Saetta M, Olivieri: Vascular component of airway remodeling in asthma is reduced by high dose of fluticasone. Am J Respir Crit Care Med 2003; 167:751–757.
4. Ikeda M, Hosoda Y, Hirose S, Okada Y, Ikeda E: Expression of vascular endothelial growth factor isoforms and their receptors Flt-1, KDR, and neuropilin-1 in synovial tissues of rheumatoid arthritis. J Pathol 2000; 191:426–433.
5. Senger DR, Galli SJ, Dvorak AM, Perruzzi CA, Harvey VS, Dvorak HF: Tumor cells secrete a vascular permeability factor that promotes accumulation of ascites fluid. Science 1983; 219:983–985.
6. De Falco S, Gigante B, Persico MG: Structure and function of placental growth factor. Trends Cardiovac Med 2002; 12:241–246.
7. Frelin C, Ladoux A, D'angelo G: Vascular endothelial growth factors and angiogenesis. Ann Endocrinol (Paris) 2000; 61:70–74.
8. Marone G, Triggiani M, Genovese A, de Paulis A: Role of human mast cells and basophils in bronchial asthma. Adv Immunol 2005; 88:97–160.
9. Schroeder JT, Lichtenstein LM, MacDonald SM: Recombinant histamine-releasing factor enhances IgE-dependent IL-4 and IL-13 secretion by human basophils. J Immunol 1997; 159:447–452.
10. Genovese A, Borgia G, Björck L, Petraroli A, de Paulis A, Piazza M, Marone G: Immunoglobulin superantigen protein L induces IL-4 and IL-13 secretion from human FcεRI+ cells through interaction with κ light chains of IgE. J Immunol 2003; 170:1854–1861.
11. Ying S, Robinson DS, Meng Q, Barata LT, McEuen AR, Buckley MG, Walls AF, Askenase PW, Kay AB: C-C chemokines in allergen-induced late-phase cutaneous responses in atopic subjects: association of eotaxin with early 6-h eosinophils, and of eotaxin-2 and monocyte chemoattractant protein-4 with the later 24-h tissue eosinophilia, and relationship to basophils and other C-C chemokines (monocyte chemoattractant protein-3 and RANTES). J Immunol 1999; 163:3976–3984.
12. de Paulis A, Prevete N, Fiorentino I, Walls AF, Curto M, Petraroli A, Castaldo V, Ceppa P, Fiocca R, Marone G: Basophils infiltrate human gastric mucosa at sites of *Helicobacter pylori* infection, and exhibit chemotaxis in response to *H. pylori*-derived peptide Hp(2–20). J Immunol 2004; 172:7734–7743.
13. de Paulis A, Montuori N, Prevete N, Fiorentino I, Rossi FW, Visconte V, Rossi G, Marone G, Ragno P: Urokinase induces basophil chemotaxis through a urokinase receptor epitope that is an endogenous ligand for formyl peptide receptor-like 1 and -like 2. J Immunol 2004; 173:5739–5748.
14. Tuccillo C, Cuomo A, Rocco A, Martinelli E, Staibano S, Mascolo M, Gravina AG, Nardone G, Ricci V, Ciardiello F, Del Vecchio Blanco C, Romano M: Vascular endothelial growth factor and neo-angiogenesis in *H. pylori* gastritis in humans. J Pathol 2005; 207:277–284.
15. McEuen AR, Buckley MG, Compton SJ, Walls AF: Development and characterization of a monoclonal antibody specific for human basophils and identification of a unique secretory product of basophil activation. Lab Invest 1999; 79:27–38.
16. Boesiger J, Tsai M, Maurer M, Yamaguchi M, Brown LF, Claffey KP, Dvorak HF, Galli SJ: Mast cells can secrete vascular permeability factor/vascular endothelial cell growth factor and exhibit enhanced release after immunoglobulin E-dependent upregulation of Fcε receptor I expression. J Exp Med 1998; 188:1135–1145.
17. Grützkau A, Krüger-Krasagakes S, Baumeister H, Schwarz C, Kögel H, Welker P, Lippert U, Henz BM, Möller A: Synthesis, storage, and release of vascular endothelial growth factor/vascular permeability factor (VEGF/VPF) by human mast cells: implication for the biological significance of $VEGF_{206}$. Mol Biol Cell 1998; 9:875–884.
18. Abdel-Majid RM, Marshall JS: Prostaglandin E_2 induces degranulation-independent production of vascular endothelial growth factor by human mast cells. J Immunol 2004; 172:1227–1236.
19. Cao J, Papadopoulou N, Kempuraj D, Boucker WS, Sugimoto K, Cetrulo CL,. Theoharides TC: Human mast cells express corticotropin-releas-

ing hormone (CRH) receptors and CRH leads to
selective secretion of vascular endothelial
growth factor. J Immunol 2005; 174:7665–7675.
20. Puxeddu I, Alian A, Piliponsky AM, Ribatti D,
Panet A, Levi-Schaffer F: Human peripheral
blood eosinophils induce angiogenesis. Int J Biochem Cell Biol 2005; 37:28–636.
21. Ferrara N, Kerbel RS: Angiogenesis as a therapeutic target. Nature 2005; 438:967–974.

Gianni Marone

Department of Clinical Immunology and Allergy, University
of Naples Federico II, Via S. Pansini 5, I-80131 Napoli, Italy, Tel.
+39 081 770-7492, Fax +39 081 746-2271, E-mail marone@un-
ina.it

Identification of Nitric Oxide Regulated Genes with Potential Roles in Signaling in Mast Cells

J.W. Coleman and D.D. Metcalfe

Laboratory of Allergic Diseases, NIAID, NIH, Bethesda, MD, USA

Summary. *Background.* Nitric oxide (NO) inhibits mast cell cytokine production as well as specific consequences of allergic inflammation; and may therefore represent a critical disease-limiting mechanism. In this study we examined if NO might regulate certain genes with potential roles in the suppression or recovery of mast cells after exposure to NO. *Methods:* Mouse bone marrow-derived mast cells (BMMC) were exposed for 2 h at 37°C to NO and RNA extracted and reverse transcribed. The resultant cDNA was labeled with Cy3-dUTP (test samples) or Cy5-dUTP (reference sample) and competitively hybridized to a spotted gene array. *Results:* Forty-five genes were significantly regulated by NO. Of particular interest, expression of dual specificity phosphatase 1 (Dusp1) was upregulated 17-fold and of heme oxygenase 1 (Hmox1) 13-fold. Western blot experiments confirmed that NO upregulated Hmox1 protein but this occurred subsequent to NO-induced changes in signaling. Furthermore, an inhibitor of Hmox1 suppressed IL-6 production by BMMC. *Conclusions:* The expression of several mast cell genes is regulated by NO. Of particular interest, NO induced expression of Hmox1 is implicated in recovery of mast cell function.

Keywords: mast cells, nitric oxide, gene expression, signaling

Introduction

Nitric oxide (NO) [1], inhibits mast cell degranulation [2], cytokine production and Fos and Jun activation [3]; as well as specific consequences of allergic inflammation [4]. NO may therefore represent a disease-limiting mechanism in allergy. The time dependence and reversibility of NO effects suggest that it acts via gene regulation. The aim of this study was to identify genes with roles in mast cell suppression or recovery after NO exposure.

Materials and Methods

Mouse bone marrow-derived mast cells (BMMC) were exposed for 2 h at 37°C to S-ni-trosoglutathione (GSNO, a natural storage form of NO), spermine–NO (SPNO, a synthetic NO source) or to control medium. RNA was extracted, reverse transcribed; and the cDNA labeled with Cy3-dUTP (test samples) or Cy5-dUTP (reference sample) and competitively hybridized to mouse spotted array set Mmbe38 ($N = 4$) [5]. Cy3/Cy5 ratios for each gene were calculated and analyzed by MicroArray DataBase (mAdb) and Significance Analysis of Microarrays (SAM) [5]. Western blot and cytokine analyses were done as described [3].

Results and Discussion

Statistical analysis of gene array data revealed 45 genes were significantly regulated by NO

Table 1. Genes in BMMC whose expression upregulated by NO. Fold = mRNA levels in cells exposed to NO relative to levels in control cells.

Fold	Gene	Description
23.7	Egr1	Early growth response 1
22.7	Jun	Jun oncogene
17	Dusp1	Dual specificity phosphatase 1
13	Hmox1	Heme oxygenase 1
5.6	Ccl4	Chemokine C-C ligand 4
5.5	Phlda1	Pleckstrin homology-like domain A1
5.3	Hod	Hypothetical protein E130218H05
4.7	Ier5	Immediate early response 5
4.6	Tnfrsf12a	Tumor necrosis factor receptor superfamily member 12a
4.5	Rgs1	Regulator of G-protein signaling 1
4.2	1810032O08Rik	RIKEN cDNA 1810032O08
4	Junb	Jun-B oncogene
4	Atf4	Activating transcription factor 4
3.7	Crem	cAMP responsive element modulator
3.4	Rabgef1	RAB guanine nucleotide exchange factor 1
3	Myd116	Myeloid differentiation primary response gene 116
2.8	Slc16a3	Solute carrier family 16 member 3
2.8	Nfkbiz	Nuclear factor kappa beta inhibitor zeta
2.7	Hk2	Hexokinase 2
2.7	Ier2	Immediate early response 2

(GSNO and SPNO combined data), a number that includes 2.2 false positive genes at a Δ value (SAM) of 0.9. Of these, 40 genes were upregulated (by 1.5–23.7-fold) and 5 downregulated (by 0.43–0.62-fold). Table 1 lists the top 20 genes upregulated. Many of these genes are known to be responsive to nitrosative stress. A proportion of these have defined roles in cell signaling pathways. For example, dual specificity phosphatase 1 (Dusp1) (MAP kinase phosphatase 1) inactivates Erk1/2 and JNK in several cell types [6]; while heme oxygenase 1 (Hmox1), via its product carbon monoxide, regulates IL-2 production by T-cells [7]. Western blot experiments confirmed that NO upregulated Dusp1 and Hmox1 at the protein level in BMMC (not shown). Hmox1 protein was induced at 6 h but not at 2 h after exposure to NO, while at 2 h NO completely blocked IgE/Ag-induced synthesis of Fos and Jun proteins (not shown). Therefore, the inhibitory effect of NO on Fos and Jun signaling occurs prior to induction of Hmox1 protein. In further experiments, incubation of BMMC with tin protoporphyrin-IX (SnPP-IX), a selective Hmox1 inhibitor, led to a concentration-dependent inhibition of IgE/Ag-induced

IL-6 production by BMMC without influencing the inhibitory actions of NO. These results suggest that induction of Hmox1 by NO is important in the recovery of cytokine responsiveness of mast cells following nitrosative stress and that Hmox1 activity is required to maintain mast cell functionality.

References

1. Swindle EJ, Metcalfe DD and Coleman JW: Rodent and human mast cells produce functionally significant intracellular reactive oxygen species but not nitric oxide. J Biol Chem 2004; 279: 48751–48759.
2. Eastmond NC, Banks EMS and Coleman JW: Nitric oxide inhibits IgE-mediated degranulation of mast cells and is the principal intermediate in IFN-γ-induced suppression of exocytosis. J Immunol 1997; 159:1444–1450.
3. Davis BJ, Flanagan BF, Gilfillan AM, Metcalfe DD and Coleman JW: Nitric oxide inhibits IgE-dependent cytokine production and Fos and Jun activation in mast cells. J Immunol 2004; 173:6914–6920.
4. Speyer CL, Neff TA, Warner RL, Guo RF, Sarma JV, Riedemann NC, Murphy ME, Murphy HS, Ward PA: Regulatory effects of iNOS on acute

lung inflammatory responses in mice. Am J Pathol 2003; 163:2319–2328.

5. http://madb.niaid.nih.gov/index.shtml

6. Camps M, Nichols A, Arkinstall S: Dual specificity phosphatases: a gene family for control of MAP kinase function. FASEB J 2000; 14:6–16.

7. Pae HO, Oh GS, Choi BM, Chae SC, Kim YM, Chung KR, Chung HT: Carbon monoxide produced by heme oxygenase-1 suppresses T-cell proliferation via inhibition of IL-2 production. J Immunol 2004; 172:4744–51.

J.W. Coleman

Department of Asthma, Allergy and Respiratory Science, King's College London, 5th Floor, Thomas Guy House, Guy's Hospital, London SE1 9RT, UK, Tel. +44 1773 820 514, E-mail john.coleman@kcl.ac.uk

Molecular Mechanisms for Regulation of the Human High-Affinity IgE Receptor β Subunit (FcεRIβ) Gene Expression

C. Ra and K. Takahashi

Division of Molecular Cell Immunology and Allergology, Advanced Medical Research Center, Nihon University Graduate School of Medical Sciences, Tokyo, Japan

Summary. *Background:* FcεRI is a key molecule for mast cell activation in allergic reactions, consisting of three subunits, one α, one β, and a homodimer of γ. There has recently been some focus on the β-chain as a dualfunctional (positive/negative) signal regulator based on the unique β-chain ITAM (immunoreceptor tyrosine-based activation motif), which contains two canonical, and one noncanonical tyrosine residues. Therefore, we considered that elucidation of regulatory mechanisms of the β-chain gene expression would make a meaningful contribution to research on the manipulation of allergic reaction.

Keywords: FcεRI, mast cell, transcriptional regulation, chromosome, allergy, GM-CSF

Methods

Genomic DNA fragments of the human FcεRI β-chain gene were tested for their transcriptional regulatory activities employing a reporter assay with luciferase activity. To identify factors constituting the complex with myeloid zinc finger/four and a half LIM-only protein 3 (MZF-1/FHL3), yeast three-hybrid screening assay was performed. To elucidate that nuclear transcription factor YC (NFYC) and histone deacetylase (HDAC) interact with the β-chain gene, chromatin immunoprecipitation (ChIP) assay was employed.

Results

For activation of the β-chain gene promoter, two Oct-1 binding sites in the 5' untranslated region were essential. The transcription factor MZF-1 repressed β-chain gene expression through an element in the fourth intron. FHL3 was a repressive cofactor for MZF-1 and together they formed a very large molecular weight complex in the nucleus. Addition of granulocyte macrophage-colony stimulating factor (GM-CSF) facilitated the formation of the MZF-1/FHL3 complex in the nucleus and reduced the β-chain gene expression through deacetylation of histones by histone deacetylases (HDACs) that are recruited to the fourth intron of the β-chain gene.

Conclusion

The repression of β-chain gene expression in the presence of GM-CSF is dependent on de-

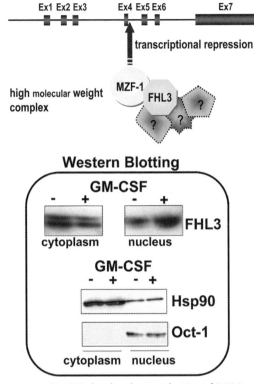

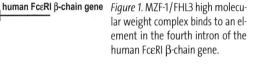

Figure 1. MZF-1/FHL3 high molecular weight complex binds to an element in the fourth intron of the human FcεRI β-chain gene.

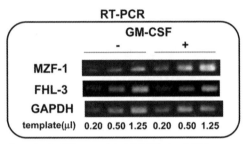

Figure 3. GM-CSF upregulated MZF-1 but not FHL3 expression. Expression levels of mRNAs for MZF-1 and FHL3 in KU812 cells cultured in the presence or absence of GM-CSF

Figure 2. GM-CSF induced nuclear translocation of FHL3 in human mast cells. Cytoplasmic and nuclear fractions from KU812 cells treated with or without GM-CSF were prepared. Total protein from each fraction was analyzed by Western blotting with anti-FHL3 antibody. As a control, total protein from each fraction was analyzed by Western blotting with anti-Oct-1 antibody. Similarly, total protein from each fraction was employed for immunoblotting with anti-Hsp90 antibody.

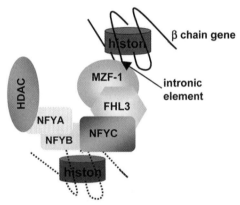

Figure 4. A model for histone deacetylation-mediated regulation of FcεRIβ gene expression.

acetylation of histones by HDACs that are recruited to the β-chain gene through the MZF-1/FHL3/NFY complex.

FcεRI is a crucial molecule for mast cell activation in an allergic reaction, consisting of three subunits, one α, one β, and a homodimer of γ. The α-chain binds IgE through its extracellular domain, while the β- and γ-chains mediate intracellular signals through ITAM. Although a functional receptor is expressed both as tetramers (αβγ2) and trimers (αγ2) in humans [1], intracellular signals [2, 3], in addition to cell surface expression of the receptor [4], have been reported to be significantly amplified by the β-chain, indicating that the β-chain increases cell activation sensitivity to stimulation by allergens. There has recently been a focus on the β-chain as a dualfunctional (positive/negative) signal regulator based on the unique β-chain ITAM, which contains two canonical and a noncanonical tyrosine residues [5, 6, 7]. These studies suggest that the β-chain is a fine regulator of FcεRI-mediated cell activation to precisely control the allergic reaction. It is, therefore, reasonable to consider that elucidation of the regulatory mechanisms of the β-chain gene expression represent a novel target for the treatment of allergy.

We analyzed the 5' noncoding region of the β-chain gene and revealed that two Oct-1 binding sites in the 5' UTR were essential for activation of the promoter [8]. Next we screened for cis-acting elements over the entire region of the human β-chain gene and identified the transcription factor MZF-1, which repressed β-chain gene expression through an element expressed in the fourth intron [9]. On one hand, FHL3, a repressive cofactor for MZF-1, formed a very large molecular weight complex in the nucleus (Figure 1) [10]. On the other hand, GM-CSF was reported to induce MZF-1 expression [11]. We have found that GM-CSF induces translocation of FHL3 from the cytoplasm to the nucleus (Figure 2) [10], suggesting that both up-regulation of MZF-1 (Figure 3) and nuclear translocation of FHL3 by GM-CSF facilitates formation of a MZF-1/FHL3 complex in the nucleus and reduces β-chain gene expression through the element in the fourth intron. Finally we revealed that FcεRI β-chain gene expression can be suppressed in the presence of GM-CSF through deacetylation of histones mediated by HDACs that are recruited to the β-chain gene through the complex including MZF-1/FHL3 (Figure 4) [12]. A greater understanding of the molecules and their interaction as they participate in the regulation of β-chain gene expression will contribute to the development of novel therapeutic and prophylactic drugs for allergy.

Acknowledgments

This work was supported in part by a Grant-in-Aid from the Ministry of Education, Culture, Sports, Science, and Technology of Japan, and grants from Nihon University and the Uehara Memorial Life Science Foundation.

References

1. Miller L, Blank U, Metzger H, Kinet JP: Expression of high-affinity binding of human immunoglobulin E by transfected cells. Science 1989; 244:334–337.
2. Lin S, Cicala C, Scharenberg AM, Kinet JP: The FcεRI β subunit functions as an amplifier of FcεRI γ-mediated cell activation signals. Cell 1996; 85:985–995.
3. Dombrowicz D, Lin S, Flamand V, Brini AT, Koller BH, Kinet JP: Allergy-associated FcεRIβ is a molecular amplifier of IgE- and IgG-mediated in vivo responses. Immunity 1998; 8:517–529.
4. Donnadieu E, Jouvin MH, Kinet JP: A second amplifier function for the allergy-associated FcεRIβ subunit. Immunity 2000; 12:515–523.
5. Furumoto Y, Nunomura S, Terada T, Rivera J, Ra C: The FcεRIβ ITAM exerts inhibitory control on MAP kinase and Ikappa B kinase phosphorylation and mast cell cytokine production. J Biol Chem 2004; 279:49177–49187.
6. Nunomura S, Gon Y, Yoshimaru T, Suzuki Y, Nishimoto H, Kawakami T, Ra C: Role of the FcεRI β-chain ITAM as a signal regulator for mast cell activation with monomeric IgE. Int Immunol 2005;17:685–694.
7. Xiao W, Nishimoto H, Hong H, Kitaura J, Nunomura S, Maeda-Yamamoto M, Kawakami Y, Lowell CA, Ra C, Kawakami T: Positive and negative regulation of mast cell activation by Lyn via the FcεRI. J Immunol 2005; 175:6885–6892.
8. Akizawa Y, Nishiyama C, Hasegawa M, Maeda K, Nakahata T, Okumura K, Ra C, Ogawa H: Regulation of human FcεRIβ chain gene expression by Oct-1. Int Immunol 2003; 15:549–556.
9. Takahashi K, Nishiyama C, Hasegawa M, Akizawa Y, Ra C: Regulation of the human high affinity IgE receptor β-chain gene expression via an intronic element. J Immunol 2003; 171:2478–2484.
10. Takahashi K, Matsumoto C, Ra C: FHL3 negatively regulates the human high affinity IgE receptor β-chain gene expression by acting as a transcriptional co-repressor of MZF-1. Biochem J 2004; 386:191–200.
11. Welker P, Grabbe J, Zuberbier T, Henz BM: GM-CSF downregulates expression of tryptase, FcεRI and histamine in HMC-1 mast cells. Int Arch Allergy Immunol 1997; 113:284–286.
12. Takahashi K, Hayashi N, Kaminogawa S, Ra C: Molecular mechanisms for transcriptional regulation of human high-affinity IgE receptor β-chain gene induced by GM-CSF. J Immunol 2006; 177:4605–4611.

Chisei Ra

Division of Molecular Cell Immunology And Allergology, Advanced Medical Research Center, Nihon University Graduate School of Medical Sciences, 30–1, Oyaguchi-Kami Machi, Itabashi-ku, Tokyo, 173-8610, Japan, Tel. +81 3 3972-8111(ext) 2720, Fax +81 3 3972-8227, E-mail fcericra@med.nihon-u.ac.jp

Integrating Control of Mast Cell Function and Allergic Responses

J. Rivera[1], T. Baumruker[5], M.A. Beaven[4], S. Brooks[1], K. Chihara[1],
Y. Furumoto[1], A. Gilfillan[2], G. Gomez[1], M. Kovarova[1], K. Mizugishi[3],
S. Odom[1], A. Olivera[1], R.L. Proia[3], N. Urtz[5], and Y. Yamashita[1]

[1]Molecular Inflammation Section, Molecular Immunology and Inflammation Branch, NIAMS,
[2]Laboratory of Allergic Diseases, NIAID, [3]Genetics of Development and Disease Branch, NIDDK
[4]Laboratory of Molecular Immunology, NHLBI, National Institutes of Health, Bethesda, MD,
USA, [5]Novartis Institute for BioMedical Research/Vienna, Brunner Str. 59, A-1235 Vienna, Austria

Summary. *Background:* Activating and inhibitory cell surface receptors on mast cells determine the outcome of a mast cells encounter with a stimulus. However new evidence suggests that, once mast cells are activated, multiple intracellular molecules play an important role in regulating the type and extent of the cellular response. Some of these molecules can play a dual role in both stimulating and inhibiting signals that impact on effector responses. *Methods:* In vitro studies on bone marrow derived cultured mast cells (BMMC) from genetically altered mice, *in vivo* anaphylaxis studies, and silencing RNA approaches on human mast cells are the principal source of data for these studies. *Results: In vitro* and *in vivo* experiments on Lyn- and Fyn-deficient mice or mast cells showed that Lyn and Fyn have primary, but not exclusive, roles as negative and positive modulators of mast cell responses. The negative role of Lyn is partly mediated by its regulation of Fyn kinase activity and its control of cellular phosphatidylinositol (3, 4, 5)-trisphosphate (PIP$_3$). Our studies demonstrate that failure to downregulate the production of PIP$_3$ results in a mast cell hyperresponsive phenotype. The importance of lipid mediators in mast cell function is further demonstrated by the close link between Lyn and Fyn activity and activation of sphingosine kinases (SphK). By producing sphingosine-1-phosphate, SphKs contribute to mast cell chemotaxis and degranulation. *Conclusion:* These studies reveal a new complexity in the regulation of mast cell responses that might contribute to allergic disease.

Keywords: FcεRI, Lyn, Fyn, IgE, mast cell, PI3K, PTEN, degranulation, sphingosine kinase

Introduction

Molecular signals are required for control of mast cell homeostasis and activation [1–4]. Dysequilibrium of these signals may be manifested in increased or unfettered mast cell responses that may lead to disease. Thus, regulatory events preceding and following engagement of the high affinity IgE receptor (FcεRI) are likely determinants of the responsiveness of a mast cell [5–10].

Herein, we describe our studies on molecular controls of mast cell responsiveness in quiescent and activated mast cells. Our findings reaffirm the role of Lyn as a dominant negative regulator in the context of cholesterol-enriched membrane micro-domains (lipid rafts) [5, 6, 9]. Moreover, we find that the phosphatase and tensin homolog deleted on chromosome 10 (PTEN) functions as "gatekeeper" of mast cell activation [11], as downregulation of PTEN expression by shRNA caused increased phosphatidylinositol (3,4,5)-trisphosphate (PIP$_3$) levels and basal cytokine production, but not spontaneous degranulation. Additionally, the requirement for the FcεRI-proximal Src PTKs, Fyn and Lyn in the generation of sphingosine-1-phosphate, an autocrine/para-crine regulator of mast cell chemotaxis and de-granulation, is established in our studies [12,13].

Results

Studies on Lyn- and Fyn-Deficient Mice and Mast Cells

Lyn-deficient mice exhibit an exaggerated al-lergic response when compared to wild type littermates [5], which is associated with in-creased IgE production and increased expres-sion of the high affinity receptor for immuno-globulin E (FcεRI) on mast cells [14, 15]. Oth-er phenotypic traits included increased levels of circulating histamine, eosinophilia, and in some cases increased mast cell numbers indi-cating an apparent activation of mast cells even in the absence of a known allergen [5, 6].

The increased mast cell activity may have multiple underlying causes. One contributor, as demonstrated by others [9, 10], is the lipid phosphatase SHIP-1, which regulates the levels of PIP_3 by dephosphorylating the 5' po-sition to generate PI (3,4)-P_2 and thereby di-minishes recruitment and activation of PIP_3-associated proteins [16]. Lyn is required for phosphorylation of SHIP-1 [9, 17] and in the absence of Lyn [9], or when Lyn-FcεRI inter-action is impaired [17], phosphorylation of SHIP-1 is defective and PIP_3 levels are in-creased. Interestingly, a similar phenotype was observed in a murine model of Smith-Lemli-Opitz disease, a disease where the gene for 7-dehydrocholesterol reductase is mutated re-sulting in cholesterol deficiency. Mast cells from these mice have reduced levels of Lyn in cholesterol-enriched membrane microdo-mains (lipid rafts), increased Fyn kinase and Akt activities, and enhanced degranulation [7]. This demonstrates a role for lipid raft-lo-calized Lyn in control of Fyn, and possibly SHIP activities. Therefore, a common feature to all models is that increased PIP_3 levels are associated with the hyperresponsive pheno-type, suggesting that PIP_3 is a key regulatory component of mast cell responsiveness.

In support of this view, the inability to pro-duce PIP_3 is associated with decreased mast cell responsiveness. Multiple approaches that inhibit the activity of PI3K, the kinase that phosphorylates PIP_2 at the 3' position to gen-erate PIP_3, have demonstrated the importance of this activity in mast cell degranulation and cytokine production [18–21]. Genetic deletion of Fyn caused a marked decrease in the pro-duction of PIP_3 [19, 22]. Fyn-deficient mast cells showed impaired actin rearrangement, defective degranulation responses and re-duced cytokine production. The latter may be a consequence of defects in the activation of c-jun N-terminal kinase (JNK) and NFκB [22]. Investigation of the underlying mecha-nism revealed that the adaptor protein Gab2 was minimally phosphorylated in these cells relative to wild type mast cells. Gab2 binds the p85 regulatory subunit of PI3K and is a key adaptor in the activation of PI3K activity in various cell types [23]. Gab2-deficient mast cells also had defective PI3K activity and both cytokine production and degranulation was impaired [24]. Similarly, a point mutation of the p110δ catalytic subunit of PI3K demon-strated the importance of this isoform in mast cell degranulation and cytokine production [21]. Mast cells expressing this mutant form of p110δ manifested a phenotype that was similar to Fyn or Gab2-deficient mast cells. This re-markable similarity suggests the possibility that p110δ is the key PI3K isoform functioning downstream of Fyn and Gab2.

Studies on PTEN-Deficient Human Mast Cells

The consequence of increased PIP_3 on cellular responses is less well understood. PTEN op-poses PI3K function by dephosphorylating the 3' position of PIP_3. PTEN is a known tumor suppressor and is a key regulator of cell growth and apoptosis [25]. PTEN knockout mice are embryonic lethal. However, $PTEN^{+/-}$ mice develop an autoimmune disorder charac-terized by increased numbers of activated T-cells and polyclonal lymphoid hyperplasia [26], demonstrating its importance in immune cell regulation.

To address the question of whether the aforementioned increase in PIP$_3$ was key in the hyper-responsive phenotype of Lyn- and SHIP-null mast cells [10, 19], we downregulated the expression of PTEN in human mast cells (HuMC) [11]. PTEN-deficiency caused a constitutive phosphorylation of Akt in HuMC in contrast to SHIP-null murine BMMC, which exhibited minimal phosphorylation of Akt [10]. After FcεRI-stimulation, Akt phosphorylation in PTEN-deficient HuMC was further increased. PTEN-deficiency also enhanced FcεRI-dependent calcium mobilization and increased degranulation through increased activation of PLCγ [11]. No differences were observed in spontaneous degranulation, demonstrating that the loss of PTEN is insufficient to initiate a constitutive degranulation response. In contrast, both IL-8 and GM-CSF were found to be constitutively secreted. This was associated with constitutive activation of the MAP kinase family members, c-jun N-terminal kinase (JNK) and p38. Phosphorylation of the transcription factor ATF2 was also induced by PTEN-deficiency. Furthermore, the PI3K inhibitor wortmannin-blocked cytokine secretion from control cells (60–90% inhibition) but did not inhibit the constitutive or stimulated secretion of cytokines from the PTEN-deficient HuMCs. Thus, PTEN-deficiency bypassed the need for FcεRI-stimulated PI3K activity.

Studies on the Activation of Sphingosine Kinase and Its Role in Mast Cells

In addition to PIP$_3$, other lipids may regulate cellular responses [27]. Sphingolipids, such as sphingomyelin, are concentrated in lipid rafts and are critically important for initiation and maintenance of diverse aspects of mast cell function (reviewed in [4]). The conversion of sphingomyelin to ceramide (Cer), sphingosine (Sph) or sphingosine-1-phosphate (S1P) provides interconvertible metabolites with distinct biological activities. Considerable focus has been placed on the role of S1P because of its requirement for thymocyte emigration and

lymphocyte recirculation [28]. Many of the S1P effects are mediated through S1P receptor family members (S1P$_{1-5}$). S1P$_1$ and S1P$_2$ receptors (R) are expressed on mast cells and are transactivated in response to FcεRI stimulation [29]. Transactivation of S1P$_1$R is important for mast cell chemotaxis whereas transactivation of S1P$_2$R contributes to mast cell degranulation [29]. SIP$_1$R is constitutively expressed in mast cells and is activated at very low ligand concentrations whereas S1P$_2$R is inducibly upregulated by FcεRI stimulation. This suggests the possibility that these receptors may regulate mast cell responses in a sequential manner, whereby the chemotactic S1P$_1$R is first engaged and in an autocrine/paracrine manner promotes mast cell chemotaxis toward its site of action. As antigen concentration increases, S1P$_2$R is upregulated (competing with S1P$_1$R) contributing to a maximal mast cell degranulation response [4, 29].

There is an intimate connection between this autocrine/paracrine regulatory loop and FcεRI stimulation as the S1P-generating kinases (sphingosine kinase 1 and 2, SphK1 and 2) appear to be linked to the FcεRI proximal kinases, Lyn and Fyn [12, 13]. Both Lyn and Fyn contribute to the activation of SphKs, with Fyn playing an essential role and Lyn having a contributory role in the early phase of SphK activation and translocation. Moreover, the two isoforms (SphK1 and SphK2) are regulated differently. SphK1 required Fyn-dependent signals that were mediated through Gab2/PI3K activation whereas SphK2 required Fyn-dependent but Gab2/PI3K-independent signals [13]. These findings reveal a bifurcation of Fyn-dependent signals that was previously unappreciated.

Conclusion

In summary, our findings demonstrate the existence of multiple signaling pathways involved in regulating FcεRI-dependent mast cell responses. Of particular note is the intimate molecular relationship between the Src kinases Lyn and Fyn and lipid mediators, like

S1P and PIP$_3$, downstream of FcεRI activation. Importantly, we are learning that lipid-mediated regulation occurs by modulating intracellular signaling pathways as well as by engagement of cell surface receptors. This dual mode of regulating FcεRI-dependent mast cell effector responses is likely to reflect the redundancy required to control mast cell activity *in vivo* and may underlie the plasticity of mast cells in different tissue.

This research was supported in part by the Intramural Research Programs of the National Institute of Arthritis and Musculoskeletal and Skin Diseases, the National Heart Lung and Blood Institute, and the National Institute of Allergy and Infectious Diseases of the National Institutes of Health.

References

1. Gilfillan AM, Tkaczyk C: Integrated signaling pathways for mast-cell activation. Nat Rev Immunol 2006; 6:218–230.
2. Galli SJ et al.: Mast cells as "tunable" effector and immunoregulatory cells: recent advances. Annu Rev Immunol 2005; 23:749–786.
3. Blank U, Rivera J: The ins and outs of IgE-dependent mast cell exocytosis. Trends Immunol 2004; 25:266–273.
4. Olivera A, Rivera J: Sphingolipids and the balancing of immune cell function: lessons from the mast cell. J Immunol 2005; 174:1153–1158.
5. Beavitt SJ et al.: Lyn-deficient mice develop severe, persistent asthma: Lyn is a critical negative regulator of Th2 immunity. J Immunol 2005; 175:1867–1875.
6. Odom S et al.: Negative regulation of immunoglobulin E-dependent allergic responses by Lyn kinase. J Exp Med 2004; 199:1491–1502.
7. Kovarova M et al.: Cholesterol-deficiency in a murine model of Smith-Lemli-Opitz Syndrome reveals increased mast cell responsiveness. J Exp Med, in press.
8. Jolly P et al.: The roles of sphingosine-1-phosphate in asthma. Mol Immunol 2002; 38:1239–1251.
9. Hernandez-Hansen V et al.: Dysregulated FcεRI signaling and altered Fyn and SHIP activities in Lyn-deficient mast cells. J Immunol 2004; 173:100–112.
10. Huber M et al.: The src homology 2-containing inositol phosphatase (SHIP) is the gatekeeper of mast cell degranulation. Proc Natl Acad Sci USA 1998; 95:11330–11335.
11. Furumoto Y et al.: Cutting Edge: Lentiviral shRNA silencing of PTEN in human mast cells reveals constitutive signals that promote cytokine secretion and cell survival. J Immunol 2006; 176:5167–5171.
12. Urtz N et al.: Early activation of sphingosine kinase in mast cells and recruitment to FcεRI are mediated by its interaction with Lyn kinase. Mol Cell Biol 2004; 24:8765–8777.
13. Olivera A et al.: IgE-dependent activation of sphingosine kinases 1 and 2 and secretion of sphingosine 1-phosphate requires Fyn kinase and contributes to mast cell responses. J Biol Chem 2006; 281:2515–2525.
14. Malveaux FJ et al.: IgE receptors on human basophils. Relationship to serum IgE concentration. J Clin Invest 1978; 62:176–181.
15. Furuichi K et al.: The receptor for immunoglobulin E on rat basophilic leukemia cells: effect of ligand binding on receptor expression. Proc Natl Acad Sci USA 1985; 82:1522–1525.
16. Cantley LC: The phosphoinositide 3-kinase pathway. Science 2002; 296:1655–1657.
17. Furumoto Y et al.: The FcεRIβ immunoreceptor tyrosine-based activation motif exerts inhibitory control on MAPK and IκB kinase phosphorylation and mast cell cytokine production. J Biol Chem 2004; 279:49177–49187.
18. Barker SA et al.: Wortmannin-sensitive phosphorylation, translocation, and activation of PLCγ1, but not PLCγ2, in antigen-stimulated RBL-2H3 mast cells. Mol Biol Cell 1998; 9:483–496.
19. Parravicini V et al.: Fyn kinase initiates complementary signals required for IgE-dependent mast cell degranulation. Nat Immunol 2002; 3:741–748.
20. Smith AJ et al.: p110β and p110δ phosphatidylinositol 3-kinase up-regulate FcεRI-activated Ca^{2+} influx by enhancing inositol 1, 4, 5-trisphosphate production. J Biol Chem 2001; 276:17213–17220.
21. Ali et al.: Essential role for the p110δ phosphoinositide 3-kinase in the allergic response. Nature 2004; 431:1007–1011.
22. Gomez G et al.: Impaired FcεRI-dependent gene expression and defective eicosanoid and cytokine production as a consequence of Fyn-deficiency in mast cells. J Immunol 2005; 175:7602–7610.
23. Gu H et al.: Cloning of p97/Gab2, the major SHP2-binding protein in hematopoietic cells, reveals a novel pathway for cytokine-induced gene activation. Mol Cell 1998; 2:729–740.

24. Gu H et al.: Essential role for Gab2 in the allergic response. Nature 2001; 412:186–190.
25. Cantley LC, Neel BG: New insights into tumor suppression: PTEN suppresses tumor formation by restraining the phosphoinositide 3-kinase/AKT pathway. Proc Natl Acad Sci USA 1999; 96:4240–4245.
26. Di Cristofano A et al.: Pten is essential for embryonic development and tumor suppression. Nat Genet 1998; 19:348–355.
27. Brown DA, London E: Structure and function of sphingolipid- and cholesterol-rich membrane rafts. J Biol Chem 2000; 275:17221–17224.
28. Matloubian M et al.: Lymphocyte egress from thymus and peripheral lymphoid organs is dependent on S1P receptor 1. Nature 2004; 427:355–360.
29. Jolly PS et al.: Transactivation of sphingosine-1-phosphate receptors by FcεRI triggering is required for normal mast cell degranulation and chemotaxis. J Exp Med 2004; 199:959–970.

Juan Rivera

NIAMS/NIH, Building 10, Room 9N228, Bethesda, MD 20892-1820, USA, Tel. +1 301 496-7592, Fax +1 301 480-1580, E-mail juan_rivera@nih.gov

Gene Expression Profiling of Human Mast Cell Lines

H. Saito[1,2], K. Oboki[2], Y. Tanimoto[3], M. Sakugawa[3], M. Tanimoto[3], and Y. Okayama[2]

[1]*Department of Allergy & Immunology, National Research Institute for Child Health & Development, Tokyo,* [2]*Research Unit for Allergy Transcriptome, Research Center for Allergy & Immunology, RIKEN Yokohama Institute, Yokohama,* [3]*Department of Internal Medicine II, Okayama University Medical School, Okayama, all Japan*

Summary. *Background:* Although human mast cell (MC) lines, i.e., LAD1, LAD2, and HMC1, are widely used, their global profiles of expressed molecules are not generally reported. *Methods:* We used Affymetrix GeneChip U133A and a hierarchical clustering method to examine the global gene expression profiles of MCs derived from three different tissues and the MC lines. FcεRIα was transfected into HMC-1 with a retrovirus vector. They were then activated through aggregation of FcεRIα. *Results:* By analyzing 3,745 differentially expressed genes of 31 different cell types, a large gene cluster consisting of approximately 1,000 genes were preferentially expressed by all MC types, LAD2, and HMC-1, while leukocytes including basophils preferentially expressed another large gene cluster. Upon challenge with anti-IgE, MCs and the MC lines released histamine, while only MCs strongly expressed some cytokine genes at loci 5q31–33 (*IL3, IL5, IL13, CSF2*) and 4q13–21 (*IL-8, CXCL3, AREG*). MCs and LAD2 expressed *CCL1, CCL3,* and *CCL4* at loci 17q12–21 by IgE-mediated activation, while LAD2 cells tended to lose the CC-chemokine-expressing capacity in a prolonged culture. Although old LAD2 constitutively expressed lower levels of *FCER1A* and higher levels of *IL13RA2*, a negative regulator of IL-4 signaling, these differentially expressed genes between fresh LAD2 and old LAD2 were only sporadically found. *Conclusion:* Although human MC lines are extremely useful in terms of availability, genes present at some loci may be differentially expressed in MCs and MC lines. Such differences should be understood before performing experiments using the MC lines.

Keywords: gene expression, LAD2 cells, HMC-1, human mast cells, microarray, transcriptome

Introduction

HMC-1 is an immature mast cell (MC) line established from a patient with mast cell leukemia and was first reported by Butterfield et al. in 1988 [1]. These cells express human MC-specific markers such as tryptase but do not express high-affinity IgE receptors (FcεRI). LAD1 and LAD2 are recently established stem cell factor (SCF)-dependent human MC lines derived from a patient with MC sarcoma. These cell lines, like primary human MCs, have intragranular histamine, tryptase, and chymase. Unlike HMC-1, LAD cell lines do not exhibit activating mutations at codon 816 of c-kit, express high-affinity IgE receptors (FcεRI), and can release mediators upon aggregation of the receptors [2]. Although these human MC lines are widely used, their global profiles of expressed molecules are not generally reported. We used Affymetrix GeneChip U133A and a hierarchical clustering method to examine the gene expression profiles of MCs derived from three different tissues and these MC lines.

Material and Methods

LAD2 cells were kindly provided by Dr. Kirshenbaum, NIAID, NIH, Bethesda, MD. The HMC-1 cell line was kindly provided by Dr.

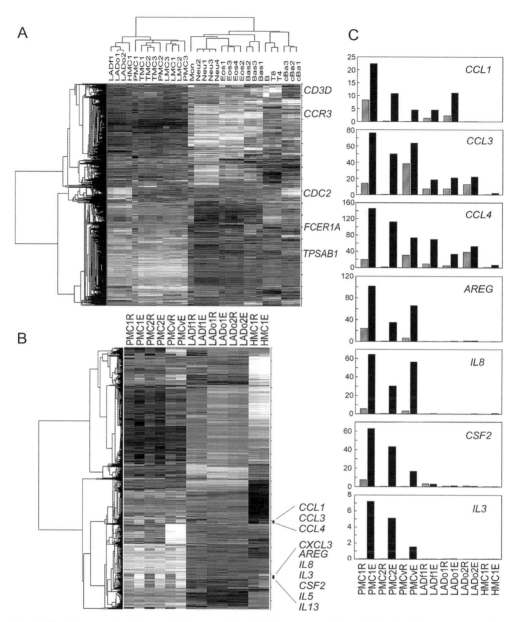

Figure 1. Clustering analysis of human MC lines and MCs. Bright bars represent transcripts having high expression levels, while dark bars represent transcripts having low expression levels. Gene symbols of some marker transcripts were shown in italic in the right hand side (A, B). Detailed experimental conditions and the corresponding Excel files are available at http://www.nch.go.jp/imal/GeneChip/CIA2006.htm. A. Clustered 3,745 genes were aligned and then numbered in the vertical axis from top to bottom (see the number in Supplementary Table 1). The cell-sample clusters were aligned in the horizontal axis from left to right, fresh LAD2 cells (cultured < 10 weeks after thawing; LADf1), old LAD2 cells (cultured > 26 weeks after thawing; LADo1, LADo2), HMC1, adult PB-derived MCs (PMC1–3), tonsil-derived MCs (TMC1–3), lung-derived MCs (LMC1–3), monocytes (Mon), neutrophils (Neu 1–4), eosinophils (Eos 1–4), basophils (Bas 1–3), B cells, CD4+ T-cells (T4), CD8+ T-cells (T8), and culture basophils (cBa 1–3). B. Clustered 1,959 genes were aligned and then numbered in the vertical axis from top to bottom (see the number in Supplementary Table 2). Several pairs of resting (R) and activated (E) MCs and MC lines were horizontally aligned. PMCv means adenovirus infected PB-derived MCs. C. The expression levels of seven representative cytokine transcripts obtained from the Figure 1B experiment are shown in the vertical axis.

Butterfield, Mayo Clinic, Rochester, MN. For transfection of human FcεRIα into HMC-1 cells, the murine leukemia virus-based retroviral vector, which contains the internal ribosome entry site of the encephalomyocarditis virus between the multiple cloning sites and the enhanced green fluorescent protein (EGFP) coding region, were employed. EGFP-positive HMC-1 cells were then clonally expanded. In some experiments, PB-derived MCs were infected with recombinant adenovirus with inserted EGFP as a mock control for a certain experiment.

Adult peripheral blood (PB)-derived MCs were obtained as previously reported [3, 4]. Briefly, MCs used in this study were obtained by culturing PB hemopoietic progenitors with SCF and IL-6 for 8–14 weeks. Lung and tonsil-derived MCs were also obtained as previously reported [3]. Various types of human leukocytes were also obtained by using the methods previously reported [4]. Cultured basophils were obtained by cultivating PB progenitors in the presence of IL-3 as reported [5]. All human subjects in this study provided written informed consent; the study was approved by the ethical review boards of all the hospitals.

For activation experiments, MCs were sensitized with myeloma-derived IgE (CosmoBio, Tokyo, Japan) at 1 μg/ml for 24 h, and then challenged with either 1 or 10 μg/ml rabbit antihuman IgE Ab (Dako Ltd. Carpinteria, CA) or the culture medium alone at 37°C for the indicated time period.

Human genome-wide gene expression was examined by using the Human Genome U133A probe array (GeneChip, Affymetrix, Santa Clara, CA), which contains the oligonucleotide probe set for approximately 22,283 transcripts as previously reported [3, 4]. The data obtained from four human MC line samples were merged with nine human MC samples and 18 leukocyte samples downloaded from supplementary data of the previous reports [3, 4] at http://www.nch.go.jp/imal/GeneChip/GeneChip.htm into one Excel file. These data were normalized with the median value. Detailed methods and all supplementary data are available at http://www.nch.go.jp/imal/GeneChip/CIA2006.htm

Results and Discussion

We selected 3,745 differentially expressed (>10 times of the maximum to minimum ratio) transcripts with high levels (>10-fold of the median) and then hierarchically clustered them. A large gene cluster consisting of approximately 1,000 genes were preferentially expressed by all MC types and the two MC lines, while primary and cultured leukocytes including basophils preferentially expressed another large gene cluster (Figure 1A, Supplementary Table 1, see http://www.nch.go.jp/imal/GeneChip/CIA2006.htm). The two MC lines and cultured basophils preferentially expressed several tens of cycle controller genes such as CDC2 (Figure 1A). When these cell cycle-related genes were omitted and the remaining transcripts were hierarchically clustered, three samples of cultured basophils were found in a common cell-type clustered branch shared with three primary basophil samples [data not shown].

Upon challenge with anti-IgE, all of MCs and the two MC lines specifically released 11–36% of their histamine content (data not shown), while only MCs expressed a set of cytokine genes at loci 5q31–33 (IL3, IL5, IL13, CSF2) and 4q13–21 (IL-8, CXCL3, AREG). MCs and LAD2 expressed CCL1, CCL3, and CCL4 at loci 17q12–21 by IgE-mediated activation, while LAD2 cells tended to lose the CC-chemokine-expressing capacity in a prolonged culture (Figure 1B, C and Supplementary Table 2, http://www.nch.go.jp/imal/GeneChip/CIA2006.htm). Although old LAD2 constitutively expressed lower levels of some activation-related genes such as FCER1A, CF59, and KCNMA1, and higher levels of negative regulators such as IL13RA2, these differentially expressed genes between fresh LAD2 and old LAD2 were only sporadically found.

Human MC lines, LAD2 cells, and HMC-1 are extremely useful in terms of availability, while genes present at some loci may be differentially expressed in MCs and MC lines.

We should understand such differences to perform experiments using the MC lines.

References

1. Butterfield JH, Weiler D, Dewald G, Gleich GJ: Establishment of an immature mast cell line from a patient with mast cell leukemia. Leuk Res 1988; 12:345–55.
2. Kirshenbaum AS, Akin C, Wu Y, Rottem M, Goff JP, Beaven MA, Rao VK, Metcalfe DD: Characterization of novel stem cell factor responsive human mast cell lines LAD 1 and 2 established from a patient with mast cell sarcoma/leukemia; activation following aggregation of FcεRI or FcγRI. Leuk Res 2003; 27:677–82.
3. Kashiwakura JI, Yokoi H, Saito H, Okayama Y: T-cell proliferation by direct cross-talk between OX40 ligand on human mast cells and OX40 on human T-cells. J Immunol 2004; 173:5247–5257.
4. Nakajima T, Iikura M, Okayama Y, Matsumoto K, Uchiyama C, Shirakawa T, Yang X, Adra CN, Hirai K, Saito H: Identification of granulocyte subtype-selective receptors and ion channels by using a high-density oligonucleotide probe array. J Allergy Clin Immunol 2004; 113:528–535.
5. Takao K, Tanimoto Y, Fujii M, Hamada N, Yoshida I, Ikeda K, Imajo K, Takahashi K, Harada M, Tanimoto M: *In vitro* expansion of human basophils by interleukin-3 from granulocyte colony-stimulating factor-mobilized peripheral blood stem cells. Clin Exp Allergy 2003; 33:1561–1567.

Hirohisa Saito

Department of Allergy and Immunology, National Research Institute for Child Health & Development, 2-10-1 Okura, Setagaya-ku 157-8535, Tokyo, Japan, Tel. +81 3 5494-7120 Ext. 4950, Fax +81 3 5494-7028, E-mail hsaito@nch.go.jp

In vivo Imaging of Activated Eosinophils in Inflamed Tissues

S. Yousefi[1], D. Simon[2], H. Nievergelt[2], and H.-U. Simon[1]

[1]*Department of Pharmacology,* [2]*Department of Dermatology, both University of Bern, Switzerland*

Summary. *Background:* It is generally accepted that the release of granule proteins and other toxic mediators from eosinophils is unwanted in noninfectious diseases since it causes tissue damage in the absence of a pathogen. However, eosinophil infiltration of tissues is not necessarily associated with eosinophil-mediated tissue damage and the development of clinical symptoms. *Objective:* To develop a method that detects activated eosinophils. *Methods:* Eosinophils and eosinophil-derived products were analyzed following fluorescence staining by confocal microscopy and image analysis under both *in vitro* and *in vivo* conditions. *Results:* We describe the phenomenon of eosinophil extracellular traps (EETs), which contain both granule and nuclear components, following eosinophil activation *in vitro*. EETs were also found in multiple different but not in all eosinophilic skin diseases. The detection of eosinophil-derived extracellular DNA appears to be a simple but powerful analytical tool suitable to detect EETs under *in vivo* conditions. *Conclusion:* The presence of EETs suggests eosinophil activation and can easily be demonstrated by the presence of eosinophil-derived extracellular DNA in tissues.

Keywords: DNA release, eosinophil activation, extracellular traps, imaging, inflammation, skin diseases

Eosinophil infiltration in nonhematopoietic organs does not exist under physiologic conditions except in the gastrointestinal tract. In contrast, under inflammatory conditions eosinophils can infiltrate virtually all organs. Eosinophil infiltration has been shown to often correlate with clinical symptoms, suggesting that eosinophils largely contribute to the pathogenesis in such inflammatory responses [1]. However, eosinophil infiltration itself does not necessarily lead to clinical symptoms, since some patients with blood and tissue eosinophilia do not show any sign of organ impairment, suggesting that the eosinophils are not activated [2]. Therefore, many efforts have been undertaken to distinguish resting from activated eosinophils. For instance, an anti-eosinophil cationic protein (ECP) monoclonal antibody (mAb) was developed that should detect the "secreted" form of ECP only [3], but subsequent studies showed that this mAb detects

both resting and activated eosinophils [4, 5]. Clearly, a marker able to detect activated eosinophils would be helpful in clinical situations, in which the pathogenic role of the eosinophil is uncertain and/or when therapeutic decisions need to be made.

To overcome the current limitations regarding the detection of activated eosinophils, we have developed an approach that allows direct observation of activated eosinophils under *in vivo* conditions. Recently, it has been shown that neutrophils can kill bacteria extracellularly by the generation of neutrophil extracellular traps (NETs), which contain not only granule proteins, but, surprisingly, also nuclear constituents [6, 7].

To check whether eosinophils are able to generate eosinophil extracellular traps (EETs), we stimulated purified blood eosinophils under *in vitro* conditions. We analyzed EETs by immunofluorescence and confocal

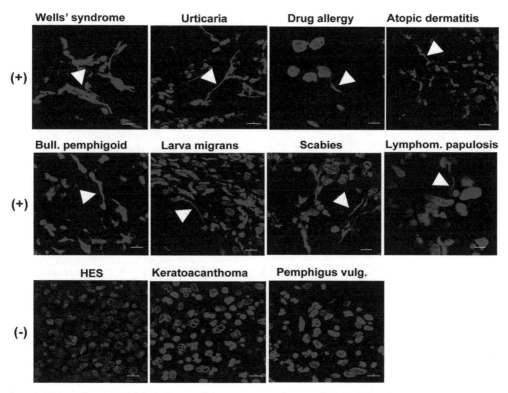

Figure 1. Evidence for eosinophil-derived extracellular DNA in many but not all eosinophilic inflammatory skin conditions. Sections were stained with PI only. All images are projections of a z stack. Some visible extracellular DNA is indicated by arrows. The bars represent 10 mm. Note that in some tissues no extracellular DNA was detected (lower panel).

microscopy. EETs were seen following 15-min priming of eosinophils with IL-5 and GM-CSF, respectively, and subsequent 15-min stimulation with C5a or PAF [8]. DNA was a major structural component of EETs. EETs contained eosinophil-specific cationic proteins, such as MBP and ECP, but not surface (CD9, CD18) or cytoplasmic (actin, caspase-3) molecules. Moreover, additional careful studies (cell death and apoptosis assays) demonstrated that the formation of EETs was not the result of cell damage.

To obtain evidence for the possible existence of EETs *in vivo*, we analyzed skin tissues from patients suffering from different eosinophilic skin diseases. The biopsies taken from these patients demonstrated large numbers of eosinophils (ECP positive cells) and no neutrophils (CD16 positive cells). We searched for the presence of EETs by simply staining sections of skin biopsies with PI (Figure 1).

Multiple EETs were observed in idiopathic (Wells' syndrome, urticaria), allergic (drug allergy, atopic dermatitis), autoimmune (bullous pemphigoid), infectious (larva migrans, scabies), and tumor-associated (lymphomatoid papulosis) eosinophilic responses, demonstrating that this *in vivo* imaging technique is simple, rapid, and sensitive, and therefore useful in a clinical setting. In contrast, no EETs were detected in benign hypereosinophilic syndrome (HES), keratoacanthoma and pemphigus vulgaris in spite of large eosinophil infiltration of these tissues. Therefore, certain clinical conditions associated with eosinophilia exist in which eosinophils are not activated.

Many attempts have been made to distinguish activated from resting eosinophils. Although many changes were observed after stimulation of eosinophils *in vitro*, there is no evidence to suggest that any of such activation markers reflects eosinophil activation under *in vivo* conditions. For instance, CD25 is up-regulated on eosinophils by IL-5 *in vitro* and also frequently expressed on these cells *in vivo* [9]. However, CD25 expression by eosinophils does not necessarily mean that the eosinophil indeed released cytotoxic intracellular material. A CD25-expressing eosinophil rather suggests that it can more easily be activated to perform such a degranulation event. The process that brings the cell in such a condition is also-called "priming" [9]. In summary, it can be concluded that markers of eosinophil priming but not of recent degranulation are currently available.

In this report, we provide evidence for a previously unrecognized function of eosinophils. We did not only show the presence of EETs in inflamed skin tissues, we also, at least partially, characterized their molecular structure. Immunofluorescence analysis using specific Abs is a suitable method for this purpose. However, many questions remain to be answered. For instance, what is the function of the EETs? Are EETs, like NETs [6], able to bind and to kill bacteria extracellularly? Are EETs important in anti-parasite or anti-viral defence mechanisms? What is the kinetic of EET formation? How much and which of the eosinophil DNA is released, etc. Therefore subsequent studies need to be performed to answer these and other important questions.

Acknowledgments
We thank Evelyne Kozlowski (Department of Pharmacology, University of Bern) for excellent technical assistance. This study was supported by grants from the Swiss National Science Foundation (grant no. 310000–112078) and Stanley Thomas Johnson Foundation, Bern.

References

1. Rothenberg ME: Eosinophilia. N Engl J Med 1998; 338:1592–1600.
2. Weller P, Bubley G: The idiopathic hypereosinophilic syndrome. Blood 1994; 83:2759–2779.
3. Tai PC, Spry CJ, Peterson C, Venge P, Olsson I: Monoclonal antibodies distinguish between storage and secreted forms of eosinophil cationic protein. Nature 1984; 309:182–184.
4. Jahnsen FL, Brandtzaeg P, Halstensen TS: Monoclonal antibody EG2 does not provide reliable immunohistochemical discrimination between resting and activated eosinophils. J Immunol Methods 1994; 175:23–36.
5. Nakajima H, Loegering DA, Kita H, Kephart GM, Gleich GJ: Reactivity of monoclonal antibodies EG1 and EG2 with eosinophils and their granule proteins. J Leukoc Biol 1999; 66:447–454.
6. Brinkmann V, Reichard U, Goosmann C, Fauler B, Uhlemann Y, Weiss DS et al.: Neutrophil extracellular traps kill bacteria. Science 2004; 303:1532–1535.
7. Martinelli S, Urosevic M, Daryadel A, Oberholzer PA, Baumann C, Fey MF et al.: Induction of genes mediating interferon-dependent extracellular trap formation during neutrophil differentiation. J Biol Chem 2004; 279:44123–44132.
8. Simon HU, Weber M, Becker E, Zilberman Y, Blaser K, Levi-Schaffer F: Eosinophils maintain their capacity to signal and release cationic protein upon repetitive stimulation with the same agonist. J Immunol 2000; 165:4069–4075.
9. Simon HU, Plötz S, Simon D, Seitzer U, Braathen LR, Menz G et al.: Interleukin-2 primes eosinophil degranulation in hypereosinophilia and Wells' syndrome. Eur J Immunol 2003; 33:834–839.

Shida Yousefi

Department of Pharmacology, University of Bern, Friedbühlstrasse 49, CH-3010 Bern, Switzerland, Tel. +41 31 632-3281, Fax +41 31 632-4992, E-mail shida.yousefi@pki.unibe.ch

Aspirin-Sensitive Rhinosinusitis

Is Associated with Reduced E-Prostanoid 2 (EP2) Receptor Expression on Nasal Mucosal Inflammatory Cells

S. Ying[1], Q. Meng[1], G. Scadding[2], A. Parikh[2], C.J Corrigan[1], and T.H. Lee[1]

[1]King's College London, MRC & Asthma UK Centre in Allergic Mechanisms of Asthma, Division of Asthma, Allergy and Lung Biology, [2]the Royal National Throat, Nose and Ear Hospital, both London, UK

Summary. *Background:* Impaired "braking" of inflammatory cell cysteinyl leukotrienes (CysLT) production by prostaglandin E2 (PGE$_2$) has been implicated in the pathogenesis of aspirin exacerbated airways disease, but the mechanism is obscure. PGE$_2$ acts via G-protein-coupled receptors, EP$_{1-4}$, but there is little information on the expression of PGE$_2$ receptors in this condition. We hypothesized that expression of one or more EP receptors on nasal mucosa is deficient in patients with aspirin-sensitive, as compared with non-aspirin-sensitive, polypoid rhinosinusitis. *Methods:* Using immunohistochemistry and image analysis, we measured the expression of EP$_{1-4}$ in nasal biopsies from patients with aspirin-sensitive ($n = 12$) and non-aspirin-sensitive ($n = 10$) polypoid rhinosinusitis and normal controls ($n = 9$). Double staining was employed to phenotype inflammatory leukocytes expressing EP$_{1-4}$. *Results:* The results showed that global mucosal immunoreactivity of EP$_1$ and EP$_2$, but not EP$_3$ or EP$_4$ was significantly elevated in aspirin-sensitive and non-aspirin-sensitive rhinosinusitis as compared with controls ($p < .03$). This was attributable principally to elevated expression on tubulin$^+$ epithelial cells and Muc-5AC$^+$ goblet cells. In contrast, the percentages of neutrophils, mast cells, eosinophils and T-cells expressing EP$_2$, but not EP$_1$, EP$_3$, or EP$_4$ were significantly reduced ($p \leq .04$) in the aspirin sensitive, as compared with non-aspirin-sensitive patients. *Conclusions:* The data suggest a possible role for PGE$_2$ in mediating epithelial repair in rhinitis and asthma. Since PGE$_2$ exerts some inhibitory actions on inflammatory leukocytes via the EP$_2$ receptor, its reduced expression in aspirin-sensitive rhinosinusitis may be partly responsible for the increased inflammatory infiltrate and production of CysLT which characterize aspirin-sensitive disease.

Keywords: aspirin, rhinosinusitis, prostaglandin E2, EP receptor, asthma

To measure expression of all four EP receptors on mucosal epithelial cells, fibroblasts and inflammatory leukocytes in nasal biopsies from patients with aspirin-sensitive and non-aspirin-sensitive chronic polypoid rhinosinusitis and normal controls, single and double immunohistochemistry were performed to identify individual cells and cell types expressing EP$_{1-4}$ receptors as previously described [1]. Global EP$_1$ expression was significantly greater in pa-tients with aspirin sensitive, but not non-aspirin-sensitive rhinosinusitis as compared with normal controls ($p = .025$), although analysis of variance between the 3 groups only just reached significance ($p = .05$). On the other hand, global expression of EP$_2$ immunoreactivity was clearly elevated in both aspirin-sensitive and non-aspirin-sensitive rhinosinusitis as compared with controls ($p = .028, .008$, respectively). Global expression of EP$_3$ and EP$_4$

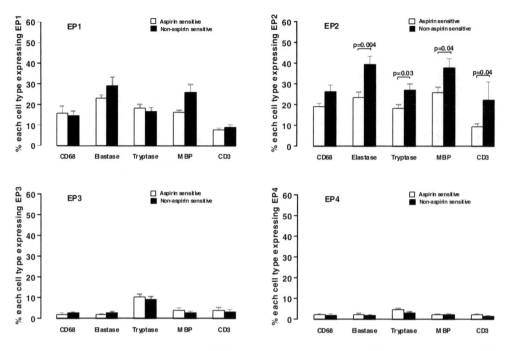

Figure 1. Percentages of inflammatory leukocytes (CD68+ macrophages, elastase⁺ neutrophils, tryptase⁺ mast cells, MBP⁺ eosinophils and CD3⁺ T-cells) expressing immunoreactivity for EP_1 (top, left), EP_2 (top, right), EP_3 (bottom, left) and EP_4 (bottom, right) in patients with aspirin-sensitive ($\square$, n = 12), and non-aspirin-sensitive polypoid rhinosinusitis (■, n = 10). Mann-Whitney U test.

immunoreactivity did not show significant variation between the three groups. Compared with normal controls, there was significantly elevated expression of EP_1, EP_2, and EP_3, but not EP_4 receptor immunoreactivity on tubulin-β⁺ ciliated columnar epithelial cells, but not in Muc-5AC⁺ goblet cells or CD90⁺ fibroblasts, between aspirin-sensitive and tolerant rhinosinusitis ($p < .04$). Significantly lower percentages of elastase⁺ neutrophils, tryptase⁺ mast cells, MBP⁺ eosinophils and CD3⁺ T-cells expressed EP_2 in the nasal mucosa of the patients with aspirin sensitive, as compared with aspirin tolerant rhinosinusitis (Figure 1). Thus, if defects in PGE_2 responsiveness exist and can be overcome by stable EP_2 agonists, this promises new avenues of treatment for asthma and rhinitis in general, and aspirin-sensitive disease in particular.

Reference

1. Ying S, O'Connor B, Meng Q, Woodman N, Greenaway S, Wong H, Mallett K, Lee TH, Corrigan C: Expression of prostaglandin E_2 receptor subtypes on cells in sputum from asthmatics and controls: effect of allergen inhalational challenge. J Allergy Clin Immunol 2004; 114:1309–1316.

Sun Ying

King's College London, MRC & Asthma UK Centre in Allergic Mechanisms of Asthma, Division of Asthma, Allergy & Lung Biology, 5th Floor Thomas Guy House, Guy's Hospital, London SE1 9RT, UK, Tel. +44 207 188 3392, Fax +44 207 403 8640, E-mail ying.sun@kcl.ac.uk

Effects of Lipid Mediators on the Activation of Human Lung Fibroblasts

S. Takafuji[1], S. Kuboshima[2], A. Ishida[3], and T. Nakagawa[3]

[1]*International University of Health and Welfare, Atami Hospital,* [2]*Tokyo Medical University,*
[3]*St.Marianna University School of Medicine, all Japan*

Summary. *Background:* Although lipid mediators such as leukotriene C4 (LTC4) and platelet-activating factor (PAF) play important roles in the pathogenesis of bronchial asthma, the effects of lipid mediators on human lung fibroblasts have not been thoroughly elucidated. We examined effects of LTC4 and PAF on eotaxin production and adhesion molecules expression by human lung fibroblasts. *Methods:* Fibroblasts were cultured with chemical mediators including LTC4 and PAF in the absence or presence of IL-4 for 48 h. At the end of the culture period, eotaxin in the supernatant was measured by ELISA. Adhesion molecules expression on fibroblasts was analyzed by flow cytometry. *Results:* IL-4 clearly enhanced eotaxin production by fibroblasts. When fibroblasts were cultured with IL-4 plus LTC4, eotaxin production was significantly enhanced in comparison with IL-4 alone. When fibroblasts were cultured with IL-4 plus PAF, eotaxin production was significantly enhanced in comparison with IL-4 alone. Also when fibroblasts were cultured with IL-4 plus PAF, vascular cell adhesion molecule (VCAM)-1 expression was clearly enhanced in comparison with IL-4 alone. *Conclusion:* These results suggest that LTC4 and PAF may increase eotaxin production and VCAM-1 expression by fibroblasts in the presence of IL-4 and that lipid mediators may induce eosinophil recruitment into airways through the activation of lung fibroblasts in the presence of IL-4 in allergic inflammation.

Keywords: fibroblast, IL-4, LTC4, PAF, eotaxin, VCAM-1, bronchial asthma

Introduction

Lipid mediators such as LTC4 and PAF play important roles in the pathogenesis of bronchial asthma. However, the effects of lipid mediators on human lung fibroblasts and the mechanism of eosinophil recruitment by those effects have not been thoroughly elucidated. On the other hand, eotaxin and VCAM-1 are important molecules in eosinophil recruitment into tissues. In this study, we examined effects of LTC4 and PAF on eotaxin production and adhesion molecules expression by human lung fibroblasts.

Materials and Methods

Human lung fibroblasts (HFL-1; American Type Culture Collection, Rockville, MD,

USA) were cultured with chemical mediators including LTC4 (Sigma, St Louis, MO, USA) and PAF (Sigma) in the absence or presence of IL-4 (Genzyme, Cambridge, MA, USA) for 48 h. At the end of the culture period, eotaxin in the supernatant was measured by ELISA (BioSource International, Camarillo, CA, USA). In addition, adhesion molecules expression on fibroblasts was analyzed by flow cytometry(Becton Dickinson, San Jose, CA, USA).

Results and Discussion

We examined the effect of IL-4 on eotaxin production by fibroblasts [1]. IL-4 (100 ng/ml) clearly enhanced eotaxin production by

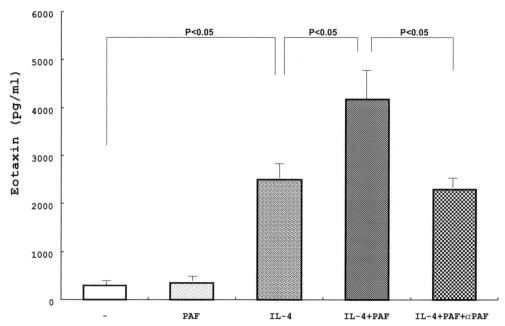

Figure 1. Effects of IL-4 and PAF on eotaxin production by fibroblasts. Fibroblasts were cultured with or without 10^{-6} M PAF, with or without 100 ng/ml IL-4, and with or without 10^{-6} M Y-24180 (PAF antagonist) for 48 h. Each column represents the mean ± SEM obtained from six experiments performed in duplicate.

fibroblasts. Next, we examined the effects of LTC4 on eotaxin production by fibroblasts [2]. LTC4 alone had no effect on eotaxin production. When fibroblasts were cultured with IL-4 plus LTC4, eotaxin production was significantly enhanced in comparison with IL-4 alone. In the presence of IL-4, the enhancement of eotaxin production by LTC4 was concentration dependent, becoming maximal at 10^{-6} M. Next, we examined the effect of PAF on eotaxin production and adhesion molecules expression by fibroblasts [3]. PAF alone had no effect on eotaxin production. When fibroblasts were cultured with IL-4 plus PAF, eotaxin production was significantly enhanced in comparison with IL-4 alone (Figure 1). In the presence of IL-4, the enhancement of eotaxin production by PAF was concentration dependent, becoming maximal at 10^{-6} M. Also when fibroblasts were cultured with IL-4 plus PAF, VCAM-1 expression was clearly enhanced in comparison with IL-4 alone. Y-24180 (PAF antagonist) clearly inhibited PAF effects on eotaxin production and VCAM-1 expression. From our results, it is possible that eosinophil recruitment by lipid mediators such as LTC4

and PAF may occur through the activation of lung fibroblasts. It has been reported that, in mice injected intraperitoneally with eotaxin, the increase of eosinophils in the lavage fluid was inhibited by 5-lipoxygenase inhibitor given before eotaxin[4]. Therefore, it is suggested that eotaxin induces eosinophil activation, which leads to lipid mediator production by eosinophils. Then, lipid mediator may activate fibroblasts, leading to further eotaxin production by fibroblasts and eosinophil recruitment. Such interaction between fibroblasts and eosinophils may induce continuous eosinophil recruitment into tissues.

In summary, this study shows that lipid mediators such as LTC4 and PAF increase eotaxin production and VCAM-1 expression by fibroblasts in the presence of IL-4. It is possible that lipid mediators may induce eosinophil recruitment into airways through the activation of lung fibroblasts in the presence of IL-4 in allergic inflammation.

Acknowledgments
We thank E. Ishii for her expert technical assistance.

References

1. Miyamasu M, Nakajima T, Misaki Y, Izumi S, Tsuno N, Kasahara T, Yamamoto K, Morita Y, Hirai K: Dermal fibroblasts represent a potent major source of human eotaxin: *in vitro* production and cytokine-mediated regulation. Cytokine 1999; 130:751–758.
2. Takafuji S, Tadokoro K, Ito K, Nakagawa T: Release of granule proteins from human eosinophils stimulated with mast-cell mediators. Allergy 1998; 53:951–956.
3. Miyakuni Y, Takafuji S, Nakagawa T: Effects of Th2 cytokines and eosinophils on stem cell factor production by lung fibroblasts. Allergol Int 2003; 52:13–19.
4. Harris RR, Komater VA, Marett RA, Wilcox DM, Bell RL: Effect of mast cell deficiency and leukotriene inhibition on the influx of eosinophils induced by eotaxin. J Leukoc Biol 1997; 62:688–691.

Shigeru Takafuji

Department of Internal Medicine, Atami Hospital, International University of Health and Welfare, 13–1 Higashikaigan-cho, Atami-City, Shizuoka, 413-0012 Japan, Tel. +81 557 81 9171, Fax +81 557 83 6632, E-mail takafuji@iuhw.ac.jp

Potentially Novel Mediators of Mast Cell-Sensory Nerve Interactions

M.-G. Lee, X. Dong, Q. Liu, O.H. Choi, and B.J. Undem

Johns Hopkins School of Medicine, Baltimore MD, USA

Summary. *Background:* Many signs and symptoms of allergic disease are due to activation or modulation of primary afferent (sensory) nerves. We hypothesize that there may be heretofore uncharacterized mediators stored in mast cells that can modify sensory nerve function. Recently, a family of G-protein coupled receptors have been identified that are expressed preferentially, if not specifically, by nociceptive type sensory nerves. The receptors are derived from *mas*-related genes and referred to as "Mrgs." They have also been termed sensory nerve specific receptors (SNSRs). We hypothesize that mast cells release mediators that can interact with certain sensory nerve containing Mrgs. *Methods:* Mrg C11 and MrgA1 (Mrg found exclusively on nociceptive type neurons in mouse sensory ganglia) were transfected into HEK-293 cells. An Increase in cytosolic calcium was used as a marker of Mrg activation. Mouse bone-marrow-derived mast cells or RBL-2H3 cells were sensitized with DNP-specific IgE and stimulated with DNP-HSA. Supernatant fluid from activated mast cells was evaluated for its ability to activate wild-type and Mrg expressing HEK-293 cells. *Results:* IgE-dependent activation of mast cells led to the release of mediator(s) that stimulated HEK cells expressing Mrg C11, but not those expressing Mrg A1. Similar results were obtained with the putative Mrg receptor agonist neuropeptide FF (NPFF). RT-PCR analysis revealed that both mouse mast cells and RBL-2H3 cells express the gene for the NPFF propeptide. *Conclusion:* The results provide support for the hypothesis that upon immunological activation, mast cells release mediator(s) that can stimulate certain Mrg receptors. A member of the RF-amide family of small peptides is a candidate for such a mediator. Mrg receptor activators may represent a novel class of mast cell mediators involved in mast cell-sensory nerve interactions.

Keywords: mast cell, mas related genes, IgE

Introduction

Many symptoms of allergic diseases are the consequence of inappropriate activation of peripheral nerves. In allergic airway disorders these symptoms include excessive coughing, itching, sneezing, increased mucus secretion, episodic reflex bronchospasm and, arguably, inappropriate dyspnea. The fact that there is a close association between mast cells and peripheral nerves may explain why allergic inflammation in particular is so adept at perturbing neurophysiology [1, 7].

Allergen-induced activation of tissue mast cells has been associated with alterations in the phenotype and physiology of nearby sympathetic, parasympathetic, enteric, and sensory nerves [8]. Some effects of mast cell activation on nerves can be explained by defined mast cell mediators such as histamine, cysleukotrienes, PGD_2, and tryptase. Other neuronal effects of mast cell activation, however, are unexplained by the release of these mediators. Even allergic itch, one of the most recognized consequences of mast-cell sensory nerve interactions, is only marginally inhibited by antagonists of histamine and other known mast cell mediators. Based on this, we hypothesize that mast cells may regulate peripheral nerve function by secreting novel neurally active mast cell mediators.

Previous studies have shown that in mouse embryos lacking the bHLH transcription factor Neurogenin1 (Ngn1), nociceptive sensory neurons in the dorsal root ganglia (DRG) fail to be generated [6]. cDNA subtractive screening on sensory ganglia from control mouse embryos vs mouse embryos lacking Ngn1 led to the discovery a large family of G-protein coupled receptors, referred to as Mas1 related genes (Mrgs), whose expression is limited to nociceptive neurons [3]. Further library screening led to the identification of a family of Mrg genes that can be grouped into several subfamilies: *MrgA*, *MrgB*, *MrgC*, and a single gene product, *MrgD*. G-protein coupled receptors of the same family were independently described in rats and humans and were referred to as "sensory neuron specific receptors" (SNSRs) [5].

While the transmembrane and intracellular domains of Mrgs are highly conserved, there appears to be considerable species heterogeneity among the agonist binding sites. There is still relatively little known about the natural agonists for the various Mrg receptors, with many Mrgs classified as orphan receptors. Among known Mrg activators, the RF-amide class of small peptides (e.g., FMRF-amide, peptide NPFF) are particularly effective at stimulating several mouse Mrg receptors [3].

Many of the sensory nerve specific Mrg receptors are coupled to Gq proteins [4]. Activation of Gq-coupled receptors can lead to activation or increases in excitability of sensory nerves [2]. Therefore mediators that act as Mrg receptor agonists could, in theory, serve as important sensory neuromodulators in tissues.

In this preliminary report we describe experiments aimed at addressing the hypothesis that mast cells release Mrg receptor agonists.

Methods and Results

We stably transfected HEK-293 cells with Mrg A1 and Mrg C11 (two Mrg receptors that are localized to pain type sensory neurons in the mouse dorsal root ganglia). The HEK cells were loaded with fura-2 so that increases in cytosolic calcium could be used as a marker of activation. Rat basophilic leukemia cells (RBL-2H3 cells) were used initially as a model of mast cells. The RBL-2H3 cells have a mast cell phenotype and degranulate upon IgE receptor cross-linking and release "mast cell" mediators. We sensitized the RBL cells with DNP-specific IgE and co-cultured the cells with wild type HEK cells or HEK cells transfected with Mrg A1 or Mrg C11 receptors. The mast cells were activated with an antigen (DNP-HSA) and the calcium response in wild-type and transfected Hek cells was monitored. We found that upon IgE-dependent activation of RBL -2H3 cells, mediator(s) were released that led to a 7-fold increase in intracellular calcium in HEK cells expressing Mrg C11 ($n = 5$, $p < .01$). By contrast antigen stimulation of RBL-2H3 cells did not lead to increases in cytosolic calcium in wild type or Mrg A1 expressing HEK cells.

In a second set of experiments we applied the supernatant fluid (100 µl) of antigen-stimulated RBL-2H3 cells to wild type and Mrg-expressing HEK cells. While the control supernatant fluid did not activate HEK cells, the antigen-stimulated supernatant fluid caused a modest activation of wild-type HEK cells (an increase of 20 ± 8 nM in peak free calcium concentration, $n = 9$). The response of Mrg C11-expressing HEK cells was approximately doubled that observed with wild type HEK cells ($p < .01$, $n = 9$). The response of Mrg A1-expressing HEK cells was not different from that of control (18 ± 3 nM).

We next carried out experiments using mouse bone marrow-derived mast cells and obtained similar results. The supernatant solutions of unstimulated mast cells did not lead to changes in cytosolic free calcium concentration in any HEK cell preparation. The supernatant from antigen-stimulated mouse bone marrow-derived mast cells caused a modest 12

± 4 nM increase in peak calcium in Mrg A-expressing HEK cells, but this was not different from the response in control HEK cells ($p >$ .1). By contrast the supernantant solutions from stimulated mast cells caused a robust increase in cytosolic free calcium concentration in Mrg C11-expressing cells (peak change of calcium = 50 ± 10 nM, $p < .05$ compared to control).

These results suggest that IgE-mediated activation of RBL-2H3 cells or mouse mast cells releases a mediator(s) that can selectively stimulate Mrg C11 but not Mrg A1. Several RF-amide ligands are known to be potent and effective activators of various Mrg receptors. The most extensively studied RF-amide is FMRF-amide (Phe-Met-Arg-Phe-amide), and the mammalian counterparts to this small peptide include NPFF and NPAF. We found that NPFF effectively stimulated the Mrg C11 expressing HEK cells ($n = 4$, $p < .01$) with an EC 50 of ~100 nM, but had little effect on native HEK cells or Mrg A1 expressing HEK cells, similar to the findings with mast cells.

We used RT-PCR to evaluate whether RBL-2H3 and mouse bone marrow-derived mast cells express the gene for the common precursor peptide for to NPFF (proNPFF(A)). We observed strong expression of mRNA in both cell types. Subsequent sequencing confirmed that the PCR product was proNPFF (A).

Discussion

G protein coupled receptors belonging to the Mrg family are localized primarily to nociceptive-type sensory neurons [3]. The ligands for many Mrg receptors have not yet been defined, but based on their G protein linkage it is reasonable to assume that their activation may have sensory neuromodulatory consequences. In the present study we transfected HEK cells with MrgC11 and MrgA1, two Mrg receptors found exclusively in mouse nociceptive sensory neurons, and used an increase in cytosolic free calcium to denote receptor activation. IgE-dependent activation of RBL-2H3 cells and mouse cultured mast cells led to the release product(s) that consistently activated

HEK cells expressing Mrg C11 but not those HEK cells expressing Mrg A1.

The finding that the RF-amide NPFF mimicked the mast cell supernatant in stimulating HEK cells expressing Mrg C11 but not MrgA1, provides circumstantial support for the hypothesis that mast cells may release a product similar to this small peptide. Further support for this hypothesis comes from the RT-PCR analysis that reveled expression by mast cells of the precursor peptide for NPFF.

The study of neuronal Mrgs is admittedly in its infancy and it is not yet clear what effect stimulating Mrg receptors has on sensory nerve function. Based on the influence of other autacoids that stimulate G-protein coupled receptors, one might expect overt activation (action potential discharge), changes in electrical excitability or possibly neuroplastic changes (e.g., changes in expression in various neuropeptide synthesizing genes at the level of the cell body) [2]. In any event the data support the preliminary hypothesis that Mrg activators may represent a novel class of mediators involved in mast cell-sensory nerve interactions.

References

1. Bienenstock J, Tomioka M, Matsuda H, Stead RH, Quinonez G, Simon GT, Coughlin MD, Denburg JA: The role of mast cells in inflammatory processes: evidence for nerve/mast cell interactions. Int Arch Allergy Appl Immunol 1987; 82:238–243.

2. Carr MJ, Undem BJ: Pharmacology of vagal afferent nerve activity in guinea pig airways. Pulm Pharmacol Ther 2003; 16:45–52.

3. Dong X, Han S, Zylka MJ, Simon MI, Anderson DJ: A diverse family of GPCRs expressed in specific subsets of nociceptive sensory neurons. Cell 2001; 106:619–632.

4. Han SK, Dong X, Hwang JI, Zylka MJ, Anderson DJ, Simon MI: Orphan G protein-coupled receptors MrgA1 and MrgC11 are distinctively activated by RF-amide-related peptides through the Galpha q/11 pathway. Proc Natl Acad Sci USA 2002; 99:14740–14745.

5. Lembo PM, Grazzini E, Groblewski T, O'Donnell D, Roy MO, Zhang J, Hoffert C, Cao J, Schmidt R, Pelletier M et al.: Proenkephalin A gene prod-

ucts activate a new family of sensory neuron-specific GPCRs. Nat Neurosci 2002; 5:201–209.

6. Ma Q, Fode C, Guillemot F, Anderson DJ: Neurogenin1 and neurogenin2 control two distinct waves of neurogenesis in developing dorsal root ganglia. Genes Dev 1999; 13:1717–1728.
7. Olsson Y: Mast cells in the nervous system. Int Rev Cytol 1968; 24:27–70.
8. Undem BJ, Kajekar R, Hunter DD, Myers AC: Neural integration and allergic disease. J Allergy Clin Immunol 2000; 106:S213–220.

Bradley J. Undem

Johns Hopkins Asthma and Allergy Center, 5501 Hopkins Bayview Circle, Baltimore MD 21224-6801, USA, Tel. +1 410 550-2131, Fax +1 410 550-2130, E-mail bundem @jhmi.edu

Purification of the Natural Peanut Allergen Ara h 1

W.-M. Becker

Research Center Borstel, Borstel, Germany

Summary: *Background:* Under nearly physiological, nondenaturing conditions Ara h 1 and Ara h 3/4 form large complexes between 160 and 500 kDa, of which Ara h 3/Arah 4 are the main components. Both allergens consist of many isoallergens and posttranslationally modified forms. All column chromatographic methods interact with such complexes. This may be one reason why purification of Ara h 1 without cross-contamination of Ara h 3/4 is so difficult. *Material and Methods:* Peanut powder was "defatted" by washes with ether and extracted with 100 mM ammonium acetate pH. 5.4. Ara h 1 was purified by affinity chromatography using immobilized Con A and alpha methyl-mannoside as eluent. The Ara h 1 containing fractions were tested with a battery of monoclonal antibodies specific to Ara 1, Ara h 3/4 and Ara h 2 and pooled. *Results:* The purified Ara h 1 forms under nondenaturing conditions complexes between 160 and 500 kDa. As shown by Western blotting under reducing conditions the purification strategy of Ara h 1 starting with an acidic extraction step was successful in that a contamination of the preparation with Ara h 3/4 was suppressed. A potential impurity at 31 kDa was identified as Ara h 1 fragments by monoclonal antibodies. *Conclusions:* Acid extraction (pH. 5.4) of peanut flour is the key step to generate suitable starting material for Ara h 1 purification. Natural Ara h 1 consists of many isoforms and forms complexes between 160 and 500 kDa.

Keywords: peanut allergen, Ara h 1, purification, glycoprotein

Introduction

Purification of immunological pure Ara h 1 from peanut extract is not trivial, since Ara h 1 consists of several isoforms [1]. Published purification approaches use only a one step strategy to isolate Ara h 1 from the extract by ion exchange chromatography [2]. However, it is difficult to prevent the Ara h 1 preparation from being contaminated by Ara h 3/Ara h 4 [3]. An other approach has been to use the ConA reactivity to Ara h 1 for purification by affinity chromatography. This approach might be restricted because of the possibility that Ara h 3/ Ara h 4 could be glycosylated containing one or two glycosylation sites .Furthermore, Ara h 1 and Ara h 3 /Ara h 4, which are isoforms, form under natural conditions large complexes between 160 and 500 kDa, of which Ara h 3/Arah 4 are the main components [3]. All column chromatographic methods interact with such complexes which may

be the reason for the difficulties of circumventing contamination with Ara h 3 /Ara h 4 in the case of Ara h 1 purification. Therefore, we tested the extraction efficacy of Ara h 1 and Ara h 3/Ara h 4 in relation to the pH of the extraction buffer.

Material and Methods

Crude peanut extract: Peanuts (*Arachis hypogaea*, Virginia) were ground under liquid N_2. 10 g peanut flour was defatted by five washes with 10 ml ether and air dried. One part peanut flour was extracted by 10 parts of 0.1 M $(NH_4)_2CO_3$, pH. 8 (weight/volume) or 0.1 M ammonium acetate pH. 5.4 over night at 4 °C. After centrifugation the supernatant was filtered using filters with descending pore size (8, 0.8, 0.45 and 0.2 µm) and dialyzed against ddH$_2$O, lyophilized and stored at –20 °C until use.

Chromatography: Chromatography techniques were carried out using a ÄKTA purifier HPLC or Äkta prime system (Amersham Pharmacia, Freiburg, Germany). Peanut protein extract (10 mg) was dissolved in 200 mM $(NH_4)HCO_3$ and loaded onto a Superdex 200 column (10/300 GL Amersham Pharmacia).

Affinity chromatography: 100 mg peanut extract was dissolved in 30 ml binding buffer pH. 7.4 (20 mM Tris, 0.5 M NaCl) and loaded on 30 ml ConA-Sepharose. The immobilized ConA was incubated with the solution which circulated through the column in a close circuit for 2 h. After a washing step the bound material was eluted with 0.5 M methyl-mannoside in binding buffer.

SDS-PAGE and Western blotting: Discontinuous SDS-PAGE followed by Western blotting was performed as described by Suhr et al. [4].As monoclonal antibodies were used: Pn-t and Pn-c (Ara h 1 specific), Pn-2 (Ara h 2 specific) and Pn-x and PEI-7B2 (kindly provided by G. Reese, PEI Langen, Germany) (Ara h 3/Ara h 4 specific).

Results and Discussion

The pH dependent extractability of Ara h 1 in comparison to Ara h 3/Ara h 4 from peanut flour with ammonium acetate buffer was tested. The best results were achieved at pH. 5.4. Under these conditions no Ara h3/Ara h 4 in contrast to Ara h 1 was virtually detectable. Thus peanut flour extracted at pH. 5.4 was the source material for starting Ara h 1 purification. At first, the extract was separated on immobilized ConA. The alpha-methyl-mannoside eluate was analyzed by Western blotting using Ara h 1, Ara h 3/Ara h 4 and Ara h 2 specific monoclonal antibodies and sera of peanut allergic patients. The preparation contained Ara h 1 as the main component and was free from Ara h 3/Ara h 4 but was still contaminated probably by breakdown products of Ara h 1 at 31 kDa. The Ara h 1-containing fraction was further purified by size exclusion chromatography on Superdex 200. The chromatogram depicts two peaks in the exclusion volume indicating complexes between 160 and 500 kDa. More than 99% of the protein content was recovered in these peaks. Western blot analysis under reducing conditions displayed a broad band of Ara h 1 at 65 kDa, faint bands of dimeric and trimeric Ara h 1 and a band at 31 kDa reactive with the Ara 1 specific monoclonal antibody. Moreover, the Ara h 1 preparation is free of Ara h 3/Ara h 4, Ara h 2, Ara h 6.

Normally, our view of allergen structure is formed by a combination ofSDS-PAGE, Western blots and 2D electrophoresis. In the context of peanut allergens under natural conditions we have to accept that Ara h 1 and Ara h 3/Ara h 4 form complexes between 160 and 500 kDa. These complexes are preserved in chromatographic separation techniques, which as a consequence are hardly suitable to cleave these complexes and separate them into single allergens. We have successfully solved the problem at the level of the extract production thereby avoiding the extraction of Ara h 3/Ara h 4 at pH. 5.4. Since natural Ara h 1 forms tight complexes between 160 and 500 kDa it is not possible to separate these complexes into single components by standard chromatographic techniques under nondenaturing conditions. The described purification strategy of Ara h 1 creates the preparation for authentic natural Ara h 1.

Acknowledgments

The author thanks S. Fox for excellent technical assistance.

References

1. Buschmann L, Petersen A, Schlaak M, Becker WM: Reinvestigation of the major peanut allergen Ara h 1 on molecular level. Monogr Allergy 1996; 32:92–98.
2. Koppelman SJ, Wensing M, Ertmann M, Knulst AC, Knol EF: Relevance of Ara h 1, Ara h 2 and Ara h 3 in peanut-allergic patients, as determined by immunoglobulin E Western blotting, basophil-histamine release and intracutaneous testing: Ara h2 is the most important peanut allergen. Clin Exp Allergy 2004; 34:583–590.
3. Koppelman SJ, Knol EF, Vlooswijk RA, Wensing

M, Knulst AC, Hefle SL, Gruppen H, Piersma S: Peanut allergen Ara h 3: isolation from peanuts and biochemical characterization. Allergy 2003; 58:1144–1151.

4. Suhr M, Wicklein D, Lepp U, Becker WM: Isolation and characterization of natural Ara h 6: evidence for a further peanut allergen with putative clinical relevance based on resistance to pepsin digestion and heat. Mol Nutr Food Res 2004; 48: 390–399.

WM Becker

FZB, Parkallee 35, D-23845 Borstel, Germany, Tel. +49 4537 188337, Fax +49 4537 188328, E-mail wbecker@fz-borstel.de

Apples Can Drive Birch-Pollen-Allergic Patients Nuts!

T-Cell Crossreactivity as a Basis for Food Allergy

B. Bohle, C. Ebner, B. Jahn-Schmid, A. Radakovics, E.M. Schimek, and B. Zwölfer

Department of Pathophysiology, Center for Physiology and Pathophysiology, Medical University of Vienna, Vienna, Austria

Summary: *Background:* Birch-pollen-allergic patients frequently develop allergic reactions to certain foods, e.g., apples, hazelnuts and celery, because these foods contain proteins highly homologous to the major birch pollen allergen, Bet v 1. Bet v 1-specific IgE antibodies crossreact with these homologs resulting in IgE-mediated immediate symptoms, such as the oral allergy syndrome, after the consumption of fresh foods. *Methods:* The T-cell response to the Bet v 1-related food allergens Mal d 1 (apple), Cor a 1 (hazelnut) and Api g 1 (celery) was characterized using allergen-specific T-cell lines and clones. Moreover, T-cell crossreactivity of food allergens with Bet v 1-specific T-cell cultures was analyzed. *Results:* The T-cell response to Bet v 1-related food allergens was found to be Th2-dominated. Mal d 1, Api g 1 and Cor a 1 contained several T-cell epitopes matching relevant T-cell-activating regions of Bet v 1. Accordingly, they induced proliferation and cytokine production of Bet v 1-specific T-cells. These T-cell-stimulatory properties of food allergens resisted simulated gastrointestinal digestion and heat processing because both treatments did not destroy relevant T-cell epitopes. Moreover, T-cell crossreactivity caused late phase reactions in the skin of birch-pollen-allergic patients with atopic dermatitis. *Conclusions:* Our data emphasize that birch-pollen-related foods represent potent stimuli of pollen-specific T-cells which can be relevant for late phase reactions in birch-pollen-allergic patients with atopic dermatitis.

Keywords: birch pollen allergy, Bet v 1, food allergy, T-cells, crossreactivity

Patients with birch pollen allergy frequently develop hypersensitivity reactions to certain foods, e.g., apples, celery, carrots and hazelnuts. These reactions are mainly caused by IgE antibodies specific for the major birch pollen allergen, Bet v 1, which crossreact with homologous proteins in these foods [1, 2]. We focused on the characterization of the T-cell response to Bet v 1-related food allergens in apple (Mal d 1), celery (Api g 1) and hazelnut (Cor a 1) [3–5]. T-cell lines and clones specific for these food allergens were generated from peripheral blood of allergic individuals. Anal-

ysis of the IL-4 and IFN-γ production in response to allergen-specific stimulation revealed that the majority of T-cells specific for these dietary proteins belonged to the Th2 subset (Figure 1). Food allergen-specific T-cell cultures applied also for T-cell epitope mapping experiments of each protein. Each food allergen contained several T-cell epitopes spreading the entire amino acid sequence (Figure 2). These epitopes were located in regions corresponding to relevant T-cell activating regions of the major birch pollen allergen and also possessed considerable ami-

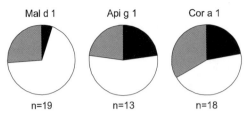

Mal d 1   Api g 1   Cor a 1

n=19   n=13   n=18

Figure 1. T-cell subset distribution of food allergen-specific T-cells. Cytokine responses of Mal d 1-, Api g 1 and Cor a 1-specific T-cell clones were evaluated after allergen-specific stimulation. TCC synthesizing more than 5 times pg/ml IL-4 than pg/ml IFN-γ were attributed to the Th2-like subset (white segments), TCC producing 5 times more pg/ml IFN-γ than pg/ml IL-4 to the Th1-like subset (black segments). TCC producing similar levels of IL-4 and IFN-γ were classified as Th0 (grey segments).

Bet v 1, Bet v $1_{142-156}$, responded to stimulation with various food allergens as the C-terminal part is highly conserved among Bet v 1-related proteins [6].

As peptides containing T-cell epitopes are short, linear peptides, they may survive gastric as well as pancreatic digestion and reach the gut-associated lymphoid immune system as immunologically active peptides. This hypothesis tempted us to stimulate Bet v 1-specific T-cell cultures with Cor a 1 and Mal d 1 incubated with pepsin for 30 min at 37 °C followed by trypsin for another 30 min at 37 °C. This simulated gastrointestinal digestion completely abolished their ability to bind IgE and to induce mediator release but did not abrogate their ability to activate Bet v 1-specific T-cells to proliferate and synthesize cytokines [7]. The latter observation was explained by the fact that several T-cell epitopes of both food allergens were not destroyed by the enzymatic digestion (Figure 3).

no acid sequence similarity with these Bet v 1-epitopes (Figure 2). Accordingly, Bet v 1-specific T-cells also proliferated and produced cytokines when stimulated with the food allergens [3–5]. In particular T-cells specific for the immunodominant T-cell epitope of

```
Bet: 1    GVFNYETETTSVIPAARLFKAFILDGDNLFPKVAPQAISSVENIEGNGGPGTIKKISFPE  60
Api: 1    GVQTHVLELTSSVSAEKIFQGFVIDVDTVLPKAAPGAYKSVE-IKGDGGPGTLKIITLPD  59
Cor: 1    GVFCYEDEATSVIPPARLFKSFVLDADNLIPKVAPQHFTSAENLEGNGGPGTIKKITFAE  60

Bet: 61   GFPFKYVKDRVDEVDHTNFKYNYSVIEGGPIGDTLEKISNEIKIVATP-DGGSILKISNKY  120
Api: 60   GGPITTMTLRIDGVNKEALTFDYSVIDGDILLGFIESIENHVVLVPTA-DGGSICKTTAIF  119
Cor: 61   GNEFKYMKHKVEEIDHANFKYCYSIIEGGPLGHTLEKISYEIKMAAAPHGGGSILKITSKY  120

Bet: 121  HTKGDHEVKAEQVKASKEMGETLLRAVESYLLAHSDAY             159
Api: 120  HTKGDAVVPEENIKYANEQNTALFKALEAYLIAN                153
Cor: 121  HTKGNASINEEEIKAGKEKAAGLFKAVEAYLLAHPDAY            159
```

Figure 2. T-cell epitopes of Bet v 1-related food allergens. T-cell lines generated from peripheral blood of allergic patients with food allergens were used for T-cell epitope mapping. Relevant T-cell activating regions are highlighted in grey the sequence of each allergen.

```
Bet 1     GVFNYETETTSVIPAARLFKAFILDGDNLFPKVAPQAISSVENIEGNGGPGTIKKISFPE   60
Cor 1     GVFCYEDEATSVIPPARLFKSFVLDADNLIPKVAPQHFTSAENLEGNGGPGTIKKITFAE   60
Mal 1     GVYTFENEFTSEIPPSRLFKAFVLDADNLIPKIAPQAIKQAEILEGNGGPGTIKKITFGE   60

Bet 61    GFPFKYVKDRVDEVDHTNFKYNYSVIEGGPIGDTLEKISNEIKIVATP-DGGSILKISNKY  120
Cor 61    GNEFKYMKHKVEEIDHANFKYCYSIIEGGPLGHTLEKISYEIKMAAAPHGGGSILKITSKY  120
Mal 61    GSQYGYVKHRIDSIDEASYSYSYTLIEGDALTDTIEKISYETKLVACGS-GSTIKSISH-Y  120

Bet 121   HTKGDHEVKAEQVKASKEMGETLLRAVESYLLAHSDAY   159
Cor 121   HTKGNASINEEEIKAGKEKAAGLFKAVEAYLLAHPDAY   159
Mal 121   HTKGNIEIKEEHVKAGKEKAHGLFKLIESYLKDHPDAY   159
```

Figure 3. Fragments of food allergens created by simulated gastrointestinal digestion contain relevant T-cell epitopes. Cor a 1 and Mal d 1 were incubated with pepsin and trypsin for 30 min at 37 °C each. Thereafter, digestion products were analyzed by liquid chromatography and mass spectrometry (LC-MS/MS). Identified peptides are marked in grey and matched several relevant T-cell epitopes of Bet v 1 (bold type).

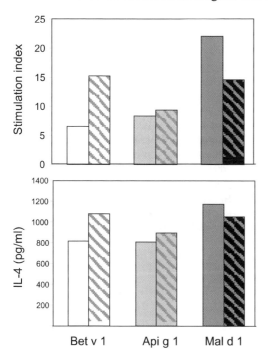

Figure 4. Bet v 1-specific T-cells are activated by cooked food allergens. Bet v 1-specific Th2 clones were stimulated with Bet v 1, Api g 1 and Mal d 1 or with each allergen after incubation for 60 min at 95 °C (hatched bars). After 48 h proliferation and IL-4 synthesis was determined. One representative example is shown.

Cooked birch-pollen-related foods are generally well tolerated by allergic patients and rarely induce immediate IgE-mediated symptoms. However, heating of proteins changes their 3-dimensional structure but not their amino acid sequence. Therefore, we speculated that cooking of birch-pollen-related food allergens may result in the loss of IgE-binding but would not affect their ability to activate allergen-specific T-cells. Mal d 1 and Api g 1 were heated for 60 minutes at 95 °C. Thermally processed allergens were then incubated with Bet v 1-specific T-cell cultures and proliferation and cytokine synthesis were determined (Figure 4). Both cooked food allergens still activated Bet v 1-specific T-cell cultures to proliferate and produce cytokines although they had completely lost their ability to bind IgE antibodies and to induce mediator release from basophils (data not shown). To substantiate these results *in vivo*, Bet v 1-monosensitized birch-pollen-allergic individuals with food allergy and atopic dermatitis were tested in double blind placebo controlled food challenges with fresh and cooked apple, celery and carrot, respectively. All patients reacted with an oral allergy syndrome and the deterioration of their eczema after consumption of fresh

foods. Ingestion of cooked foods triggered a comparable worsening of atopic eczema as fresh foods in the absence of oral allergy syndromes [8].

In summary, we could demonstrate that i) Bet v 1-homologs in foods are potent stimuli of pollen-specific T-cells *in vitro* and *in vivo*; ii) neither cooking nor gastrointestinal enzymes destroy T-cell epitopes in Bet v 1-related food allergens that are crossreactive with pollen-specific T-cells; and iii) T-cell crossreactivity between Bet v 1 and its food-homologs is independent from IgE crossreactivity. These immunological findings are of *in vivo* relevance because ingestion of birch-pollen-related food can induce T-cell mediated late phase reactions without the occurrence of immediate IgE-mediated symptoms. Therefore, the general view that cooked pollen-related foods can be consumed without allergological consequences should be reconsidered.

References

1. Ebner C, Hirschwehr R, Bauer L, Breiteneder H, Valenta R, Ebner H, Kraft D, Scheiner O: Identification of allergens in fruits and vegetables: IgE

crossreactivities with the important birch pollen allergens Bet v 1 and Bet v 2 (birch profilin). J Allergy Clin Immunol 1995; 95:962–969.

2. Wensing M, Akkerdaas JH, van Leeuwen WA, Stapel SO, Bruijnzeel-Koomen CA, Aalberse RC, Bast BJ, Knulst AC, van Ree R: IgE to Bet v 1 and profilin: crossreactivity patterns and clinical relevance. J Allergy Clin Immunol 2002; 110:435–442.

3. Fritsch R, Bohle B, Vollmann U, Wiedermann U, Jahn-Schmid B, Krebitz M, Breiteneder H, Kraft D, Ebner C: Bet v 1, the major birch pollen allergen, and Mal d 1, the major apple allergen, cross-react at the level of allergen-specific T-helper-cells. J Allergy Clin Immunol 1998; 102:679–686.

4. Bohle B, Radakovics A, Jahn-Schmid B, Hoffmann-Sommergruber K, Fischer GF, Ebner C: Bet v 1, the major birch pollen allergen, initiates sensitization to Api g 1, the major allergen in celery: evidence at the T-cell level. Eur J Immunol 2003; 33:3303–3310.

5. Bohle B, Radakovics A, Luttkopf D, Jahn-Schmid B, Vieths S, Ebner C: Characterization of the T-cell response to the major hazelnut allergen, Cor a 1.04: evidence for a relevant T-cell epitope not crossreactive with homologous pollen allergens. Clin Exp Allergy 2005; 35:1392–1399.

6. Jahn-Schmid B, Radakovics A, Luttkopf D, Scheurer S, Vieths S, Ebner C, Bohle B: Bet v 1$_{142-156}$ is the dominant T-cell epitope of the major birch pollen allergen and important for crossreactivity with Bet v 1-related food allergens. J Allergy Clin Immunol 2005; 116:213–219.

7. Schimek EM, Zwolfer B, Briza P, Jahn-Schmid B, Vogel L, Vieths S, Ebner C, Bohle B: Gastrointestinal digestion of Bet v 1-homologous food allergens destroys their mediator-releasing, but not T-cell-activating, capacity. J Allergy Clin Immunol 2005; 116:1327–1333.

8. Bohle B, Zwolfer B, Heratizadeh A, Jahn-Schmid B, Dall'Antonia A, Keller W, Zuidmeer L, van Ree R, Werfel T, Ebner C: Cooking birch-pollen-related food: divergent consequences for IgE- and T-cell-mediated reactivity in vitro and in vivo. J Allergy Clin Immunol 2006; 118:242–249.

Barbara Bohle

Medical University of Vienna, Center for Physiology and Pathophysiology, Dept. of Pathophysiology, Waehringer Guertel 18–20, AKH-3Q, A-1090 Wien, Austria, Tel. +43 1 40400-5114, Fax +43 40400-5130, E-mail barbara.bohle @meduniwien.ac.at

Mass Spectroscopic Analysis of Natural and Recombinant Preparations of Pollen (Birch, Grass, Olive) and House Dust Mite Allergens

P. Briza[1], A.M. Erler[1], M. Wallner[1], M. Susani[2], H. Fiebig[3], W.M. Becker[4], M. Villalba[5], R. Monsalve[6], L.D. Vailes[7], M. Chapman[7], R. van Ree[8], F. Ferreira[1], and the CREATE consortium

[1]University of Salzburg, Austria, [2]Biomay AG, Vienna, Austria, [3]Allergopharma, Reinbek, Germany, [4]Forschungszentrum Borstel, Germany, [5]Universidad Complutense de Madrid, Spain, [6]ALK-Abello, Madrid, Spain, [7]Indoor Biotechnologies, Cardiff, UK, [8]Sanquin Research, Amsterdam, The Netherlands

Summary: One of the aims of the European Union CREATE project is to analyze natural and recombinant major allergens from birch pollen (Bet v 1), grass pollen (Phl p 1, Phl p 5), olive pollen (Ole e 1) and house dust mite (Der f 1, Der f 2, Der p 1, Der p 2) regarding their physico-chemical and immunological properties. On the basis of this and other analyses, allergen preparations will be identified that meet the requirements to become certified reference material for allergenic products. Here, we present the mass spectrometric investigation of the recombinant allergens and their natural counterparts from the CREATE project.

Keywords: tandem mass spectrometry, allergens, CREATE project

Diagnosis and immunotherapy of allergic diseases are based on the use of aqueous extracts of natural allergen sources. These extracts usually are highly complex, consisting both of allergenic and nonallergenic compounds. Ratios of major and minor allergens in extracts may vary between different production batches. Even more important are the possible variations of allergen contents of extracts produced by different manufacturers, due to different pretreatment of the source material and extraction protocols. In present standardization protocols, the allergenic potency of extracts is determined either by *in vivo* testing in allergic volunteers, or by radioallergosorbent (RAST) or similar tests, using pooled sera of allergic individuals. It has to be emphasized that standardization is done within a company using in-house references, and all companies on the market use their own methods and protocols, making it difficult to compare the allergenic properties of different products. The aim of the CREATE project, funded by the European Commission and consisting of a multidisciplinary consortium consisting of allergen manufacturers, biotech companies, regulatory bodies, clinicians and research laboratories, is the analysis of natural and recombinant major allergens from birch pollen (Bet v 1), grass pollen (Phl p 1, Phl p 5), olive pollen (Ole e 1) and house dust mite (Der f 1, Der f 2, Der p 1, Der p 2) regarding their physico-chemical and immunological properties. On the basis of these and other analyses, allergen preparations will be identified that meet the requirements to become certified reference material for allergenic products [1]. Here we want to present the methodology for the mass spectrometric investigation of the recombinant allergens and their natural counterparts from the CREATE project.

We use a Micromass Q-Tof Global Ultima tandem mass spectrometer (Waters) with electrospray ionization (ESI), consisting of a quadrupole for mass filtering, a collision quadrupole for peptide fragmentation and a time-of-flight mass spectrometer (Tof-MS) for mass analysis. Samples dissolved in a water/acetontrile/formic acid mixture are either directly infused to the MS using a pico-spray ionization inlet, or separated by online coupled capillary HPLC prior to MS analysis. While direct infusion is mostly used for mass determination of intact proteins, HPLC separation is mandatory for the analysis of proteolytic peptides obtained from complex protein mixtures, like aqueous extracts of allergen sources.

How are proteins identified by tandem mass spectrometry (MS/MS)? Before HPLC separation, samples are digested with specific proteases. This can be done either with bands excised from a SDS gel, or with complex protein mixtures without prior separation. Trypsin is preferentially used for digestion, since it cleaves proteins highly specific at the carboxyl side of lysine and arginine residues. The resulting peptides are doubly charged at acidic pH. One positive charge resides on the N-terminal amino acid, the other charge is located to the side chain of the C-terminal arginine or lysine. Because of the charge state, it is possible to distinguish signals from tryptic peptides from signals of other compounds present in the sample and background peaks. A further advantage of doubly charged tryptic peptides is that fragmentation patterns are relatively easy to interpret. We use the ProteoExtract diges-

tion kit by Calbiochem both for in-solution and in-gel digests. HPLC separation of the peptides involves two steps. First, the sample is loaded onto the precolumn (Waters Symmetry300). At that stage, precolumn and main column are not connected and salts and other substances not binding to the column material are removed. At the second stage, precolumn and main column (Waters Atlantis) are connected and peptides are eluted with an acetonitrile gradient. During the development of the gradient, the eluate is continuously monitored for peptides by Tof-MS. As soon as the software detects doubly charged ions, the quadrupole is activated to select the peptide in question that is subsequently fragmented in the collision cell by collision with argon atoms. Fragment ions in turn are analyzed in the Tof-MS. Since fragmentation occurs preferentially at the peptide bond, fragment spectra can be used to deduce the amino acid sequence of a peptide. After two to five seconds, quadrupole and collision cell are deactivated and monitoring for tryptic peptides continues. In this way it is possible to obtain from one HPLC run both data about peptide masses and peptide sequence. Finally the raw data are processed and analyzed using the ProteinLynx software (Waters). By comparing both peptide masses and peptide fragment spectra with protein data bases, it is possible to unequivocally identify proteins in the sample. Data bases used can be both public, like SwissProt or TREMBL, or custom made, consisting e.g., of unpublished sequences provided by the CREATE consortium. Peptides not identified by data base search are sequenced de novo. This way, it is possible to identify new isoforms of allergens. ProteinLynx is also capable of identifying protein modifications that might have occurred during the production or purification process. The various steps of mass spectrometric analysis of proteins are summarized in Figure 1. The application of mass spectrometry in proteomic research was reviewed by Aebersold and Mann [2].

Using the methodology described above, we analyzed several samples provided by the CREATE consortium. 14 and 3 isoforms were detected in a preparations of natural Bet v 1

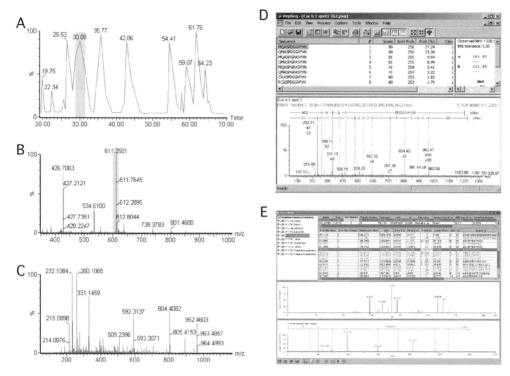

Figure 1. Example of mass spectrometric analysis of tryptic peptides derived from allergen preparations. (A) Base Peak Intensity chromatogram of the HPLC eluate indicating eluting peptides during development of the acetonitrile gradient. (B) Intact mass spectra of peptides eluting from the column at 30 minutes. (C) Collision induced fragment spectrum of the peptide with the m/z value of 611.25. The sequence of this peptide can be determined either by *de novo* sequencing (D) or by data base search (E).

and Phl p 5, respectively. Sequences were confirmed of recombinant preparations of Bet v 1 and Der f 1. We discovered that the signal peptide at the N-terminus of recombinant Der p 1 was not properly processed. Finally, in one preparation of recombinant Bet v 1 we could identify a chemical modification of the N-terminus that occurred during the purification procedure.

Acknowledgments

This work was supported by EU-grant GRD2-2000-30032.

References

1. van Ree R, and the CREATE partnership: The create project: EU support for the improvement of allergen standardization in Europe. Allergy 2004; 59:571–574
2. Aebersold R, Mann M: Mass spectrometry based proteomics. Nature 2003; 422:198–207.

Peter Briza

Department of Molecular Biology, University of Salzburg, Hellbrunnerstraße 34, A-5020 Salzburg, Austria, Tel. +43 662 8044-5769, Fax +43 662 8044-183, E-mail peter.briza@sbg.ac.at

Identification of the Major Components of the Dust Mite Proteome and the Full Repertoire of Its Allergens

F.T. Chew

Allergy and Molecular Immunology Laboratory, Department of Biological Sciences, Lee Hiok Kwee Functional Genomic Laboratories, National University of Singapore

Summary: *Background:* Very little is known about the mite proteome apart from the allergens that have been characterized. Knowledge of the other components may be useful in enhancing our understanding of host allergic responses, mite control, monitoring and biology. *Methods:* To understand its underlying components, proteins from *Dermatophagoides* spp. were separated by 2-D gel electrophoresis and coomassie-stained spots were subjected to tandem mass spectrometry (MS-MS). The peptide mass fingerprints (PMF) and MS-MS sequences were then compared to *in silico* fingerprints generated from our in-house mite expressed sequence tag (EST) database to identify the proteins. *Results:* One hundred of the most abundant spots were identified. Many of these appear as protein isoforms – matching the same sequence contig composing of various homologs; among them are the group 1, 2, 5, 7, 10, 13, and 20 mite allergens. Careful analysis indicated that about 32 of the top 100 proteins in the proteome were allergens. Other known allergens did not appear as abundant proteins. Further analysis indicate that many of the major proteins are novel with unknown functions, while others show homology to putative gene products from *Drosophila*, common structural, biosynthetic or metabolic proteins such as actins, cuticle-like proteins, esterases, kinases, and ferritin. Using the EST database, we identified more than 40 groups of antigens with sequence similarities to allergenic components. *Conclusion:* The database was not only useful in assisting the identification of the major proteins but also indicating potentially the full repertoire of allergens present in dust mites.

Keywords: dust mite proteins, allergens, expressed sequence tag (EST), proteomics

Introduction

House dust mites are among the most important source of allergens in the indoor environment. To-date, more than 20 groups of house dust mite allergens has been identified (www.allergen.org). Nevertheless, very little is essentially known about the make up of the mite proteome apart from these allergens. As mites are "nongenome sequenced" organisms, proteomic studies on them are a challenging task. We demonstrate here that a combination of both genomic and proteomic technologies can enable us to identify the majority of the major abundant components in the mite proteome and in turn allow us to identify the full spectrum of it's allergenic components [1]. This strategy can thus be applied to the other sources of allergens and we have in fact demonstrated this not only among the different species of mites [2–6] but also for cockroaches [7], tropical pollen [8] and fungal species [9].

Materials and Methods

The procedure of processing the proteins and analysis have been described in detail elsewhere [10]. Briefly, purified life *Dermatophagoides* spp. mites were grounded in liquid nitrogen and thereafter extracted using a trichloroacetic acid extraction procedure. The proteins were then separated using 2-dimensional gel electrophoresis and the gel was then commasie stained to visualize the protein spots. The top 100 protein spots were then subjected in-gel tryptic digestion followed by mass spectrometric analysis. The peptide mass fingerprints (PMF) and MS-MS sequences were then compared to *in silico* fingerprints generated from our in-house mite expressed sequence tag (EST) database to identify the proteins [1].

Results and Discussion

The standardization of allergenic crude extracts for diagnosis and treatment of allergic diseases have been hampered by the fact that we do not have a well defined "component list" of what goes into the extract. This has resulted in variability not only due to the source of extracts but also in batch-to-batch productions [11–13]. To begin listing its "components," we initiated a proteomic and genomic characterization of the dust mite extract. This however is hampered by the fact that we have limited dust mite specific gene sequences in the public databases. Without such sequences, it would be difficult to pursue large scale protein identification as mass spectrometric analysis of the peptides is dependent on the availability of genomic or sequence data for comparison. With the expressed sequence tag database however, we were able to match the majority of the abundant proteins to this database and confirm several of them using de novo tandem mass spectrometric sequencing [14]. The major component in the dust mite proteome seems to be made up of multiple forms of a cuticle-like protein localized to the epithelial layer of the mite body [10, 14]. The major dust mite allergens (particularly, the group 1, 2, 5, 7, 10, 13, and 20 mite allergens) made up approximately 30 of the top 100 major protein spots identified. Other major components include several novel proteins with no known sequence homology and function – which may be mite specific, while others show homology to putative gene products from *Drosophila*, common structural, biosynthetic or metabolic proteins such as actins, esterases, kinases, several classes of proteases, ferritin and several other metabolic enzymes.

Of particular interest however to allergology is the list of allergenic components present. Apart from the described group 1–20 mite allergens already listed in www.allergen.org, we have found several paralogous proteins which share some sequence homology to known allergens but share structural homology with them. These include the paralogues to the dust mite group 5 allergens (putatively now called dust mite group 21) [15–17] as well as the paralogues to the group 2 allergens (submitted to the WHO IUIS allergen nomenclature committee and tentatively called the dust mite group 22) [18]. In addition, paralogues to the group 7 and 13 allergens have also been identified [19–20]. In addition, we were also able to identify dust mite allergen homologs to other organisms such as cockroaches, tree or pollen (*Juniperus ashei, Juniperus virginiana* and *Prunus avium, Hevea brasiliensis*), yeast (*Malassezia* spp.), chicken (*Gallus gallus*), yellow jacket venom, fungi (*Alternaria alternata, Cladosporium herbarum, Penicillium citrinum, Candida albicans* and *Coprinus comatus*), and fruit (*Actnidia chinensis*). These allergens were identified as heat shock protein 70, heat shock protein 90, profilin, enolase, ovomucoid precursor and ovalbumin, phospholipase A1, ribosomal protein P2, alcohol dehydrogenase, thioredoxin, hexosaminidase, cyclophilin, Mn superoxide dismutase, lipid-transfer proteins, thaumatin-like proteins and actinadain-like allergen homologs and many were also shown to be IgE binding [21–26].

This study demonstrates that proteome identification can still be performed on a non-genome sequenced organism using PMF and tandem MS-MS with the help of expressed sequence tags. In combination with the genomic analysis, we have identified more than 40 groups of dust mite allergens, believed to be the majority, if not the full spectrum, of the dust mite allergens present in the environment.

Acknowledgments

Our work on house dust mite allergens have been supported by the Biomedical Research Council (BMRC) of the Agency for Science, Technology and Research (A*STAR) in Singapore.

References

1. Angus AC, Ong ST, Chew FT: Sequence tag catalogs of dust mite-expressed genomes: utility in allergen and acarologic studies. Am J Pharmacogenomics 2004; 4:357–369.

2. Chew FT, Ong ST, Wang WL, Kuay KT, Lee BW, Tsai LC, Lim SH: Preliminary profile of the dust mite genomes: an expressed sequence tag (EST) analysis of *Dermatophagoides farinae* and *Blomia tropicalis* genes. The 57th American Academy of Allergy and Immunology Annual Meeting. New Orleans, Louisiana, USA 2001. J Allergy Clin Immunol 2001; 107:56.

3. Reginald K, Haroon-Rashid L, Sew YS, Tan SH, Chew FT: Identification of putative *Tyrophagus putrescentiae* allergens with sequence homology to other known allergens by expressed sequence tagging. XXIth European Academy of Allergology and Clinical Immunology Annual Meeting (EAACI). Naples, Italy 2002. Allergy 2002; 57 (Suppl. 73):286–287.

4. Gao YF, Chew FT: Large scale screening of putative allergen genes from *Acarus siro*. The 60th American Academy of Allergy and Immunology Annual Meeting. Denver, USA 2003. J Allergy Clin Immunol 2003; 111:326.

5. Reginald K, Gao YF, Lim YP, Chew FT: The expressed sequence tag catalog and allergens of dust mite, *Suidasia medanensis*. Abstract book of the XXIIIth European Academy of Allergology and Clinical Immunology Annual Meeting (EAACI). Amsterdam, The Netherlands 2004; 614:185–186.

6. Ramjan SFR, Loo AHB, Lim YP, Chew FT: Catalogue of the major transcripts of the storage mite, *Aleuroglyphus ovatus*: revealing the putative allergenic repertoire. The 62th American Academy of Allergy and Immunology Annual

Meeting. San Antonio, USA 2005. J Allergy Clin Immunol 2005; 115:351.

7. Toh GT, Tan SH, Chew FT: Utilization of expressed sequence tags for identification of *Periplaneta americana* allergens. The XXIIth European Academy of Allergology and Clinical Immunology Annual Meeting (EAACI). Paris, France 2003. Allergy 2003; Suppl. 73:A1469.

8. Chew FT, Tan SH, Harikrishna K, Liew CF, Tan HTW, Lee BW: Initial collection of expressed sequence tags of the oil palm (*Elaeis guineensis Jacq.*) pollen – identification of pollen allergen homologs. XVII International Congress of Allergology and Clinical Immunology. Sydney, Australia 2000. Allergy Clin Immunol International 2000; Suppl. 2:181.

9. Joshi SS, Wong FL, Tan TK, Chew FT: Screening for putative allergenic and pathogenesis-related components in *Curvularia lunata*: an expressed sequence tag approach. XVIII International Congress of Allergology and Clinical Immunology. Vancouver, Canada 2003. Allergy Clin Immunol International 2003; Suppl. 1:192–193.

10. Batard T, Hrabina A, Bi ZX, Chabre H, Lemoine P, Couret MN, Faccenda D, Villet B, Harzic P, André F, Goh SY, André C, Chew FT, Moingeon P: Production and proteomic characterization of pharmaceutical-grade *Dermatophagoides pteronyssinus* and *Dermatophagoides farinae* extracts for allergy vaccines. Int Arch Allergy Immunol 2006; 140:295–305.

11. Esch RE. Manufacturing and standardizing fungal allergen products. J Allergy Clin Immunol 2004; 113:210–215.

12. Grier TJ, Hazelhurst DM, Duncan EA, West TK, Esch RE: Major allergen measurements: sources of variability, validation, quality assurance, and utility for laboratories, manufacturers, and clinics. Allergy Asthma Proc 2002; 23:125–131.

13. Reginald K, Bi XZ, Ong ST, Chew FT: Profiling of crude allergen extracts using SELDI mass spectrometry for rapid standardization. The 60th American Academy of Allergy and Immunology Annual Meeting. Denver, USA 2003. J Allergy Clin Immunol 2003; 111:242.

14. Bi XZ, Ong ST, Chew FT: Identification, cloning and expression of a major component of the house dust mite proteome, a putative cuticle-like protein, via peptide mass fingerprinting, tandem mass spectrometry and contiguous expressed sequence tag alignments. The 60th American Academy of Allergy and Immunology Annual Meeting. Denver, USA 2003. J Allergy Clin Immunol 2003; 111:165.

15. Gao YF, Tan XJ, Ong ST, Bi XZ, Shang HS, Wang DY, Chew FT: Characterization of two paralogous genes showing identities to Group 5 allergens in house dust mite *Dermatophagoides farinae*. Abstract book of the XXIIIth European Academy of Allergology and Clinical Immunology Annual Meeting (EAACI). Amsterdam, The Netherlands 2004; 610:184–185.

16. Gao YF, Bi XZ, Shang HS, Wang DY, Chew FT: Molecular cloning and characterization of a group 5 paralogue from *Blomia tropicalis*. The 62th American Academy of Allergy and Immunology Annual Meeting. San Antonio, USA 2005. J Allergy Clin Immunol 2005; 115:362.

17. Gao Y, Wang DY, Chew FT: Co-sensitization not due to cross-reactivity between paralogs of group 5 allergens from *Blomia tropicalis* and *Dermatophagoides farinae*. The 63th American Academy of Allergy and Immunology Annual Meeting. Miami, Florida, USA 2006. J Allergy Clin Immunol 2006; 117:119.

18. Tan CL, Reginald K, Chew FT: Genomic organization and characterization of group 2 allergen paralogs from *Dermatophagoides farinae*. The 63th American Academy of Allergy and Immunology Annual Meeting. Miami, Florida, USA 2006. J Allergy Clin Immunol 2006; 117:120.

19. Ong ST, Ong SY, Shang HS, Gulzar Mohd R, Mari A, Wang DY, Chew FT: Paralogous forms of the Group 7 allergens from dust mite, *Dermatophagoides farinae*. Abstract book of the XXIIIth European Academy of Allergology and Clinical Immunology Annual Meeting (EAACI). Amsterdam, The Netherlands 2004; 612:185.

20. Ong ST, Gulzar Mohd R, Lua BL, Wang WL, Kuay KT, Mahakittikun V, Baratawidjaja KG, Lim SH, Mari A, Tsai LC, Chew FT: Identification of paralogous forms of the dust mite group 13 fatty acid binding proteins from *Dermatophagoides farinae* and *Blomia tropicalis*: under-recognition of group 13 allergens as an important dust mite allergen. The 61th American Academy of Allergy and Immunology Annual Meeting. San Francisco, USA 2004. J Allergy Clin Immunol 2004; 113:228.

21. Ong ST, Angus AC, Tsai LC, Lim SH, Chew FT: Molecular cloning and characterization of an ovalbumin (Gal d 2) homolog in house dust mite, *Dermatophagoides farinae*. The 60th American Academy of Allergy and Immunology Annual Meeting. Denver, USA 2003. J Allergy Clin Immunol 2003; 111:324–325.

22. Shang HS, Kuay KT, Wang WL, Lim SH, Chew FT: Allergenicity of homologs to fungal, pollen, food and insect allergens in dust mite, *Blomia tropicalis*: identification of new classes of pan-allergens. XVIII International Congress of Allergology and Clinical Immunology. Vancouver, Canada 2003. Allergy Clin Immunol International 2003; Suppl. 1:32.

23. Bi XZ, Chew FT: Molecular, proteomic and immunological characterization of isoforms of arginine kinase, a cross-reactive invertebrate pan-allergen, from the house dust mite, *Dermatophagoides farinae*. The 61th American Academy of Allergy and Immunology Annual Meeting. San Francisco, USA 2004. J Allergy Clin Immunol 2004; 113:226.

24. Lai FY, Loo AHB, Ramjan SFR, Reginald K, Shang HS, Chew FT: Pan-allergenicity of profilins – tests using recombinant protein homologs. Abstract book of the XXIIIth European Academy of Allergology and Clinical Immunology Annual Meeting (EAACI). Amsterdam, The Netherlands 2004; 581:176–177.

25. Angus AC, Xiong SQ, Mari A, Wang DY, Chew FT: Identification of a full length IgE-binding thaumatin-like protein from the storage mite, *Glycyphagus domesticus*. Abstract book of the XXIIIth European Academy of Allergology and Clinical Immunology Annual Meeting (EAACI). Amsterdam, The Netherlands 2004; 611:185.

26. Joshi SS, Gan HY, Chew FT: Cross comparison between the IgE binding profiles of cyclophilins from human, mouse, dust mites and fungi. The 63th American Academy of Allergy and Immunology Annual Meeting. Miami, Florida, USA 2006. J Allergy Clin Immunol 2006; 117:120.

Fook Tim Chew

Department of Biological Sciences, Lee Hiok Kwee Functional Genomics Laboratories, Allergy and Molecular Immunology Laboratory, National University of Singapore (NUS), Science Drive 4, Singapore 117543, Tel. +65 65161685, Fax +65 68722013, E-mail dbscft@nus.edu.sg

Nitration of Allergens: Another Pollution Effect to Be Concerned About

Y.K. Gruijthuijsen[1], I. Grieshuber[1], A. Stöcklinger[1], U. Tischler[1], T. Fehrenbach[2], M.G. Weller[2], L. Vogel[3], S. Vieths[3], U. Pöschl[2*], and A. Duschl[1]

[1]Department of Molecular Biology, University of Salzburg, Salzburg, Austria, [2]Institute of Hydrochemistry, Technical University of Munich, Munich, Germany, [3]Paul Ehrlich Institute, Langen, Germany, *Present address: Max Planck Institute for Chemistry, Mainz, Germany

Summary: *Background:* In considering environmental pollutants it is not sufficient to analyze only the emitted substances, since many of them can be modified after emission, both in the environment and after incorporation into the body. The observation of nitrated proteins present in urban environments with high NO_2 and ozone raises the possibility that these gases may influence allergy indirectly via the nitration of allergens. In this case NO_2 would affect human health even if it is not inhaled. *Methods:* The allergens Ovalbumin and Bet v 1 were nitrated by reaction with tetranitromethane, resulting in the generation of 3-nitrotyrosine. Effects of both allergens were analyzed in BALB/c mice. Ovalbumin was also studied using spleen cells from DO11.10 mice, and human sera were tested for binding of IgE to Bet v 1. *Results:* We found that nitrated versions of both allergens were more powerful than the unmodified versions in inducing allergic parameters, including T-cell proliferation, IL-5 production and serum levels of IgE. Also, sera from human patients with Bet v 1 allergy showed higher IgE binding to nitrated than to unmodified Bet v 1. *Conclusions:* Our data suggest that nitrated allergens, which can be demonstrated in the environment, lead to more severe allergic responses. Since sera from Bet v 1 allergic patients showed enhanced binding to nitrated Bet v 1, it is likely that these patients have indeed previously been exposed to Bet v 1 in nitrated form.

Keywords: allergen, modification, nitration, mouse model, environmental pollution

Introduction

Nitration of tyrosine residues contained in endogenous proteins occurs for example in inflammation, cellular stress and aging. Protein nitration may also happen in the environment, due to high levels of NO_2 and O_3 present especially during summer smog conditions. It was not known that these pollutants are able to affect proteins, until Franze et al. in 2005 published the finding that proteins get nitrated on tyrosine residues by simple exposure to urban air [1]. Among the nitrated proteins identified was Bet v 1, which raises the possibility that nitration of inhaled allergens may affect the immune response.

Results and Discussion

We have investigated the immunogenic and allergenic properties of *in vitro*-nitrated allergens. Ovalbumin and recombinant Bet v 1 were used in unmodified and in nitrated forms, where the allergens contained 3–4 residues of 3-nitrotyrosine per protein molecule.

Upon stimulation with nitrated vs. unmodified allergen splenocytes from DO11.10 mice showed enhanced proliferation and increased production of IL-5 and IFN-γ. It should be noted that the Ovalbumin epitope recognized by the T-cell receptor from DO11.10 cells contains no tyrosines [2]. It is clear from this and other data discussed be-

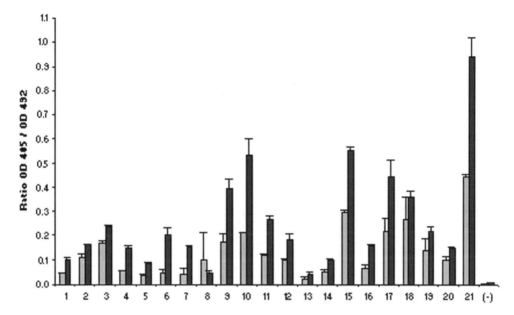

Figure 1. An ELISA for binding of specific IgE to allergen shows higher binding of specific IgE to nitrated Bet v 1 (black bars) compared to untreated Bet v 1 (grey bars) in 20/21 randomly selected samples. A pool of sera from nonallergic controls had no IgE against either protein (–).

low that 3-nitrotyrosine acts not just as a new B-cell epitope.

Similar results were obtained using splenocytes from BALB/c mice sensitized with either Ovalbumin or Bet v 1 in unmodified or nitrated form. Proliferation and cytokine production were enhanced by using the appropriate allergens in nitrated form. Furthermore, sera of mice sensitized with nitrated allergens (ovalbumin or Bet v 1) showed elevated levels of specific IgE, IgG_1, and $IgG_{2A,}$ compared to sera from mice sensitized with unmodified allergens. The effects on IFN-γ production and IgG_{2A} levels indicate that the enhancement of immune reactions is not exclusive for the allergic branch. However, allergens can of course be expected to specifically induce allergic sensitivity. Human sera from birch pollen-allergic individuals were analyzed by ELISA for presence of IgE specific for nitrated Bet v 1. Fig 1 shows higher binding of specific IgE to nitrated compared Bet v 1 compared to untreated Bet v 1 in 20 of 21 patients with allergy against Bet v 1.

In light of these findings, it is likely that protein nitration of allergens enhances allergic responses, which may contribute to an increased prevalence of allergic diseases in polluted urban environments. Since sera from Bet v 1 allergic patients showed enhanced binding of IgE to nitrated compared to unmodified Bet v 1 these patients seem to have been exposed previously to nitrated birch pollen allergen. The likely source of previously encountered nitrated allergen is modification of allergens in the environment by gaseous pollutants.

Acknowledgments

We thank T. Hawranek and M. Wallner for supplying human sera and human IgE-antibodies, P. Hammerl and R. Weiss for help with the mouse models, and R. Niessner for support. This work was financially partly supported by the European Union (MAAPHRI QLK-CT-2002–02357 (A.D.) and European commission, FP6 Contract No. 003956 (A.D.)), by the priority program "Biosciences and Health" of the University of Salzburg (A.D.), and by the BMBF-AFO2000 project CARBAERO (U.P.).

References

1. Franze T, Weller MG, Niessner R, Pöschl U: Protein nitration by polluted air. Environ Sci Technol 2005; 39:1673–1678.
2. Murphy KM, Heimberger AB, Loh DY: Induction by antigen of intrathymic apoptosis of CD4⁺ CD8⁺ TCRlo thymocytes *in vivo*. Science 1990; 250:1720–1723.

Albert Duschl

Department of Molecular Biology, University of Salzburg, Hellbrunner Strasse 34, A-5020 Salzburg, Austria, Tel. +43 662 8044-5731, Fax +43 662 8044-5751, E-mail albert. duschl@sbg.ac.at

Modulation of the IgE Response by Blocking Membrane-IgE

S. Feichtner[1], D. Infuehr[1], S. Lenz[1], D. Schmid[1], R. Crameri[2], and G. Achatz[1]

[1]*Department of Molecular Biology, Salzburg, Austria*, [2]*SIAF, Davos, Switzerland*

Summary: *Background:* Transgenic mouse experiments in our lab clearly showed that the transmembrane domain of mIgE is indispensable for T-cell dependent IgE secretion and that the cytoplasmic domain not only determines the absolute amount of IgE produced, but also influences the quality of the immunoglobulins. Thus, if mIgE is the prerequisite for the later production of secreted IgE, targeting mIgE bearing B-cells with anti-mIgE specific antibodies would be a promising systemic therapeutic approach. *Results:* In order to investigate the biological mechanism behind an anti-IgE therapy, we used the extra membrane proximal domain (EMPD) of mIgE, as target sequence for generating anti mIgE antibodies with the capacity to inhibit IgE synthesis in the murine system. So far, we were able to isolate two specific single chain antibodies and one specific anti EMPD-monoclonal antibody, showing high specificity for the EMPD-region in ELISA and flow cytometry. Immunization experiments with recombinant Bet v 1 and anti-EMPD in parallel showed a reduction of specific IgE antibodies by more than 90%. *Conclusion:* Treatment with anti-secreted-IgE antibodies leads primarily to a decrease of serum IgE levels. As a consequence the number of high-affinity IgE receptors on mast cells and basophils decreases, leading to a lower excitability of the effector cells. The biological mechanism behind this reduction remains speculative and has to be evaluated carefully. A possible explanation for the reduction of serum IgE may be that these antibodies can also interact with membrane bound IgE on B-cells, leading to a clearance of the mIgE population. Our hypothesis suggests that cross linking mIgE receptors by anti-EMPD antibodies without the appropriate T-cell help leads to direct clonal deletion and/or clonal anergy of the total mIgE B-cell population.

Keywords: mIgE, anti-IgE, systemic IgE therapy

Introduction/Results/Conclusion

Immunoglobulin E is present in very low amount (nano- to microgram per ml range) in serum of nonatopic individuals, and has a very short half life, compared to the other immunoglobulins. However, IgE plays the most important role in allergic disorders.

IgE consists of two light chains and two ε-heavy chains with variable (V) and constant (C) region domains and exists in a secreted (sIgE) or membrane-bound form (mIgE). The mIg transmembrane segment of the membrane-bound form is 25 amino acids long separated in a 6 amino acids transmembrane part and a 19 amino acids long, isotype specific, extracellular membrane proximal domain (EMPD), which differs in length and variability among the other isotypes.

To smoothen the typical symptoms of allergic disorders in humans, several antigen specific and systemic treatments were developed. Conventional immunotherapy with total extracts of allergenic sources [1] often are not effective and go in parallel with anaphylactic reactions. Another strategy is the generation of therapeutic antibody responses against IgE through vaccination with chimaeric IgE-like molecules [2] or a systemic treatment with the monoclonal antibody Omalizumab, which be-

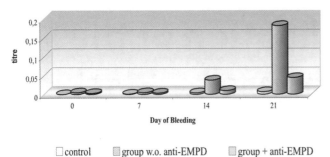

Figure 1. Bet v 1-specific IgE.

□ control   ▨ group w.o. anti-EMPD   ▢ group + anti-EMPD

longs to the group of anti-IgE-antibodies. This anti IgE antibody specifically targets the CH3 domain of circulating IgE which in turn prevents IgE from binding to FcεRI. As a result, titers of circulating free IgE are reduced and the late-phase responses are inhibited [3]. However, therapy insensitive patients of the current anti IgE therapy warrant a development of a new anti-IgE concept, based on the targeting of the mIgE antigenreceptor *in vivo*.

Transgenic mouse experiments in our lab [4, 5] showed that the transmembrane domain of mIgE was indispensable for T-cell-dependent IgE secretion and that the cytoplasmic domain not only determined the absolute amount of IgE produced, but also influenced the quality of the immunoglobulins. Thus, if mIgE is important for the quantity and quality of sIgE, B-cells expressing mIgE receptors could be a reasonable target for an anti IgE therapy [6]. Because of its isotype specificity the EMPD region of mIgE has been used as target sequence for generating anti mIgE antibodies with the capacity to inhibit IgE synthesis by crosslinking the IgE antigen receptor.

For monoclonal antibody production we decided to use female ΔM1M2 BALB/c mice [4], which do not express membrane bound immunoglobulins. The EMPD peptide of mouse IgE was coupled to Keyhole Limpet Hemocyanin (KLH) using standard protocols and the conjugate emulsified with Alum was used for intranodal and intraperitoneal immunization. Lymph node cells and spleen cells of anti EMPD positive mice were harvested and fused with the mouse B-lymphoma cell line Ag-8. One positive anti EMPD Hybridoma clone of IgG$_1$ isotype was selected, cultivated

in roller bottles and purified using Äkta prime HiTrap Protein G columns.

To prove the capacity of the anti-EMPD antibody to bind surface expressed mIgE antibodies, we incubated the mIgE expressing cell line JW813 with the unlabeled purified anti-EMPD antibody. The anti EMPD-antibody recognizes mIgE on the surface of the mIgE expressing cell line JW813/4.

Afterwards, three groups of five female BALB/c mice each were immunized according to the presented scheme. The control mouse group received no immunizations at all. Reference group one received Bet v 1 (20 μg recombinant Bet v 1) at day 0, 7, and 14. The EMPD group additionally received anti-EMPD i.p. (100 μg of the anti-IgE-EMPD) every three days (6 times). One control mouse was not immunized at all. Bleeding of the mice was performed at day 0, 7, 14, and 21. For specific ELISA measurements, Nunc maxisorp Immunoplates were coated with 500 ng recombinant Bet v 11 per well. Sera were diluted 1:10, 1:30 and 1:90 in 2% milkpowder PBS and incubated o.n. at 4 °C. For detection, the rat anti-mouse IgE (alkaline phosphatase labeled, Southern Biotechnology) was diluted 1:2000 and incubated for 2 h at RT. Absorption measurement (OD) was read out at 405–492 nm. Parallel application of anti EMPD leads to a reduction of specific IgE by 80% at day 21, reflecting the *in vivo* functionality of the anti-EMPD antibody in a passive immunization approach (Figure 1).

Currently available nonanaphylactogenic anti-IgE antibodies permit interruption of the allergic pathway at an early and central level by efficiently and selectively blocking IgE effector functions mediated by FcεRI as well as FcεRII-bearing effector cells. These antibodies block IgE mediated cell activation and inhibit new IgE production by IgE switched B-cells without affecting the production of other antibody classes. Clinical trials in patients with allergic rhinitis and allergic asthma reveal that selective neutralization and inhibition of IgE is associated with the inhibition of IgE mediated reactions. These studies will also encourage further investigations, which focus on the selective targeting of mIgE bearing B-cells, thus inhibiting IgE synthesis before IgE production starts.

The presented monoclonal anti IgE antibody clearly demonstrates that the idea of blocking mIgE is a practicable approach for systemic anti IgE therapies in the future.

Acknowledgments

Animal experiments were conducted in accordance with guidelines provided by the Austrian law on experimentation with live animals. The work was supported by the Austrian Science Foundation FWF grant P-19017-B13 as well as the Austrian National Bank OENB grant: 11710.

References

1. Durham SR, Walker SM, Varga EM, Jacobson MR, O'Brien F, Noble W, Till SJ, Hamid QA, Nouri-Aria KT: Long-term clinical efficacy of grass-pollen immunotherapy. N Engl J Med 1999; 341:468–475.
2. Vernersson M, Ledin A, Johansson J, Hellman L: Generation of therapeutic antibody responses against IgE through vaccination. Faseb J 2002; 16:875–877.
3. Fahy JV, Fleming HE, Wong HH, Liu JT, Su JQ, Reimann J, Fick RB Jr., Boushey HA: The effect of an anti-IgE monoclonal antibody on the early- and late-phase responses to allergen inhalation in asthmatic subjects. Am J Respir Crit Care Med 1997; 155:1828–1834.
4. Achatz G, Nitschke L, Lamers MC: Effect of transmembrane and cytoplasmic domains of IgE on the IgE response. Science 1997; 276:409–411.
5. Luger E, Lamers M, Achatz-Straussberger G, Geisberger R, Infuhr D, Breitenbach M, Crameri R, Achatz G: Somatic diversity of the immunoglobulin repertoire is controlled in an isotype-specific manner. Eur J Immunol 2001; 31:2319–2330.
6. Infuhr D, Crameri R, Lamers R, Achatz G: Molecular and cellular targets of anti-IgE antibodies. Allergy 2005; 60:977–985.

Gernot Achatz

Department of Molecular Biology, Division Allergy and Immunology, Hellbrunnerstraße 34, A-5020 Salzburg, Austria, Tel. +43 662 8044-5764, Fax +43 662 8044-183, E-mail gernot.achatz@sbg.ac.at

Artemisia and Ambrosia Hypersensitivity

Cosensitization or Corecognition? A Study Using Recombinant Weed Pollen Allergens

N. Wopfner[1], R. Asero[2], P. Gruber[1], G. Gadermaier[1], and F. Ferreira[1]

[1]*Department of Molecular Biology, Division of Allergy and Immunology, University of Salzburg, Austria,* [2]*Ambulatorio di Allergologia, Clinica San Carlo, Paderno Dugnano, Italy*

Summary: Various clinical and serological studies showed that sensitization to ragweed and mugwort pollen are often associated and this poses relevant clinical problems in patients for whom specific immunotherapy is warranted. Therefore, the goal of this study was to determine whether the concomitant ragweed and mugwort pollen hypersensitivity is the result of cosensitization or of corecognition by using purified recombinant allergens. Sensitization to ragweed and mugwort pollen was assessed by skin prick test (SPT) in all patients reporting allergic symptoms in August and September. IgE reactivity of sera from 42 patients to ragweed and mugwort pollen extract as well as to several recombinant ragweed (Amb a 1, Amb a 5, Amb a 6, Amb a 8, Amb a 9, and Amb a 10) and mugwort (Art v 1, Art v 4, Art v 5, Art v 6, and 3 EF-hand calcium-binding protein) allergens was detected by dot-blot and ELISA. In vitro, 90% of ragweed allergic patients reacted with Amb a 1. Reactivity to other ragweed allergens ranged between 20 and 35%. 46% of the mugwort-sensitized patients recognized Art v 1, 25% reacted to Art v 4, Art v 5 and Art v 6, and 7% recognized the 3-EF hand calcium binding protein. Immunoblot inhibition experiments showed that preincubation with ragweed pollen extract did not significantly decrease IgE reactivity to mugwort allergens. Therefore we concluded that patients showing both ragweed and mugwort positive SPT and/or RAST are in fact cosensitized and may need specific immunotherapy with extracts of both mugwort and ragweed pollen.

Keywords: mugwort, ragweed, cross-reactivity, immunotherapy, weed pollen allergy, recombinant allergens

Ragweed (*Ambrosia artemisiifolia*) and mugwort (*Artemisia vulgaris*) belong both to the great botanical family of *Compositae* and are the most important allergic plants in this botanical group. Although the geographical distribution of ragweed was more restricted to North America it is interesting to follow the spread of ragweed in the last ten to fifteen years in Europe and the rapid increase of allergic sensitization to ragweed pollen. Especially in the area north of Milan ragweed pollen has become the second cause of respiratory allergy after grass pollen [1]. Furthermore it is worth noting that the impressive increase in ragweed hypersensitivity has been paralleled by a sim-ilar increase in the prevalence of positive skin prick test (SPT) with mugwort pollen. Mugwort has always been present in this area, but few patients were found to be mugwort-sensitive before the appearance of ragweed and even less reported mugwort-induced symptoms. The concomitant sensitization to *Artemisia* and *Ambrosia* poses relevant clinical problems in patients for whom specific immunotherapy is warranted because of the nearly identical flowering periods in this area [2, 3]. Some studies [4, 5] concluded that in addition to profilin, mugwort and ragweed pollen contain a number of cross-reactive allergens, including the major mugwort allergen Art v 1.

In contrast, other studies concluded that Ambrosia and Artemisia pollen allergens show little or no cross-reactivity [6]. The main clinical question remains whether patients hypersensitive to both ragweed and mugwort should undergo specific immunotherapy with extracts from one particular pollen or from both.

In this study, recombinant weed pollen allergens were used to dissect sensitization patterns of mugwort and ragweed allergic patients. To determine whether ragweed and mugwort pollen hypersensitivity is the result of cosensitization or of corecognition IgE reactivity of sera from 42 patients (26 Amb+/Art+, 14 Amb+/Art–, and 2 Amb–/Art+) was analyzed in dotblot and ELISA experiments. For this purpose ragweed and mugwort pollen extract as well as several purified recombinant ragweed (Amb a 1, Amb a 5, Amb a 6, Amb a 8, Amb a 9, and Amb a 10) and mugwort (Art v 1, Art v 4, Art v 5, Art v 6, and 3-EF hand calcium-binding protein) allergens were incubated with serum IgE from the three different patients groups. A high percentage (46%) of Amb+/Art+ patients reacted to Art v 1, the major mugwort pollen allergen. Cross-reactivity to an Art v 1-homologous protein in ragweed seems not to be the case as immunoblot inhibition experiments showed a persistent IgE reactivity to mugwort allergens after absorption of sera with whole ragweed pollen extract. About 25% reacted to Art v 4, Art v 5, and Art v 6, and 7% recognized the 3-EF hand calcium-binding protein. Furthermore, in vitro 90% of the patients reacted to Amb a 1, the major ragweed allergen and the reactivity to other ragweed allergens ranged between 20% and 35%. From those patients that showed reactivity with Amb a 1, only six recognized Art v 6, the Amb a 1-homolog in mugwort. As previously reported [4, 7, 8], between 20% and 35% of the mugwort- and ragweed-sensitized patients displayed IgE antibodies to the panallergens profilin (Art v 4 and Amb a 8) and calcium-binding proteins (Art v 5, Amb a 9, Amb a 10). It is worth noting that all patients recognizing Art v 4 ($n = 8$, 20%) cross-reacted with ragweed profilin (Amb a 8). In contrast, cross-reactivity between the ragweed and mugwort calcium-binding allergens was not complete. These results are in accordance with the fact that sequence similarity between calcium-binding allergens is variable and mostly confined to the EF-hand calcium-binding motifs. Thus, it is possible that IgE antibodies directed to regions outside the EF-hands of one calcium-binding allergen might not bind to homologous proteins found in other pollen.

In conclusion, our results indicated that (i) there is very limited cross-reactivity between Amb a 1 and the homolog Art v 6 in mugwort pollen and between Art v 1 and its homolog in ragweed; (ii) the major allergens Amb a 1 from ragweed and Art v 1 from mugwort can thus be considered as markers for ragweed and mugwort sensitization, respectively. We concluded that patients showing both ragweed and mugwort positive SPT and/or RAST are in fact cosensitized. Therefore, patients with severe allergic symptoms in August and September should undergo specific immunotherapy with both pollen extracts mugwort and ragweed.

Acknowledgments

This work was supported by the grant S8802 from the Austrian research Council (FWF).

References

1. Asero R, Qualizza R, Schilke ML, Sillano V, Zanoletti T: Studio multicentrico sulla prevalenza delle pollinosi nella città e nella provincia di Milano: 1990–95. Giorn It Allergol Immunol Clin 1998; 8:241 (Abstract).
2. Caramiello R: Compositae, Artemisia. Giorn It Allergol Immunol Clin 1991; 1:461–466.
3. Gallesio MT: Compositae, Ambrosia. Giorn It Allergol Immunol Clin 1991; 1:467–471.
4. Hirschwehr R, Heppner C, Spitzauer S, Sperr WR, Valent P, Berger U, Horak F, Jager S, Kraft D, Valenta R: Identification of common allergenic structures in mugwort and ragweed pollen. J Allergy Clin Immunol 1998; 101:196–206.
5. Mutschlechner S, Mari A, Van Ree R, Didier-laurent A, Ebner C, Ferreira F, Wopfner N: Patterns of Art v 1 recognition in mugwort- and ragweed-sensitized patients. XXII Congress of the EAACI. Paris, 2003:384.
6. Weber RW: Patterns of pollen cross-allergenicity. J Allergy Clin Immunol 2003; 112:229–239.
7. Niederberger V, Hayek B, Vrtala S, Laffer S, Twar-

dosz A, Vangelista L, Sperr WR, Valent P, Rumpold H, Kraft D, Ehrenberger K, Valenta R, Spitzauer S: Calcium-dependent immunoglobulin E recognition of the apo- and calcium-bound form of a cross-reactive two EF-hand timothy grass pollen allergen, Phl p 7. Faseb J 1999; 13:843–856.
8. Wopfner N, Willeroider M, Hebenstreit D, van Ree R, Aalbers M, Briza P, Thalhamer J, Ebner C, Richter K, Ferreira F: Molecular and immunological characterization of profilin from mugwort pollen. Biol Chem 2002; 383:1779–1789.

Fátima Ferreira

Department of Molecular Biology, Christian Doppler Laboratory for Allergy Diagnosis and Therapy, University of Salzburg, Hellbrunnerstraße 34, A-5020 Salzburg, Austria, Tel. +43 662 8044-5734, Fax +43 662 8044-183, E-mail fatima.ferreira@sbg.ac.at

Cytokine Responses in Peanut Nonallergic Adults Are Dominated by Th2-Like Responses in the Absence of Detectable Th1 Function

T.B. Thottingal[1,2], F.E.R. Simons[1,2], S. Waserman[1,3], G.A. Bannon[4], W. Burks[5], and K.T. HayGlass[1,2]

[1]AllerGen NCE and [2]CIHR National Training Program in Allergy and Asthma Research, University of Manitoba, Winnipeg, Canada, [3] McMaster University, Hamilton Canada, [4]University of Arkansas for Medical Sciences, Little Rock, USA, [5]Duke University, Durham, NC, USA

Summary: *Background:* The nature of the peanut specific immunoregulatory response in nonallergic humans is poorly understood. *Methods:* Using primary culture, the prevalence and nature of peanut-driven, T-cell dependent cytokine responses in 30 adults who eat peanut without exhibiting symptoms was assessed. *Results:* Peanut-specific IL-5, IL-13 responses were common in peanut-tolerant individuals but putatively protective Th1 immunity was undetectable. *Conclusion:* Clinical tolerance to dietary peanut is maintained despite the presence of Th2 responses and absence of detectable peanut specific Th1 recall responses.

Keywords: food allergy, cytokine, chemokine, tolerance, immune regulation

Introduction

Peanuts are the most common triggers of food allergic reactions with fatal outcome in children and adults of the developed world [1, 2]. Immunoregulatory responses that develop in humans upon natural peanut exposure are little understood [3]. Most studies largely or exclusively focus on individuals with confirmed peanut allergy [4–7]. Here, we sought to define peanut Ag-specific T-cell recall responses in adults who are naturally peanut exposed but who consistently fail to exhibit allergic symptoms. Increased understanding of immune responses associated with spontaneous, typically lifelong, unre-sponsiveness could provide important insight for future development of improved diagnostic approaches, prevention and therapy of food allergies.

Methods

Participants

Following local Research Ethics Board approval, written informed consent was obtained from all participants. 30 adults, 18–40 years old, for whom a detailed history consistent with a lack of clinical reactivity to peanut, ever, were studied.

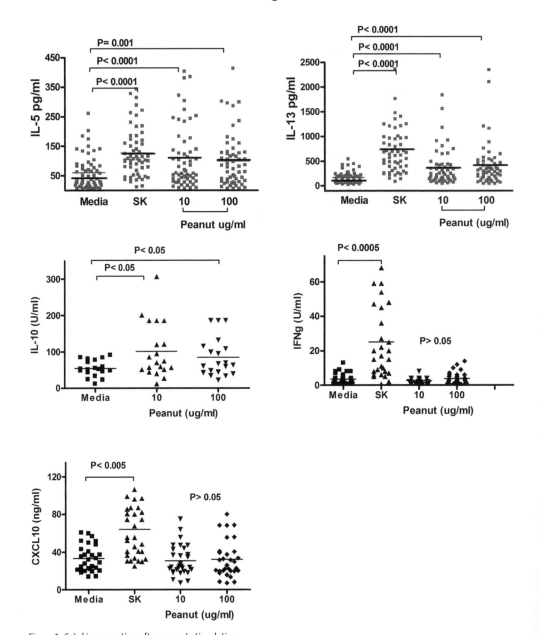

Figure 1. Cytokine secretion after peanut stimulation.

Cell Culture and Analysis

50 mL blood was collected in EDTA containing tubes, PBMC were isolated [8] (viability >95%) and cultured (5×10^5 cells/well 37 °C for 1, 3, 5, 7, and 9 days) in 96 well round-bottom microwell plates with roasted peanut Ag [9] or bacterial recall Ag, streptokinase. Supernatants were assessed by ELISA [8, 10].

Validated Wilcoxon matched pairs were used for statistical analysis.

Results

In initial studies, we identified optimal conditions for induction and analysis of peanut driven, MHC class II-dependent cytokine responses in short term primary culture directly ex vivo (Thottingal et al., manuscript submitted). To assess peanut-driven immunity among peanut allergy history-negative individuals, a panel of immunoregulatory cytokines was quantified in response to short term stimulation of PBMC directly ex vivo with peanut or streptokinase. In Figure 1, Th1-like responses are readily detected with recall antigen streptokinase, but are consistently undetectable to peanut. Similarly, CXCL10, tightly associated with IFN-γ production [10] is also undetectable in the peanut-stimulated response. This population of environmentally peanut-exposed but clinically nonallergic adults is not immunologically anergic, as it expressed readily detectable Th2-like responses upon peanut stimulation. These were blocked by inclusion of anti-CD4 mAb or CTLA4-Ig in culture and were not evident in cord blood mononuclear cells (not shown). Thus, they exhibit the characteristics of classical Ag-driven T-cell activation, demonstrating the presence of Ag-specific T-cell recall responses that are dominated by Th2 rather than Th1-biased immunity. We subsequently examined IL-10 production in a subset of individuals (for which supernatants were available) because expression of this immunosuppressive cytokine is frequently associated with regulation of adaptive immunity. Peanut-specific IL-10 responses were readily detected in peanut Ag-driven cultures of peanut nonallergic individuals.

Discussion

Despite often extreme efforts, complete avoidance of allergenic molecules is impossible in daily life. The immune responses of those who spontaneously develop desirable clinical outcomes (tolerance) are important to understand if we are to develop effective prophylactic and therapeutic interventions for food allergy. We demonstrate here that, as for inhalant Ag-specific responses in nonallergic individuals [8, 10], readily quantified Ag-specific, CD4 T-cell dependent cytokine production is common in clinically tolerant individuals. Such *clinical* unresponsiveness is clearly distinct from *immunological* unresponsiveness for common environmental Ags. However, the pattern of responses evoked by this food Ag in nonallergic individuals differs markedly from that seen with house dust mite, cat, grass pollen or streptokinase stimulation. In detailed kinetic analyses over d.1–9 of culture, production of type 1 cytokine (IFN-γ) and chemokine (CXCL10) responses were consistently undetectable to peanut stimulation. Whether this reflects differences due to the nature of the stimulating Ag, the route of exposure (airway vs gut) or different means of eliciting and maintaining clinical tolerance to inhalant vs dietary Ags remains unclear. The data suggest that enhanced IL-10, rather than tightly controlled and presumably undesirable Th1 immunity in the gut, may play a role in such clinical tolerance. A wide variety of cells including DC, monocytes and/or certain Treg populations can produce IL-10. Direct comparison of the frequency and intensity of peanut Ag driven IL-10 responses in peanut allergic vs peanut nonallergic adults will be required and is currently in progress. Clearly, more attention to defining the nature and frequency of regulatory responses that control tolerance vs IgE sensitization, and progression in a subset of individuals to life threatening anaphylaxis, is important.

Acknowledgments

We thank AllerGen NCE, the CIHR, the Manitoba Institute of Child Health and CAAIF/Anaphylaxis Canada for support.

References

1. Flinterman AE, Pasmans SG, Hoekstra MO, Meijer Y, van Hoffen E, Knol EF, Hefle SL, Bruijnzeel-Koomen CA, Knulst AC: Determination of no-observed-adverse-effect levels and eliciting doses in a representative group of peanut-sensitized children. J Allergy Clin Immunol 2006; 117:448–454.

2. Lehmann K, Schweimer K, Reese G, Randow S, Suhr M, Becker WM, Vieths S, Rosch P: Structure

and stability of 2S albumin-type peanut allergens: implications for the severity of peanut allergic reactions. Biochem J 2006; 395:463–472.

3. Sicherer SH, Leung DY: Advances in allergic skin disease, anaphylaxis, and hypersensitivity reactions to foods, drugs, and insects. J Allergy Clin Immunol 2005; 116:153–163.

4. Lewis SA, Grimshaw KE, Warner JO, Hourihane JO: The promiscuity of IgE binding to peanut allergens, as determined by Western blotting, correlates with the severity of clinical symptoms. Clin Exp Allergy 2005; 35:767–773.

5. Turcanu V, Maleki SJ, Lack G: Characterization of lymphocyte responses to peanuts in normal children, peanut-allergic children, and allergic children who acquired tolerance to peanuts. J Clin Invest 2003; 111:1065–1072.

6. Castro RR, Shreffler WG, Pei-Chi LS, Sampson HA: Characterization of T-cell responses in peanut-allergic patients by polychromatic flow cytometry. J Allergy Clin Immunology 2004; 113:251.

7. Scott-Taylor TH, Hourihane JB, Harper J, Strobel S: Patterns of fold allergen-specific cytokine production by T lymphocytes of children with multiple allergies. Clin Exp Allergy 2005; 35:1473–1480.

8. Li Y, Simons FER, HayGlass KT: Environmental antigen-induced IL-13 responses are elevated among subjects with allergic rhinitis, are independent of IL-4, and are inhibited by endogenous IFN-γ synthesis. J Immunol 1998; 161:7007–7014.

9. Pons L, Palmer K, Burks W: Toward immunotherapy for peanut allergy. Cur Opin All and Clin Immunol 2005; 5:558–562.

10. Campbell JD, Gangur V, Simons FE, HayGlass KT: Allergic humans are hyporesponsive to a CXCR3 ligand-mediated Th1 immunity-promoting loop. FASEB J 2004; 18:329–331.

K.T. HayGlass

AllerGen NCE and CIHR National Training Program in Allergy and Asthma Research, University of Manitoba, Winnipeg, Canada, E-mail Hayglass@cc.umanitoba.ca

Recombinant Hybrid Molecule Consisting of rPhl p 1, 2, 5, and 6

Is it the Best Combination for Grass Pollen Diagnosis in a Group of French Patients?

G. Pauli[1], C. Metz-Favre[1], B. Linhart[2], A. Purohit[1], F. de Blay[1], and R. Valenta[2]

[1]Hôpitaux Universitaires de Strasbourg, France, [2]Medical University of Vienna, Austria

Summary: *Background:* In a previous study we have shown that over 50% of grass allergic patients recognized Phl p 5, 2, and 4. We also demonstrated by skin prick testing the *in vivo* activity of recombinant hybrid molecule (HM) consisting of rPhl p 1, 2, 5, and 6 in a group of French patients. We compared in the same population the detection of specific IgE against a natural grass pollen extract, this hybrid molecule and a battery of recombinant allergens. *Methods:* 35 French grass pollen allergic patients were tested by ELISA for the presence of specific IgE against the natural crude grass pollen extract (9 species, Allergon), the hybrid molecule and rPhl p 1, 2, 5, 6, 7, 12, and 13. Specific IgE levels were considered positive at a level superior to 0.1. *Results:* We found a significant correlation between HM specific IgE and natural grass pollen extract IgE ($r = 0.972$, $p < .001$). More patients were positive with the HM (97.1% against 88.6%), with a high geometric mean of specific IgE levels (1.27 against 0.91). IgE binding frequency against rPhl p 1, 2, and 5 roughly corresponded to those reported earlier but the frequency against nPhl p 4 increased from 58 to 77%, while the rPhl p 6 binding frequency of sensitization was 65.7%. Moreover the 3 highest specific IgE levels were observed for rPhl p 1, 5 and 4. *Conclusions:* Both *in vivo* and *in vitro* studies confirm that the HM is an accurate tool for diagnosis. The choice of a limited number of recombinant allergens has to take into account the sensitivity profile of a given geographic population.

Keywords: recombinant grass pollen allergens, hybrid molecule, Human sensitization profiles

Introduction

Grass pollen is the most frequent pollinic allergen involved in sensitization (8.3% of the children included in ISAAC study in Strasbourg). In a previous study we were able to show that over 50% of grass allergic patients recognized Phl p 1, Phl p 2, Phl p 4, Phl p 5 [1]. A hybrid molecule was engineered by PCR-based mending and expression of the cDNAs coding for the 4 major grass pollen allergens (Phl p 1, Phl p 2, Phl p 5, Phl p 6) [2]. We first demonstrated that this hybrid molecule permitted *in* *vivo* and *in vitro* diagnosis of grass pollen allergy in 32 patients [3]. In the same patients we studied the sensitization profiles against 8 individual timothy grass pollen allergens in order to assess if the combination used in the hybrid molecule was optimal for this French population.

Material

35 patients (21 men), mean age: 28 years (18–55) were included. All patients were liv-

ing in Alsace and presented rhino-conjunctivi-
tis with or without asthma over the grass pollen season (May and June). They were all positive to grass pollen crude extracts which is a
mixture of three different grass pollen species
(*Phleum pratense, Dactylis glomerata, Lolium
perenne*, Stallergènes Laboratories) by using
skin prick-tests.

Individual grass pollen IgEs were determined by ELISA using 7 recombinant timothy
grass pollen allergens (rPhl p 1, rPhl p 2,
rPhl p 5, rPhl p 6, rPhl p 7, rPhl p 12,
rPhl p 13) and one natural allergen (nPhl p 4),
as well as specific IgEs against the hybrid molecule and the crude grass pollen extract used
for skin tests. Specific IgE levels were considered positive at a level > 0.1.

Results

Comparison Between Specific IgEs Against the Hybrid Molecule and Crude Grass Pollen Extract

A significant correlation between hybrid molecule specific IgEs and natural grass pollen extract specific IgEs was found ($r = 0.98$, $p <
.0001$, Figure 1).

Frequencies of Sensitization to a Panel of 8 Individual Timothy Grass Pollen Allergens

The frequencies of sensitization are shown in
Figure 2. The highest frequencies were observed with rPhl p 1, rPhl p 5, nPhl p 4,
rPhl p 6 and rPhl p 2 (respectively 100%,
83%, 77%, 57%, 48%). These results confirm
previous studies performed in populations living in Southern Europe [4, 5]. IgE binding frequencies for rPhl p 1, 2, 4, 5 in this study were
also compared with a previous study performed in our center: they hardly showed any
difference for rPhl p 1 or rPhl p 2 but were
higher for nPhl p 4 and rPhl p 5 with an increase of 20% (Figure 3).

From a quantitative point of view, the highest
specific IgE levels were observed for rPhl p 1
(mean: 0.94) and rPhl p 5 (mean: 1.44).

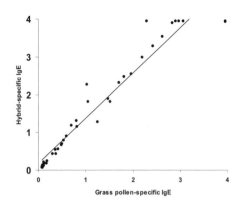

Figure 1.

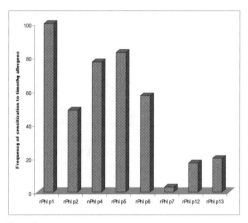

Figure 2.

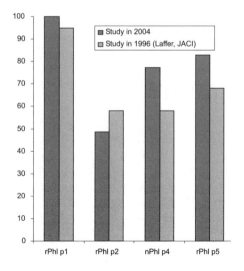

Figure 3.

nPhl p 4 was the third most frequent allergen recognized by the patients' IgEs: 77% of the population was concerned, whereas only 48% recognized rPhl p 2 and 57% rPhl p 6.

Nevertheless, several studies indicate that the biological activity of Phl p 4 is very low in contrast with group 2 grass pollen allergens which are strong elicitors of cutaneous and nasal inflammation.

Conclusions

This *in vitro* study confirms that the allergens included in the hybrid molecule allowed grass-pollen allergy diagnosis, even though it does not include all major grass pollen allergen especially Phl p 4 which sensitize 77% of the population of this geographic area.

References

1. Laffer S, Spitzauer S, Susani M, Pairleitner H, Schweiger C, Grönlund H, Menz G, Pauli G, Ishii T, Nolte H, Ebner C, Sehon A, Kraft D, Eichler H, Valenta R: Comparison of recombinant timothy grass pollen allergens with natural extract for diagnosis of grass pollen allergy in different populations. J Allergy Clin Immunol 1996; 98:652–658.

2. Linhart B, Hartl A, Jahn-Schmid B, Verdino P, Keller W, Krauth MT, Valent P, Horak F, Wiedermann U, Thalhamer J, Ebner C, Kraft D, Valenta R: A hybrid molecule resembling the epitope spectrum of grass pollen for allergy vaccination. J Allergy Clin Immunol 2005; 115:1010–1016.

3. Metz-Favre C, Linhart B, Purohit A, de Blay F, Valenta R, Pauli G: A single recombinant hybrid molecule consisting of the major Timothy grass pollen allergens to replace natural pollen extracts for skin test diagnosis. J Allergy Clin Immunol 2005; 115:271.

4. Rossi RE, Monasterolo G, Monasterolo S: Measurement of IgE antibodies against purified grass-pollen allergens (Phl p 1, 2, 3, 4, 5, 6, 7, 11, and 12) in sera of patients allergic to grass pollen. Allergy 2001; 56:1180–1185.

5. Mari A: Skin test with a timothy grass (Phleum pratense) pollen extract vs. IgE to a timothy extract vs. IgE to rPhl p 1, rPhl p 2, nPhl p 4, rPhl p 5, rPhl p 6, rPhl p 7, rPhl p 11, and rPhl p 12: epidemiological and diagnostic data. Clin Exp Allergy 2003; 33:43–51.

Gabrielle Pauli

Département de Pneumologie, Hôpital Lyautey, Hôpitaux Universitaires de Strasbourg, B.P. 426, F-67091 Strasbourg Cedex, France, E-mail gabrielle.pauli@chru.strasbourg.fr

Epitope Mapping and Characterization of the Binding Specificity of Monoclonal Antibodies Directed Against Allergens of Grass Group 1

A. Petersen[1], G. Schramm[2], A. Kramer[3], K. Grobe[4], and W.-M. Becker[1]

[1]*Molecular and Clinical Allergology, Research Center Borstel, Borstel,* [2]*Cellular Allergology, Research Center Borstel, Borstel,* [3]*Institute for Medical Immunology (Charité), Berlin,* [4]*Westfälische Wilhelms University, Münster, all Germany*

Summary: *Background:* Grass group 1 allergens consist of potent IgE-binding components which are found in all grass species. For studies of allergen extracts and for use as diagnostic markers we examined the epitope requirements for three monoclonal antibodies (mAbs) HB7, IG12 and Bo14 in detail. *Methods:* To determine the epitopes of the three mAbs we performed a screening of recombinantly produced group 1 allergen fragments. Further delimiting investigations were done by the PEPSCAN and SPOT technique using synthesized overlapping decapeptides covering the complete Phl p 1 molecule. Definition of the epitopes was performed with synthesized peptides spanning the respective epitopes and mutating each amino acid position by the 20 possible amino acid residues. By competition ELISA we analyzed whether the mAbs competed with patients' IgE for binding sites. *Results:* The epitopes of Phl p 1-directed mAbs were located on three different regions on the allergen. In case of HB7, we could encircle the epitope to the 27 N-terminal amino acids employing a set of recombinant fragments. The epitopes of IG12 and Bo14 could be limited to amino acid residues 48–53 and 225–232, respectively, and their exact epitope structure was studied by amino acid exchanges. None of the antibodies revealed an inhibitory influence on IgE binding. *Conclusion:* The results demonstrate clearly definable linear epitopes for the mAbs IG12 and Bo14, while the HB7 epitope seems to span a wider region probably due to conformational segments. These studies will help designing assays for monitoring and isolating group 1 allergens by affinity chromatography.

Keywords: epitope mapping, grass pollen allergen, monoclonal antibody

Hypersensitivity to pollen is the most common allergy of type I. Up to 95% of grass pollen allergic patients reveal IgE antibodies against the group 1 allergens, which have a molecular mass of about 30 kDa and are found in all grass species. High sequence homology causes on one hand a similar immunological reactivity of group 1 pollen allergens, on the other hand a structural microheterogeneity among the group 1 molecules within one grass species [1]. Monoclonal antibodies (mAbs) can serve as useful tools for setting up assays to monitor and characterize allergen structures in detail and to isolate a particular allergen from crude extracts. However, their suitability first needs to be proven.

We analyzed the three most promising mAbs HB7, IG12, and Bo14, which recognize

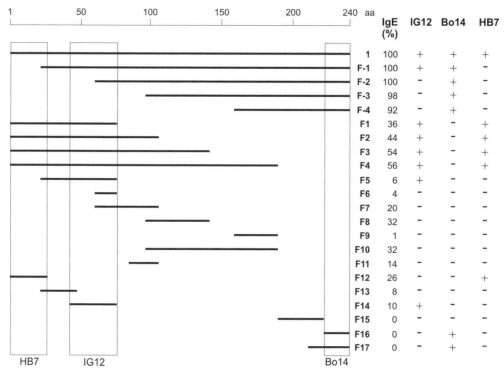

Figure 1. Schematic map of recombinant fragments on Hol l 1 to localize the epitopes of the monoclonal antibodies. Minimal fragments harbouring the epitopes of the monoclonal antibodies are highlighted.

group 1 allergens under native conditions in an ELISA as well as after denaturing conditions after SDS-PAGE and Western blotting. While HB7 and IG12 are IgG₁ antibodies, Bo14 belongs to the IgM class.

For a rough estimation of the epitopes we used Hol 1 1 fragments expressed as fusion proteins with a maltose-binding tag, an attempt which had been successfully used to localize IgE-binding epitopes [2]. Here, we analyzed the reactivity of the monoclonal antibodies by Western blotting.

Figure 1 shows the results in a schematic diagram. The boxed regions indicate the minimal segments of the allergen which were detectable by the panel of recombinant fragments: HB7 bound to amino acids 1–27 (F12), IG12 to 42–76 (F14) and Bo14 to 221–240 (F16).

For a more precise determination of B-cell epitopes, decapeptides with an increment of three amino acids were synthesized to activated polypropylene pins with a spacer consisting of 1,6-diaminohexane and β-alanine utilizing

9-fluorenylmethoxycarbonyl amino acids (Fmoc) according to the PEPSCAN technology ([3]; Chiron Mimotopes Peptide Systems, Clayton Victoria, Australia). By this technique we were able to limit the epitopes for IG12 and Bo14 to the peptides KPPFKGMT (48–55) and KDVIPEGW (224–232), respectively. No peptide was detected by HB7 indicating that wider regions and/or conformational segments of the allergen are involved in the binding.

Because of the structural variability of the group 1 allergens and the isoforms among each grass species, we wanted to determine the exact target sequence requirements for the mAbs HB7 and IG12. Therefore, the defined epitope regions were synthesized by mutating each amino acid position by the 20 possible amino acid residues.

Figure 2 demonstrates the defined epitope regions obtained by the SPOT technique (similarly performed to the PEPSCAN but spotted and synthesized on a membrane [4]). From the binding patterns we can deduce that, e.g., the proline residue in position 50 can be ex-

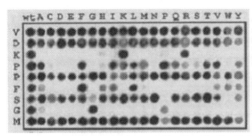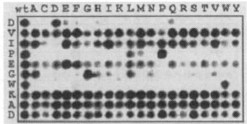

Figure 2. Epitope analysis for the monoclonal antibodies IG 12 (left) and Bo 14 (right). Peptides spanning the respective epitopes were synthesized by the SPOT technique and each amino acid position was mutated by the 20 possible amino acid residues.

changed by any other amino acid residue without loss of IG12 binding, while in position 48 the lysine residue cannot be exchanged except by arginine. From these results we now can explain, why the IG12 antibody does not bind to maize pollen: Zea m 1 (P58738) differs to the group 1 allergens of other grass species by a lysine → leucine exchange in the corresponding position.

In order to determine, whether the binding of the mAbs interfere with patients' IgE, we performed an ELISA inhibition test. Since the addition of increasing serum concentrations did not reduce the binding of all three mAbs, we can be sure that none of the antibodies binds to an IgE-reactive epitope.

From the 3D structure of Phl p 1 [5] the binding regions of the three mAbs can be estimated. All the epitopes are located on the surface of the molecule indicating that they are accessible.

Since the three mAbs bind to distant epitopes on the group 1 molecules, they can serve as valuable tools to build up a two side binding assay to quantify the important group 1 allergens in extracts. The IgG₁ mAbs HB7 and IG12 were also successfully used for Phl p 1 isolation from crude timothy pollen extract.

The use of the three consecutive methods is a suitable strategy to precisely determine epitopes on target molecules. While IG12 and Bo14 bind to linear epitopes, HB7 probably binds to a larger epitope, possibly forming a conformational segment.

References

1. Petersen A, Schramm G, Bufe A, Schlaak M, Becker WM: Structural investigations of the major allergen Phl p I on the complementary DNA and protein level. J Allergy Clin Immunol 1995; 95:987–994.
2. Schramm G, Bufe A, Petersen A, Haas H, Schlaak M, Becker WM: Mapping of IgE-binding epitopes on the recombinant major group I allergen of velvet grass pollen, rHol l 1. J Allergy Clin Immunol 1997; 99:781–787.
3. Geysen HM, Rodda SJ, Mason TJ, Tribbick G, Schoofs PG: Strategies for epitope analysis using peptide synthesis. J Immunol Methods 1987; 102:259–274.
4. Reineke U, Kramer A, Schneider-Mergener J: Antigen sequence- and library-based mapping of linear and discontinuous protein-protein-interaction sites by spot synthesis. Curr Top Microbiol Immunol 1999; 243:23–36.
5. Fedorov AA, Ball T, Leistler B, Valenta R, Almo SC: Crystal structure of Phl p 1, a major timothy grass pollen allergen, Structural Genomics Research Consortium (Nysgrc), 2002/10/16, 1N10, mmdbId21806.

Arnd Petersen

Molecular and Clinical Allergology, Research Center Borstel, Parkallee 22, D-23845 Borstel, Germany, Tel. +49 4537 188-497, Fax +49 4537 188-686, E-mail apetersen@fz-borstel.de

Relevance of Carbohydrate Determinants in Differentiating True Latex Allergy from Asymptomatic IgE Reactivity

M. Raulf-Heimsoth[1], U. Jappe[2], H.Y. Yeang[3], S.A.M. Arif[3], H.P. Rihs[1], A.L. Lopata[4], M.F. Jeebhay[5], and T. Brüning[1]

[1]*Berufsgenossenschaftliches Forschungsinstitut für Arbeitsmedizin (BGFA), Ruhr-University, Bochum, Germany,* [2]*Department of Dermatology, Venerology, University Heidelberg, Germany,* [3]*Rubber Research Institute of Malaysia (RRIM), Kuala Lumpur, Malaysia,* [4]*Division of Immunology, IIDMM-Allergy Section, NHLS, University of Cape Town, South Africa,* [5]*Occupational and Environmental Health Research Unit, University of Cape Town, South Africa*

Summary: *Background:* IgE-binding to cross-reacting carbohydrate determinants (CCDs) has already been described for several plant proteins, but their relevance for latex allergy is yet to be determined. Important natural rubber latex (NRL) allergens, such as Hev b 2 and Hev b 13 are glycosylated proteins. Discrimination between true latex allergy and clinically insignificant IgE sensitization still possesses a diagnostic challenge. *Methods:* The IgE reactivity to single NRL allergens and horseradish peroxidase (HRP) used as a marker of CCDs was analyzed with the UniCAP-system using sera from subjects demonstrating NRL-specific IgE. These included 72 latex-allergic HCWs, 89 patients with allergy to hymenoptera venom and 32 workers of a seafood processing company. *Results:* Six of the 72 HCW sera with clinically significant NRL allergy had elevated specific IgE to HRP. Although more than 80% of the HCW sera recognized native Hev b 2, the binding of NRL-specific IgE antibodies was inhibited by HRP appreciably only in two cases. 30 of 32 seafood workers' sera from latex-sensitized workers displayed comparable specific IgE responses to HRP and NRL. The reactivity to the recombinant allergens was low. The prevalence of Hev b 2-specific IgE was about 90% and most of the Hev b 2-specific IgE-values were similar to the HRP-values. Inhibition of NRL-specific IgE-binding with HRP was >80%. Furthermore, in patients with hymenoptera venom allergy and latex sensitization the specific IgE responses to the recombinant allergens were caused by the IgE-binding to the maltose-binding protein. There was a good correlation between NRL-specific and HRP-specific IgE response in the patient group with hymenoptera venom allergy ($r^2 = 0.84$). In this group the NRL-specific IgE-binding was completely abolished in the presence of HRP. *Conclusion:* Our data indicate that reactivity to CCDs such as HRP could be used as an *in vitro* screening tool for differentiating true latex allergy from clinically insignificant elevated specific IgE to NRL.

Keywords: latex allergy, carbohydrate determinants, allergen profile, asymptomatic IgE reactivity

IgE-binding to cross-reacting carbohydrate determinants (CCDs) has already been described for several plant proteins [1, 2], but their rele-vance for latex allergy is yet to be determined. Important natural rubber latex (NRL) aller-gens, such as Hev b 2 and Hev b 13, are glycosylated proteins. Hev b 2, e.g., has β-1,3 glucanase activity and the heterogeneous glycosylation of the As residues could be a source of the multiple allergenicity of natural Hev b 2 [3]. Previously we demonstrated that the recombinant form of Hev b 2 produced in *E. coli* was not able to bind specific IgE [4], therefore the glycan chains seem to be important for the IgE-reactivity. Although the risk for developing a latex allergy is declining in high-risk groups in western countries, sensitization outside of the medical field was observed. Discrimination between true latex allergy and clinically insignificant IgE sensitization still possesses a diagnostic challenge. Therefore, the single latex allergen profile of patients with true latex allergy and asymptomatic latex IgE reactivity and their IgE binding to different CCD reagents were determined.

The IgE reactivities to NRL (k82), single native (nHev b 2 and nHev b 13 prepared at the Rubber Research Institute in Malaysia,) and recombinant NRL allergens (produced at the BGFA), horseradish peroxidase (HRP with MMXF^3-chains; Ro400) and bromelain (with MUXF^3-chains; k202) used as markers of CCDs were analyzed with the ImmunoCAP test. Sera (n = 197) from subjects demonstrating NRL-specific IgE were tested. This collective included 72 health care workers (HCW) with clinically relevant latex allergy, 89 patients with allergy to hymenoptera venom (IgE-double positive for honeybee (HB) and yellow jacket (YJ)) [5] and 37 workers of a seafood processing company (only one worker had work-related skin symptoms and he used latex gloves).

In special cases inhibition experiments were performed with NRL (k82) ImmunoCAP as solid phase and 10 µl of HRP (10 mg/ml; Sigma, Taufkirchen, Germany) added to 50 µl patient serum as inhibitor.

Different latex sensitization profiles were measured in HCW with clinically significant NRL allergy, seafood workers with asymptomatic IgE reactivity to NRL and patients with allergy to hymenoptera venom and sIgE to NRL.

Major allergens (< 50% of IgE response) in the group of HCW were Hev b 2, Hev b 5, Hev

6.01 and Hev b 13. Although more than 75% of the HCW sera recognized native glycosylated Hev b 2 or nHev b 13, only six out of the 72 HCW sera (8.3%) had elevated specific IgE to HRP and bromelain. The specific IgE responses of the six sera to the two CCD-reagents were in the same range (sIgE to HRP: 1.48 kU/L; 0.41–7.95 kU/L; sIgE to bromelain: 2.6 kU/L; 0.51–7.79 kU/L), but different compared to the NRL-specific IgE responses (8.5 kU/L; 0.78 – > 100 kU/L). The prevalence of Hev b 2-specific IgE was about 90% in the group of seafood workers (nHev b 2 specific IgE: 2.28 kU/L; < 0.35–10.8 kU/L) and similar to the IgE response to NRL-specific IgE (2.44 kU/L; 0.75–20.8 kU/L). The reactivity to the recombinant allergens was low and in five of these sera IgE responses to the MBP-ImmunoCAP (the fusion protein being part of the recombinant allergens) were measured. 94% of the sera displayed comparable specific IgE responses to HRP (3.01 kU/L; < 0.35–15.5 kU/L) and bromelain (2.5 kU/L; <0.35–12.1 kU/L). nHev b 2-specific IgE-values correlated well to HRP – (r^2 = 0.85), and to a lesser extend to the bromelain-values (r^2 = 0.58). Nine out of 89 sera of patients with hymenoptera venom allergy and latex sensitization were tested for their specific latex allergen profile. In most of the cases the specific IgE responses to the recombinant allergens were caused by the IgE-binding to the MBP. The specific IgE-reactivity to bromelain and to HRP was 77.8%. There was a good correlation between NRL-specific and HRP-specific IgE response in this complete group (r^2 = 0.84).

Inhibition of NRL-specific IgE-binding with CCD reagents was performed in a subgroup of the seafood workers and in HCWs with specific IgE response to CCD reagents. In all representative sera of the seafood worker group the specific IgE response to NRL was completely abolished in the presence of CCDs reagents. In contrast, with the HCW sera only in two cases the NRL-specific IgE response was inhibited to more than 50%.

Our data indicate that reactivity to CCDs reagents such as HRP and bromelain could be used as an *in vitro* screening tool for differentiating true latex allergy from clinically insignificant elevated IgE to NRL. In the case of glycosylated allergens like Hev b 2 peptide as well as carbohydrate epitopes exist in the same molecule. In patients with a clear NRL-induced latex allergy the peptide epitopes are relevant, whereas in patients originally sensitized to other allergens, the carbohydrate epitopes are recognized. In addition, subsequent reciprocal inhibition is an essential diagnostic method to specify cross-reacting specific IgE results.

References

1. van Ree R: Carbohydrate epitopes and their relevance for the diagnosis and treatment of allergic diseases. Int Arch Allergy Immunol 2002; 129:189–197.
2. Malandain H: IgE reactive carbohydrate epitopes – Classification, cross-reactivity and clinical impact. Eur Ann Allergy Clin Immunol 2005; 37:122–128, 247–256.
3. Yagami T, Osuna H, Kouno M, Haishima Y, Nakamura A, Ikezawa Z: Significance of carbohydrate epitopes in a latex allergen with β-1,3-glucanase activity. Int Arch Allergy Immunol 2002; 129:27–37.
4. Raulf-Heimsoth M, Rihs HP, Brüning T: Latex: a new target for standardization. In J Löwer, WM Becker, S Vieths (Eds.), Regulatory control and standardization of allergenic extracts, 10th International Paul Ehrlich Seminar. Frankfurt a.M.: Sperlich 2003; 94:107–115.
5. Jappe U, Raulf-Heimsoth M, Hoffmann M, Burow G, Hübsch-Müller C, Enk A: *In vitro* hymenoptera venom allergy diagnosis: improved by screening for cross-reactive carbohydrate determinants and reciprocal inhibition. Allergy 2006; 61:1220–1229.

Monika Raulf-Heimsoth

Berufsgenossenschaftliches Forschungsinstitut für Arbeitsmedizin (BGFA), Institut der Ruhr-Universität Bochum, Haus X, Allergologie/Immunologie, Bürkle-de-la-Camp-Platz 1, D-44789 Bochum, Germany, Tel. +49 234 302-4582, Fax +49 234 302-4610, E-mail raulf@bgfa.de

Immunoglobulin Free Light Chains in Hypersensitivity Reactions: Need for Crosslinking by Antigens

F.A. Redegeld, S.C. Berndsen, B. Blokhuis, and M. Kool

Department of Pharmacology and Pathophysiology, Utrecht Institute for Pharmaceutical Sciences, Utrecht University, The Netherlands

Summary: *Background:* Recently, we have shown that FLC can play a crucial role in the induction of contact sensitivity and nonatopic asthma. Our current working model proposes that antigen-specific FLC sensitize mast cells through specific receptors on the cell surface. Following a second contact with the cognate antigen, surface-bound FLC are cross-linked leading to mast cell activation. In current study, we investigated whether cross-linking of FLC is indeed necessary to induce hypersensitivity responses. *Methods:* Passive cutaneous anaphylaxis (PCA): PCA1: Mice were intradermally sensitized with dinitrophenol(DNP)-specific FLC or IgE. 20 h after sensitization, mice were intravenously challenged with multivalent antigen (DNP-human serum albumin (35:1)) and ear swelling responses were measured. In a second group, mice were challenged in presence of a molar excess of monovalent antigen (DNP-alanine). PCA2: Mice were intradermally sensitized with two different Der p 2-specific FLC or with either one of the FLC preparations alone. 20 h later, mice were systemically challenged with recDer p2 or house dust mite extract and ear swelling responses were measured. *Results:* PCA1: Mice sensitized with DNP-specific FLC and systemically challenged with DNP-HSA develop a rapid ear swelling response with maximal swelling at 30 min after challenge. When the sensitized mice were challenged with DNP-HSA in combination with monovalent hapten DNP-alanine, no significant swelling was observed. Also no ear swelling was present in mice challenged with DNP-alanine only. Similar results were obtained in the IgE-sensitized animals. PCA2. Passive sensitization of mice with the two different Der p 2-specific FLC followed by challenge with house dust mite extract or recDer p 2 resulted in a rapid development of ear swelling. Both FLC were necessary to elicit this ear swelling response, because sensitization with either of the Der p 2-specific FLC alone did not result in a ear swelling response after challenge. *Conclusions:* In presence of a molar excess of monovalent antigen, no crosslinking is expected and no swelling was induced. Elicitation of ear swelling by Der p 2 needed the presence of at least two FLC directed to different epitopes on this allergen. In conclusion, these experiments clearly demonstrate that crosslinking of FLC is necessary to induce cutaneous ear swelling responses.

Keywords: mast cell, immunoglobulin free light chain, hypersensitivity reaction, crosslinking, house dust mite

Introduction

In previous work we have demonstrated that antigen-specific immunoglobulin free light chains can elicit immediate type hypersensitivity-like reactions [1–4]. The immunoglobulin free light chain-induced response has typical features equivalent to an IgE-dependent immediate reaction: i.e., mast cell activation, liberation of mast cell mediators, induction of increase in vasopermeability and edema formation [1, 3]. No such signs of immediate hy-

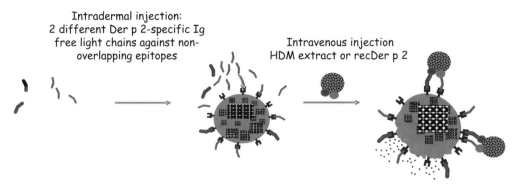

Figure 1. Schematic outline of passive cutaneous anaphylaxis reaction induced by Der p 2-specific immunoglobulin free light chains. Two Der p 2-specific immunoglobulin free light chains recognizing different, nonoverlapping epitopes were injected intradermally. At 20 h after sensitization, mice were systemically challenged with house dust mite extract (HDM) or recombinant Der p 2 (recDer p 2). Ear swelling was measured directly after challenge.

persensitivity responses occurred in W/Wv animals, demonstrating the mast cell dependency of the reaction. In vitro studies showed binding of free light chains to mast cells [1]. Experiments in common γ chain-deficient animals excluded the possibility that Fc receptors for IgE or IgG were involved in the immunoglobulin free light chain-mediated responses [1]. Current evidence therefore suggests that immunoglobulin free light chains act via unique receptors to elicit mast cell activation. Present study was conducted to investigate if crosslinking of immunoglobulin free light chains is necessary for the induction of immediate hypersensitivity responses.

Methods

PCA1: Mice were intradermally sensitized with dinitrophenol (DNP)-specific FLC or IgE. 20 h after sensitization, mice were intravenously challenged with multivalent antigen (DNP-human serum albumin, 35:1) and ear swelling responses were measured with an engineer's micrometer. In a second group, mice were challenged in presence of a molar excess of monovalent antigen (DNP-alanine).

PCA2: Mice were intradermally sensitized with two different Der p 2-specific FLC or with either one of the FLC preparations alone (kindly donated by R. Aalberse, The Netherlands). 20 h later, mice were systemically challenged with recDer p2 or house dust mite ex-

tract and ear swelling responses were measured (see Figure 1).

All animal experiments were approved by the Animal Ethics Committee of the Utrecht University.

Results

PCA1: Mice sensitized with DNP-specific FLC and systemically challenged with DNP-HSA develop a rapid ear swelling response with maximal swelling at 30 min after challenge. When the sensitized mice were challenged with DNP-HSA in combination with monovalent hapten DNP-alanine, no significant swelling was observed. Also no ear swelling was present in mice challenged with DNP-alanine only. Similar results were obtained in the IgE-sensitized animals.

PCA2: Passive sensitization of mice with the two different Der p 2-specific FLC followed by challenge with house dust mite extract or recDer p 2 resulted in a rapid development of ear swelling. Both FLC were necessary to elicit this ear swelling response, because sensitization with either of the Der p 2-specific FLC alone did not result in a ear swelling response after challenge.

Conclusions

This study provides evidence that crosslinking of immunoglobulin free light chains is needed for the elicitation of an immediate hypersensitivity response in the skin. We found that mice sensitized with DNP-specific immunoglobulin free light chains when i.v. challenged with multivalent antigen (DNP-HSA) developed a rapid cutaneous edema formation. In presence of a molar excess of monovalent antigen (DNP-alanine), no crosslinking is expected and indeed no swelling was induced. Exactly similar results were found in mice sensitized with DNP-specific IgE [5, 6].

In another set of experiments it was shown that elicitation of ear swelling by Der p 2 needed the presence of at least two immunoglobulin free light chains directed to different and nonoverlapping epitopes of Der p 2 (polyclonal passive sensitization). When only one of Der p 2-specific free light chains was used for sensitization, no significant and sustained ear swelling was observed (monoclonal passive sensitization). This experiment shows that induction of a hypersensitivity response by a protein antigen needs the binding through a minimum of two immunoglobulin free light chains recognizing different epitopes on the allergen molecule.

In conclusion, immediate hypersensitivity reactions elicited by immunoglobulin free light chains need crosslinking by multivalent antigen (in case of hapten-specific free light chains) or the presence of polyclonal immunoglobulin free light chains recognizing different allergen epitopes (in case of protein-specific free light chains). This requirement for crosslinking seems equivalent to the mechanism of IgE-mediated hypersensitivity.

References

1. Redegeld FA, Van Der Heijden MW, Kool M, Heijdra BM, Garssen J, Kraneveld AD, Loveren HV, Roholl P, Saito T, Verbeek JS, Claassens J, Koster AS, Nijkamp FP: Immunoglobulin-free light chains elicit immediate hypersensitivity-like responses. Nat Med 2002; 8:694–701.
2. Redegeld FA, Nijkamp FP: Immunoglobulin free light chains and mast cells: pivotal role in T-cell-mediated immune reactions? Trends Immunol 2003; 24:181–185.
3. Kraneveld AD, Kool M, van Houwelingen AH, Roholl P, Solomon A, Postma DS, Nijkamp FP, Redegeld FA: Elicitation of allergic asthma by immunoglobulin free light chains. Proc Natl Acad Sci USA 2005.
4. van der Heijden M, Kraneveld A, Redegeld F: Free immunoglobulin light chains as target in the treatment of chronic inflammatory diseases. Eur J Pharmacol 2006; 533:319–326.
5. Metzger H: Transmembrane signaling: the joy of aggregation. J Immunol 1992; 149:1477–1487.
6. Holowka D, Baird B: Antigen-mediated IGE receptor aggregation and signaling: a window on cell surface structure and dynamics. Annu Rev Biophys Biomol Struct 1996; 25:79–112.

Frank Redegeld

Division of Pharmacology and Pathophysiology, Department of Pharmaceutical Sciences, Faculty of Sciences, Utrecht University, PO BOX 80082, 3508 TB Utrecht, The Netherlands, Tel. +31 30 2537355, Fax +31 30 2537420, E-mail f.a.m.redegeld@uu.nl

Vacuolar Serine Proteases from *Cladosporium herbarum* and *Alternaria alternata*

B. Simon-Nobbe[1], V. Pöll[1], V. Wally[1], H.-D. Shen[2], F. Lottspeich[3], T. Hawranek[4], R. Lang[4], W. Hemmer[5], R. Jarisch[5], and M. Breitenbach[1]

[1]*Department of Cell-Biology, University of Salzburg, Salzburg, Austria,* [2]*Department of Medical Research and Education, Taipei Veterans General Hospital, Taipei, Taiwan, ROC,* [3]*Max Planck Institute of Biochemistry, Department of Protein-Analytics, Martinsried, Germany,* [4]*Private Medical Paracelsus University Salzburg, Department of Dermatology, Salzburg, Austria,* [5]*Floridsdorf Allergy Centre, Vienna, Austria*

Summary: *Background: Cladosporium herbarum* and *Alternaria alternata* represent together with several Penicillium and Aspergillus species the major causes of fungal allergy. Several allergens have been cloned from these molds so far. Beyond these there are some molecules as are enolases, serine proteases, and ribosomal proteins, which have been isolated from various fungi, showing IgE-cross-reactivity and representing so-called fungal pan-allergens. *Methods:* Uni-ZAP XR cDNA expression libraries from *C. herbarum* and *A. alternata* have been screened with a cDNA coding for Pen o 18, the vacuolar serine protease from *Penicillium oxalicum. Results:* A full-length clone of 1661 bp coding for the vacuolar serine protease of *C. herbarum* has been isolated. Five out of 26 sera (19.2%) specifically reacted with Cla h 9, the vacuolar serine protease of *C. herbarum*. Screening of the *A. alternata* cDNA expression library resulted in a partial clone of 790 bp. In IgG-immunoblots Cla h 9 reacted with two moAbs, which have been shown to be reactive with serine proteases from several Penicillium and Aspergillus species. *Conclusions:* Vacuolar serine proteases have been isolated from *C. herbarum* and *A. alternata.* Cla h 9 might be useful together with enolase and the major allergen Mannitol-Dehydrogenase for a molecule based diagnostic and therapeutic approach. Our preliminary data indicate that Cla h 9 is IgE- and IgG-cross-reactive with fungal serine proteases from Penicillium and Aspergillus species.

Keywords: vacuolar serine protease, *Cladosporium herbarum, Alternaria alternata,* allergen, mold, fungi, recombinant, allergy, pan-allergen

Introduction

Fungal species are well known causative agents of Type I allergy. Up to now allergens from approximately 20 species belonging to the classes of ascomycetes, basidiomycetes and deuteromycetes have been isolated and characterized. In the last 15 years about 90 fungal allergens have been cloned. Within these allergens there are several proteins, which have been isolated from several sources representing potential fungal pan-allergens. Candidate molecules are enolases, heat shock proteins, ribosomal proteins and serine proteases [1–4] since all of them have been isolated from at least three different genera and moreover extensive IgE-cross-reactivity has been demonstrated.

110   Allergens

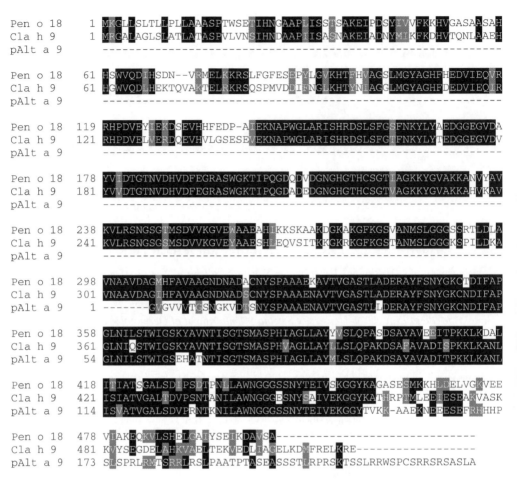

Figure 1. Sequence alignment of three fungal vacuolar serine proteases. The full-length coding sequences of the vacuolar serine proteases from *P. oxalicum* (GenBank No. AF243425) and *C. herbarum* (GenBank No. AY787775) and the partial sequence of *A. alternata* were aligned. Identical residues are shown in a black box, whereas similar residues are highlighted with a grey box.

Serine proteases are well-known fungal allergens. Alkaline and vacuolar serine proteases have been isolated from several Aspergillus, Penicillium, Rhodotorula and Epicoccum species [4–6]. Vacuolar serine proteases have been shown to be preproproteins undergoing N-terminal and sometimes also C-terminal cleavage resulting in mature proteins of 31–34 kDa [5, 7]. From IgE-immunoblots done with *C. herbarum* and *A. alternata* extract we knew that there exist IgE-reactive proteins in the molecular weight range of 35 kDa, which have not been cloned so far. Therefore we wanted to test whether one of these proteins corresponds to a vacuolar serine protease.

Material and Methods

Uni-ZAP XR cDNA expression libraries of *C. herbarum* and *A. alternata* were screened using the coding sequence of Pen o 18 (GenBank Accession number AF243425), the vacuolar serine protease from *Penicillium oxalicum*, as a probe. Positive clones were sequenced on both strands. In order to test the IgE-reactivity of *C. herbarum* vacuolar serine protease the coding sequence without the hydrophobic leader sequence (residues 1–16), as was predicted by SignalP 3.0 (http://www.cbs.dtu.dk/services/SignalP/), was subcloned as 6xHis fusion protein in the pHIS-Parallel2 vector [8]. After expression of the

6xHis-fusion protein it was purified by Ni^{2+}-chelate-affinity chromatography and used for IgE-immunoblots. Additionally, IgG-immunoblots were performed with two monoclonal antibodies (FUM20 and PCM39), which previously have been shown to be reactive with the alkaline serine proteases from *A. fumigatus*, *A. flavus* and the vacuolar serine proteases from *P. citrinum*, *P. chrysogenum*, and *P. oxalicum* [9].

Results

The screening of a *C. herbarum* library with Pen o 18 as DNA-probe resulted in a full-length clone (GenBank Accession number, AY787775). The isolated clone comprises a length of 1661 bp, has got a calculated isoelectric point of 5.84 and a molecular weight of 55.11 kDa. Comparing the coding sequence with GenBank database entries confirmed that the respective clone corresponds to a vacuolar serine protease (Figure 1). The amino acid sequences of the vacuolar serine proteases from *C. herbarum* and *P. oxalicum* are 67.9% identical. Investigation of the IgE-reactivity of the 6xHis tagged *C. herbarum* vacuolar serine protease with 26 sera from *C. herbarum* allergic patients, who either had a positive SPT or a RAST-class greater than 3, revealed a positive reaction in five out of 26 sera (19.2%). The allergen was termed Cla h 9 by the WHO-IUIS allergen nomenclature sub-committee. Additionally 6xHis-Cla h 9 was tested with the serum of a person with a proven Penicillium allergy having specific antibodies against Pen ch 13, the alkaline serine protease of *P. chrysogenum*. We could show that the given serum specifically reacts with 6xHis-Cla h 9 indicating cross-reactivity between Cla h 9 and Pen ch 13. IgG-immunoblots of 6xHis-Cla h 9 were done with two monoclonal antibodies (FUM20 and PCM39), which have been generated against culture medium and/or crude extract from *P. citrinum* and *A. fumigatus*. Previously, it was demonstrated that these moAbs are cross-reactive with the vacuolar serine proteases from *P. notatum*, *P. oxalicum* and *A. fumigatus* [9]. We could show

that FUM20 and PCM39 also cross-react with 6xHis-Cla h 9.

Using Cla h 9 as a probe an *A. alternata* cDNA expression library was screened resulting in an N-terminal truncated partial clone of 790 bp.

Discussion

Vacuolar serine proteases have been isolated from *C. herbarum* and *A. alternata*. In case of *C. herbarum* the vacuolar serine protease represents a new allergen, which complements the panel of recombinant *C. herbarum* allergens which are at hand for a molecule based diagnostic and/or therapeutic approach. Based on our data from IgE- and IgG-immunoblots, where a serum of a *P. chrysogenum* allergic patient on the one hand and two monoclonal antibodies reactive with Penicillium- and Aspergillus serine proteases on the other hand were tested, it is very likely that the vacuolar serine proteases from *C. herbarum*, various Penicillium species, and *A. fumigatus* are cross-reactive. Thus two more fungal vacuolar serine proteases have been identified making the vacuolar serine protease a fungal pan-allergen.

Acknowledgment

This work was supported by a grant from the Austrian Science Fund (FWF) (S8812) given to Birgit Simon-Nobbe. We are grateful to P. Sheffield for providing us the pHIS-Parallel2 vector.

References

1. Simon-Nobbe B, Probst G, Kajava AV, Oberkofler H, Susani M, Crameri R, Ferreira F, Ebner C, Breitenbach M: IgE-binding epitopes of enolases, a class of highly conserved fungal allergens. J Allergy Clin Immunol 2000; 106:887–895.
2. Zhang L, Muradia G, De Vouge MW, Rode H, Vijay HM: An allergenic polypeptide representing a variable region of hsp 70 cloned from a cDNA library of Cladosporium herbarum. Clin Exp Allergy 1996; 26:88–95.

3. Achatz G, Oberkofler H, Lechenauer E, Simon B, Unger A, Kandler D, Ebner C, Prillinger H, Kraft D, Breitenbach M: Molecular cloning of major and minor allergens of Alternaria alternata and Cladosporium herbarum. Mol Immunol 1995; 32:213–227.
4. Shen HD, Tam MF, Chou H, Han SH: The importance of serine proteinases as aeroallergens associated with asthma. Int Arch Allergy Immunol 1999; 119:259–264.
5. Chou H, Tam MF, Lee SS, Tai HY, Chang CY, Chou CT, Shen HD: A vacuolar serine protease (Rho m 2) is a major allergen of Rhodotorula mucilaginosa and belongs to a class of highly conserved pan-fungal allergens. Int Arch Allergy Immunol 2005; 138:134–141.
6. Bisht V, Arora N, Singh BP, Pasha S, Gaur SN, Sridhara S: Epi p 1, an allergenic glycoprotein of Epicoccum purpurascens is a serine protease. FEMS Immunol Med Microbiol 2004; 42:205–211.
7. Shen HD, Wang CW, Lin WL, Lai HY, Tam MF, Chou H, Wang SR, Han SH: cDNA cloning and immunologic characterization of Pen o 18, the vacuolar serine protease major allergen of Penicillium oxalicum. J Lab Clin Med 2001; 137:115–124.
8. Sheffield P, Garrard S, Derewenda Z: Overcoming expression and purification problems of RhoGDI using a family of expression vectors. Protein Expr Purif 1999; 15:34–39.
9. Lin WL, Chou H, Tam MF, Huang MH, Han SH, Shen HD: Production and characterization of monoclonal antibodies to serine proteinase allergens in Penicillium and Aspergillus species. Clin Exp Allergy 2000; 30:1653–1662.

Birgit Simon-Nobbe

University of Salzburg, Department of Cell-Biology, Division of Genetics, Hellbrunnerstr. 34, A-5020 Salzburg, Austria, Tel. +43 662 8044-5791, Fax +43 662 8044-144, E-mail birgit. simon@sbg.ac.at

Pollen Pave Their Way

Th2 Micromilieu Generated by Pollen-Associated Lipid Mediators (PALMs)

C. Traidl-Hoffmann[1], V. Mariani[1], M. Thiel[1], S. Gilles[1], M.J. Müller[2], J. Ring[3], T. Jakob[4], and H. Behrendt[1]

[1]Division of Environmental Dermatology and Allergy GSF/TUM, ZAUM-Center for Allergy and Environment, Technische Universität Munich, [2]Julius von Sachs Institute, University of Würzburg, Germany, [3]Department of Dermatology and Allergy, Technical University, Munich, [4]Allergy Research Group, University Medical Center, Freiburg, all Germany

Summary: We recently demonstrated that pollen liberate bioactive lipid mediators with chemical and functional similarities to leukotriens and prostaglandins – the pollen associated lipid mediators (PALMs). The prostaglandin-like mediators were characterized as dinor isoprostanes, the phytoprostanes, derived from linolenic acid while the leukotrien-like lipids are probably monohydroxylated products of linolenic and linoleic acid. Notably, mediators from pollen lead to functional and phenotypical maturation of monocyte derived dendritic cells. Furthermore, PALMs block the LPS/CD40L induced IL-12 production in human dendritic cells leading to a Th2 pattern in the ensuing T-cell response. In addition, we investigated the effects of water soluble factors from birch pollen grains (*Bet.*-APE) on chemokine release from dendritic cells. Here, the LPS-induced release of Th1 chemokines (CXCL10, CCL5) was reduced while the Th2-chemokines (CCL17 and CCL22) were enhanced by *Bet.*-APE. These protein and mRNA data were confirmed by functional studies showing that *Bet.*-APE blocked the migration of Th1 cells and favored the chemotaxis of Th2 cells toward dendritic cells (compared to LPS-stimulated DCs). In summary, our results demonstrate that pollen associated lipid mediators (PALMs) act as important regulatory mediators which may generate a Th2 promoting micromilieu leading to generation and infiltration of Th2 cells into pollen-exposed tissue of predisposed individuals.

Keywords: pollen, allergy, lipid mediators, phytoprostanes

Introduction

Allergists and immunologists immediately and often exclusively connect pollen with the release of allergens and allergic diseases. This is most unfortunate because, first of all, pollen grains primarily bear a natural mission. This natural mission is the unitary adaptive function to reach a receptive stigma and to deliver two haploid nuclei to the recipient ovary in order to transmit genetic information from the male parent to the offspring [1, 2]. The "allergen-view" of pollen prevented us for a long time from discovering other important mediators released from pollen.

Atopic diseases are characterized by a predominance of T-helper-cell type 2 (Th2) biased immune responses to environmental allergens. It is well established that allergen specific Th2 cells are the key orchestrators of allergic reactions, initiating and propagating inflammation through the release of a number of Th2 cytokines. While the importance of Th2 cells in allergy is well accepted, little is known about the mechanisms that control the initial Th2 polarization in response to exogenous allergens.

As professional antigen-presenting cells, dendritic cells (DCs) form the link between innate and adaptive immunity crucial for the initiation and maintenance of T-cell-mediated immune responses [3]. They reside in the periphery in an immature state, taking up and processing pathogens or allergens, which upon maturation they present to T-cells in the draining lymph nodes. The trafficking of immature DCs to sites of inflammation and of mature DCs to the T-cell area of secondary lymphoid organs is regulated by the expression of different chemokines and chemokine receptors [4].

Dendritic cells produce IL-12 – one of the crucial Th1-polarizing cytokines – upon activation by pathogen associated molecular patterns such as LPS [5] or by T-cell derived signals such as CD40 ligation [6]. However, simultaneous presence of endogenous signals such as IL-10, TGF-β, corticosteroids, vitamin D_3, or PGE_2 can convert DC from Th1- to Th2-skewing antigen presenting cells [7]. Recent studies demonstrate that also exogenous factors such as lipids produced by parasites can modulate DC function for the purposes of evading host immunity [8].

As mentioned above, in the context of allergy, pollen grains have simply been regarded as allergen carriers, and little attention has been devoted to nonprotein compounds of pollen. Notably, lipids are major components of pollen excine and exsudate. In both dry- and wet-type stigmas, lipids are thought to be responsible for pollen hydration [9] and the cell-cell recognition required for hydration [10].

In addition, long chain unsaturated fatty acids in pollen, such as linolenic acid, serve as precursors for the biosynthesis of several plant hormones such as dinor isoprostanes, recently termed phytoprostanes [11]. Phytoprostanes are formed nonenzymatically via autooxidation in plants and structurally resemble prostaglandins and isoprostanes in humans [12].

We recently demonstrated that pollen, under physiological exposure conditions, release not only allergens but also bioactive lipids that activate human neutrophils and eosinophils *in vitro* [13, 14, 15]. Now we are able to extend these data on the impact of pollen associated lipid mediators on dendritic cell function.

Results and Discussion

It is commonly believed that allergic sensitization starts when an allergen contacts the surface of an antigen-presenting cell in mucosal or skin epithelia of susceptible individuals. Most studies dealing with this aspect use allergen extracts as stimulus. Under natural exposure conditions, however, the mucosal membranes and the skin are exposed either to whole pollen grains or to pollen-derived particles. Thus, it is important to investigate the impact of the whole pollen grain on human health. We recently demonstrated that pollen grains secrete significant amounts of lipids that show structural and functional similarities to eicosanoids. Whether these definable lipids function in the variable and complex reproductive process at stigmatic surfaces remains to be not altogether clear. However, their highly rapid release from pollen grains [13] makes them ideal candidates in these pollen-stigma negotiations.

Concerning their effects on human health, the cross-reactivity to eicosanoids known to affect the human innate and adaptive immune system prompted us to further investigate the effects of aqueous pollen extracts and their constituents.

In the early seventies, Siegel and Shermann were the first to describe pollen interactions with cells of the immune system [16]. We were able to extend these observations by investigating the outcome of granulocyte – pollen interactions. Our data clearly show that pollen grains (birch and grass) activate neutrophils [14] and eosinophils [15] leading to the release of myeloperoxidase and eosinophilic cationic protein, respectively. This is particularly relevant since such interaction seems to occur in an IgE-independent manner. Firstly, this indicates that, alongside the adaptive immune system, innate mechanisms may also contribute to recognition of allergens within the respiratory tract and secondly, that these mechanisms may occur in allergic and nonallergic individuals .

Apart from the effects of PALMs on neutrophils and eosinophils we investigated the impact of PALMs on human monocyte derived dendritic cells. Interestingly, exposure of DCs with

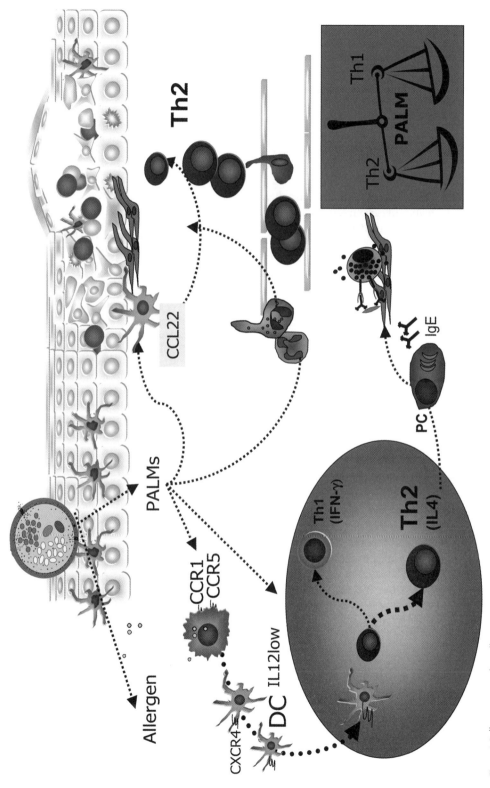

Figure 1. Pollen are more than allergen carriers.

LPS-depleted aqueous birch pollen extracts (*Bet.*-APE) resulted in moderate DC activation as documented by selective upregulation of HLA-DR surface expression. At a functional level, *Bet.*-APE-induced DC maturation resulted in an enhanced allostimulatory activity as demonstrated by enhanced proliferative responses of naïve allogeneic Th cells. In addition, *Bet.*-APE treatment of DCs induced a dose dependent inhibition of the LPS- or CD40L- mediated IL-12 p70 production, while IL-6, IL-10 and TNF-α production was not impaired [17]. Thus, water soluble factors released from pollen grains are capable of selectively modulating various DC functions, including the inhibition of activation-induced IL-12 release.

By means of GC-MS analysis of *Bet.*-APE, we demonstrate the presence of E_1-, F_1-, A_1/B_1-phytoprostanes and show that E_1-phytoprostanes – similar to *Bet.*-APE – dose-dependently inhibit IL-12 production and induce an increased Th2 polarizing capacity of human DCs.

In addition, we examined the effects of aqueous birch pollen extracts (*Bet.*-APE) on chemokine-receptor expression and chemokine production by human monocyte derived DCs. *Bet.*-APE strongly induced expression and function of CXCR4, and reduced CCR1 and CCR5 expression on immature DCs. In addition, DC treatment with *Bet.*-APE significantly reduced LPS-mediated production of CXCL10/IP-10, CCL5/RANTES, induced CCL22/MDC and did not significantly change release of CCL17/TARC. At a functional level, *Bet.*-APE increased the capacity of LPS-stimulated DCs to attract Th2 cells, while the capacity to recruit Th1 cells was reduced [18]. In summary, our results demonstrate that pollen itself release regulatory mediators which generate a Th2 promoting micro milieu with preferential recruitment of Th2 cells to the site of pollen exposure (Figure 1).

References

1. Mascarenhas JP: The male gametophyte of flowering plants. Plant Cell 1989; 7:657–664.
2. Stanley RG, Linskens HF (Eds.). Pollen. Biology – Biochemistry – Management. Berlin: Springer-Verlag 1974.
3. Jakob T, Traidl-Hoffmann C, Behrendt H: Dendritic cells – the link between innate and adaptive immunity in allergy. Curr Allergy Asthma 2002; 2:93–95.
4. Dieu MC, Vanbervliet B, Vicari A, Bridon JM, Oldham E, Ait-Yahia S, Briere F, Zlotnik A, Lebecque S, Caux C: Selective recruitment of immature and mature dendritic cells by distinct chemokines expressed in different anatomic sites. J Exp Med 1998; 188:373–386.
5. Macatonia SE, Hosken NA, Litton M, Vieira P, Hsieh CS, Culpepper JA, Wysocka M, Trinchieri G, Murphy KM, O'Garra A: Dendritic cells produce IL-12 and direct the development of Th1 cells from naive CD4$^+$ T-cells. J Immunol 1995; 154:5071–5079.
6. Cella M, Scheidegger D, Palmer-Lehmann K, Lane P, Lanzavecchia A, Alber G: Ligation of CD40 on dendritic cells triggers production of high levels of interleukin-12 and enhances T-cell stimulatory capacity: T-T help via APC activation. J Exp Med 1996; 184:747–752.
7. Kalinski P, Hilkens CM, Wierenga EA, Kapsenberg ML: T-cell priming by type-1 and type-2 polarized dendritic cells: the concept of a third signal. Immunol Today 1999; 20:561–567.
8. Angeli V, Faveeuw C, Roye O, Fontaine J, Teissier E, Capron A, Wolowczuk I, Capron M, Trottein F: Role of the parasite-derived prostaglandin D2 in the inhibition of epidermal Langerhans cell migration during schistosomiasis infection. J Exp Med 2001; 193:1135–1147.
9. McConn M, Browse J: The critical requirement of linolenic acid is pollen development, not photosynthesis, in an Arabidopsis mutant. Plant Cell 1996; 8:403–416.
10. Fiebig A, Mayfield JA, Miley NL, Chau S, Fischer RL, Preuss D: Alteration in DER6, a gene identical to CUT1, differentially affect long-chain lipid content on the surface of pollen and stems. Plant Cell 2000; 12:2001–2008.
11. Mueller MJ: Radically novel prostaglandins in animals and plants: the isoprostanes. Chem Biol 1998; 5:R323–333.
12. Thoma I, Loeffler C, Sinha AK, Gupta M, Krischke M, Steffan B, Roitsch T, Mueller MJ: Cyclopentenone isoprostanes induced by reactive oxygen species trigger defence gene activation and phytoalexin accumulation in plants. Plant J 2003; 34:363–375.
13. Behrendt H, Kasche A, Ebner von Eschenbach C, Risse UJ, Huss-Marp J, Ring J: Secretion of proinflammatory eicosanoid-like substances

precedes allergen release from pollen grains in the initiation of allergic sensitization. Int Arch Allergy Immunol 2001; 124:121–125.

14. Traidl-Hoffmann C, Kasche A, Jakob T, Huger M, Plötz C, Feussner I, Ring J, Behrendt H: Lipid mediators from pollen act as chemoattractants and activators of polymorphonuclear granulocytes. J Allergy Clin Immunol 2002; 109:831–838.
15. Plötz SG, Traidl-Hoffmann C, Feussner I, Kasche A, Feser A, Ring J, Jakob T, Behrendt H: Chemotaxis and activation of human peripheral blood eosinophils induced by pollen-associated lipid mediators. J Allergy Clin Immunol 2004; 113:1152–1160.
16. Siegel I, Shermann WB: Pollen-white cell interactions. J Allergy 1970; 45:133–145.
17. Traidl-Hoffmann C, Mariani V, Hochrein H, Kark K, Wagner H, Ring J, Mueller MJ, Jakob T, Behrendt H: Pollen-associated phytoprostanes inhibit dendritic cell interleukin-12 production and augment T helper type 2 cell polarization. J Exp Med 2005; 201:627–636.
18. Mariani V, Gilles S, Jakob T, Thiel M, Müller M, Ring J, Behrendt H, Traidl-Hoffmann C: Immunomodulatory mediators from pollen enhance the migratory capacity of dendritic cells and licence them for Th2 attraction. J Immunol 2007; 178:7623–7631.

Claudia Traidl-Hoffmann

Division of Environmental Dermatology and Allergy GSF/TUM, ZAUM-Center for Allergy and Environment, Technische Universität Munich, Biedersteinerstr. 29, D-80802 Munich, Germany, Tel. +49 89 4140-3472, Fax +49 89 4140-3453, E-mail Claudia.traidl-hoffmann@lrz.tum.de

More Than 50% of Positive Challenges with Foods Are Associated with Late Eczematous Reactions in Atopic Dermatitis

S. Ottens, K. Breuer, M. Alter, A. Kapp, and T. Werfel

Department of Dermatology, Hannover Medical School, Germany

Summary: It is well-known that foods such as cow's milk and hen's eggs often cause immediate reactions in sensitized infants with AD, whereas pollen-related foods are of greater importance in older patients. The relevance of food allergy for the course of eczema is poorly defined. In this study we evaluated the outcome of oral food challenges and focused on late eczematous skin reactions after 6 to 24 h. We analyzed 268 double-blind placebo-controlled food challenges (DBPCFC) to cow's milk, hen's egg, wheat and soy in 151 children with AD (median age 2 years). 37% of the challenges were related to a clinical reaction. Isolated late eczematous reactions were observed in 15% of positive challenges. 37% of the positive challenges were associated with late eczematous responses which followed immediate-type reactions. The parents' histories of food-induced eczema and specific IgE were often false positive.

In conclusion, more than 50% of positive reactions to foods are associated with late eczematous reactions. Because of the poor reliability of the patients' histories and food-specific IgE tests alternative diagnostic tools for the detection of food induced eczema have to be evaluated.

Keywords: atopic dermatitis, food allergy, oral provocation, eczema

Introduction

Atopic dermatitis (AD) is a chronic inflammatory skin disease, which commonly begins in early infancy, runs a course of exacerbations and remissions and is associated with a characteristic distribution and morphology of skin lesions. There is substantial evidence that foods like cow's milk and hen's egg are major provocation factors for the flares of AD in infancy, while inhalant allergens and pollen-related foods are of greater importance in adults [1–5].

The prevalence of food allergy in infants with AD was reported in a range between 20% and 80% in various studies, and may be estimated at 30% [6,7]. Hen's egg, cow's milk, soy and wheat account for about 90% of allergenic foods in children with AD [6, 8]. Immediate-type responses to these foods are well characterized in children with AD, but there are only few trials studying true late eczematous responses, which need 6–48 h to develop and may occur only after repetitive ingestion of food [9].

Due to the limited reliability of the personal history and of food-specific IgE, double-blind placebo-controlled food challeng-

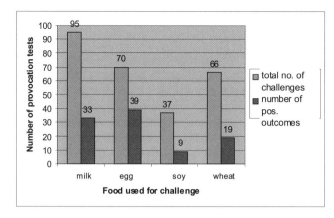

Figure 1. 268 food challenge tests with cow's milk, hen's egg, wheat gluten or soy milk were performed in 151 children with AD in a double blind, placebo controlled manner as described previously [9].

es (DBPCFCs) have been regarded as the gold standard for the diagnosis of food allergy-related diseases since 1976 (May 1976). However, late eczematous reactions to foods have only rarely been evaluated in larger series of patients with atopic dermatitis [10].

In order to investigate the importance of food for the induction of eczematous allergic reactions to foods in 151 children with AD we analyzed the results of DBPCFC retrospectively.

Materials and Methods

The results of DBPCFC were analyzed retrospectively. The food challenges were performed in 151 children aged 1–10 years (median 2 years) with mild-to-severe AD who visited the Department of Dermatology and Allergology of the Hannover Medical University as outpatients during 1998–2005. Severity of AD was determined according to the SCORAD, which is a scoring system combining extent, severity and subjective symptoms [11].

The suspected foods were avoided for 4 weeks prior to DBPCFC upon instruction by a dietitian. Local therapy with mild corticosteroids and emollients remained stable during the challenge. Antihistamines were withdrawn at least 72 h prior to the challenge. Verum and placebo were given to each patient on 2 consecutive days in random order, with a free interval of 1 day between placebo and verum challenge. The sequence of challenges was determined by the dietitian. A verum: placebo ratio of 2:1 was used. The amount of challenged food was adapt-

ed to a normal daily intake. A reaction was considered as "immediate" if occurring within 6 h upon ingestion of the last dose, thereafter as late reaction. In case of an immediate reaction that was more severe than a localized urticaria or erythema (i.e., angiedema, generalized urticaria/erythema, nausea, vomiting, rhinitis or bronchial obstruction) oral antihistamines and rectal corticosteroids were administered. An increase of 10 SCORAD points or more was considered as a significant deterioration of eczema (late eczematous reaction).

Clinical Outcome of Oral Challenge Tests

268 food challenge tests with cow's milk, hen's egg, wheat gluten or soy milk were performed in 151 children with AD. In total 98 (37%) out of 268 of the verum challenges resulted in an allergic reaction, with provocations to hen's egg showing the highest proportion of positive results (see Figure 1). 95 provocations had been performed with cow's milk protein, 70 provocations had been performed with hen's egg protein, 37 with soy protein and 66 with wheat. Isolated immediate reactions accounted for forty-seven (48%) out of 98 positive reactions. Fifteen (15%) reactions were isolated late eczematous reactions, all observed after 24 h. Thirty-six (37%) of the positive reactions immediate symptoms were followed by a late eczematous reaction. In total 52% of all showed a delayed eczematous reaction. Interestingly, 14 patients who reacted with noneczematous ("immedi-

ate") first showed reactions after 2 h or later. The highest percentage of isolated eczematous reactions was observed after challenge with wheat (42%).

Immediate Reactions

83 out of the 98 positive reactions resulted in immediate reactions (isolated/combined with late eczematous reactions). No severe anaphylactic reactions were observed.

Late Eczematous Reactions

51 (52%) of the 98 positive reactions resulted in late eczematous reactions (either isolated or in combination with immediate reactions). All late reactions appeared after a period of 24 h following the first food intake. In most cases a deterioration of the eczema presented as a flare up of preexisting lesions. No late gastrointestinal or respiratory reactions were observed. 15 isolated eczematous reactions occurred. Eight out of the 15 reactions occurred after challenge with wheat.

Conclusion

Food-induced eczema should not be neglected by the allergologist: On the one hand food can be a relevant trigger factor of persistent moderate to severe atopic dermatitis, on the other hand unnecessary diets which are not based on a proper diagnoses may lead to malnutrition and additional psychological stress in patients suffering from atopic dermatitis. Eczematous reactions to food can only be diagnosed by a thorough diagnostic procedure, taking into account the patient's history, the degree of sensitization and the clinical relevance of the sensitization. The latter has often to be proven by oral food challenges. Upon oral provocation the status of the skin should be evaluated with an established score (e.g., SCORAD, EASI) after 24 h and later because otherwise worsening of eczema will be missed. Due to our data, more than 50% of positive reactions to foods are associated with late eczematous reactions. Due to the poor reliability of the patients' histories and

food-specific IgE tests alternative diagnostic tools for the detection of food induced eczema should be evaluated in the future.

References

1. Sampson HA: Update on food allergy. J Allergy Clin Immunol 2004; 113:805–819.
2. Reekers R, Beyer K, Niggemann B et al.: The role of circulating food antigen-specific lymphocytes in food allergic children with atopic dermatitis. Br J Dermatol 1996; 135:935–941.
3. Reekers R, Schmidt P, Kapp A, Werfel T: Evidence of a lymphocyte response to birch pollen related food antigens in atopic dermatitis. J Allergy Clin Immunol 1999; 104:466–472.
4. Werfel T, Ahlers G, Schmidt P, Boeker M, Kapp A: Detection of a κ-casein specific lymphocyte response in milk-responsive atopic dermatitis. Clin Exp Allergy 1996; 26:1380–1386.
5. Werfel T, Ahlers G, Schmidt P, Boeker M, Kapp A, Neumann C: Milk-responsive atopic dermatitis is associated with a casein-specific lymphocyte response in adolescent and adult patients. J Allergy Clin Immunol 1997; 99:124–133.
6. Burks AW, James JM, Hiegel A et al.: Atopic dermatitis and food hypersensitivity reactions. J Pediatr 1998; 132:132–136.
7. Sampson HA: The immunopathogenic role of food hypersensitivity in atopic dermatitis. Acta Derm Venereol Suppl (Stockh) 1992; 176:34–37.
8. Niggemann B, Sielaff B, Beyer K, Binder C, Wahn U: Outcome of double-blind, placebo-controlled food challenge tests in 107 children with atopic dermatitis. Clin Exp Allergy 1999; 29:91–96.
9. Werfel T, Breuer K: Role of food allergy in atopic dermatitis. Curr Opin Allergy Clin Immunol 2004; 4:379–385.
10. Breuer K, Heratizadeh A, Wulf A, Baumann U, Constien A, Tetau D, Kapp A, Werfel T: Late eczematous reactions to food in children with atopic dermatitis. Clin Exp Allergy 2004; 34: 817–824.
11. Stalder JFTA, Atherton DJ, Bieber T et al.: Severity scoring of atopic dermatitis: the SCORAD index. Dermatology 1993; 186:123–129.

Prof. Dr. med. Thomas Werfel

Department of Dermatology, Hannover Medical School, Ricklinger Str. 5, D-30449 Hannover, Germany, Tel. +49 511 9246-276, Fax +49 511 9246-440, E-mail werfel.thomas@mh-hannover.de

Elevated Histamine Release in Chimeric IgE/IgG1 Antigen Receptor Knock-in-Mice

G. Achatz-Straussberger[1], S. Königsberger[1], A. Karnowsky[2],
M. Lamers[2], and G. Achatz[1]

[1]Department of Molecular Biology, Division Allergology and Immunology, Salzburg, Austria
[2]MPI for Immunobiology, Freiburg, Germany

Summary. *Background:* The classical allergic reaction starts seconds or minutes after antigen contact and is committed by antibodies of IgE isotype, leading to reactions of type I hyper-reactivity. In allergic individuals IgE antibodies trigger allergic responses through allergen-mediated cross-linkage of effector cells followed by mediator release. *Methods:* A step forward in the analysis of the tight regulation of IgE was achieved with the construction of a "knock-in" mouse with composite and chimeric poly(A) sites influencing the posttranscriptional regulation. *Results:* Exchange of the tail of membrane IgE carrying B cells from epsilon to gamma1 type resulted in higher secreted IgE titers and an increased histamine release in RBL-assays. *Conclusion:* Factors that influence the alternative polyadenylation are largely unknown. However, because expression of mIgE is essential for recruitment of IgE-producing cells in the immune response, clarification of this issue is of great importance. IgE regulation is evident on the level of DNA recombination (switch), transcription and RNA processing, but also posttranslational and post-transcriptional processes may influence the expression of membrane-bound IgE and therefore must be presumed.

Keywords: IgE titer, mediator release, regulatory mechanism

Introduction

Compared to other Ig isotypes, total IgE serum levels are kept very low not only under steady-state conditions, but also after immunizations. Many independent negative as well as positive known mechanisms are responsible for this fact: The very short half-life [1] of serum IgE which contrasts with the other immunoglobulin classes that form a substantial component of serum proteins. The negative feedback mechanism committed by CD23, the low affinity receptor of IgE [2], which additionally keeps IgE titer at a safe and low level. Published experiments from our laboratory [3, 4]

have shown very clearly the importance of the IgE antigen receptor (mIgE) which plays a significant role in the maturation process and the expansion of antigen-specific IgE B cells. At least, our *in vitro* data demonstrate an influence of an inefficient processing of the mRNA transcripts for the membrane form of IgE [5, 6]. The data show that a fundamental difference between IgE and other Igs lies in a poor expression of mRNA for mε. Deletion of the internal polyadenylation signal results in a quantitative shift toward synthesis of mRNA for mε, indicating that this polyadenylation signal is preferentially used. These data also show that the low levels of mRNA for mε cannot be explained by a preferential degradation. Exchanging the 3'UTR of the ε gene for that of the μ gene also causes a shift toward the expression of mRNA for mε, confirming that the most likely explanation for the results is the poor processing of mRNA for mε at the deviant polyadenylation signals in the 3'UTR of the ε gene.

This thesis predicts that an "improvement" of the main 3' polyadenylation signal (AAGAAA) would normalize the ratio of mRNA for sε and mε. Indeed, exchanging the second signal hexamer (AAGAAA) for a consensus hexamer (AATAAA), but without changing the context of the hexamer, led to a 10-fold change in the ratio of mRNA for sε and mε in favor of mε [6]. This was confirmed when we calculated the number of transcripts for or sε and mε relative to those for the house keeping gene TBP. A tenfold increase in the transcript numbers for mε was seen without affecting those for sε.

By constructing a mouse line expressing an IgE antigen receptor chimeric for its transmembrane and cytoplasmic tail [5], we have now investigated *in vivo* the direct influence of the processing efficiency of the transcript coding for the membrane form of IgE and its effect on the later recruitment of IgE secreting cells.

Methods

β-hexosaminidase Release Assay from RBL-2H3 Basophils

β-hexosaminidase is an enzyme that is released during degranulation of mast cells together with other mediators as histamine. 4-MUG (4-methyl umbelliferyl-N-acetyl-beta-D-glucosaminide) serves as substrate for β-hexosaminidase, detectable by fluorescence spectroscopy. RBLs were plated at 4×10^4 cells in 100 μl medium per well in FALCON 96 well flat bottom plates. Adhesion occurred over night at 37°C and 7% CO_2. Undiluted and various other serum dilutions were prepared and added to the cultured RBL-2H3 basophils. After 2 h of incubation at 37°C and 7% CO_2, supernatant was carefully removed. Cells were washed twice with 200 μl Tyrode/BSA buffer. For stimulation 100 μl antigen solution in Tyrode/BSA buffer (0.3 μg/ml recombinant protein) was added and incubated for further 30 min at mentioned conditions. 100% release of some control wells was induced by adding 10 μl of 10% trition X-100. After 5 min of centrifugation at 1200 rpm, 50 ml of supernatant was removed and transferred to a new plate. 50 ml of assay solution were added to 50 ml supernatant and incubated for a further 1 h. The reaction was stopped by adding 100 ml glycine buffer. The fluorescence was measured at the bottom at the extension of 360nm and the emission of 465nm. The gain was adjusted manually at 60.

Results and Discussion

All immunoglobulins are expressed in two forms, the membrane bound and the secreted form. In general immunoglobulins use the consensus AATAAA for their polyadenylation addition sites, with one exception, the membrane bound form of IgE, which uses three cryptic polyA sites (AGTAAA, AAGAAA, ATTAAA). This means a really dramatic reduction of the polyadenylation efficiency at best 75%, but at worst case to 10%. Karnowski et al. [5, 6] concluded that low mIgE expression at least in part is caused by a poor processing of the pre-mRNA. Thus, the differentiation state of the cell and therewith the composition of the polyadenylation/cleavage complex definitively plays an important role. These factors seem to change the use of the internal polyadenylation site (polyA site for secreted IgE), without affecting the efficiency of the external site (polyA site for membrane bound IgE). The ratio of transcripts for the secreted and the membrane form of immunoglobulin reflects the usage of either polyadenylation signal. Posttranscriptional processing of the transcript coding for the membrane form of IgE, thus influences the signal transduction and the later recruitment of IgE secreting plasma cells, which in general are factories for the production of neutralizing antibodies in response to invading pathogens.

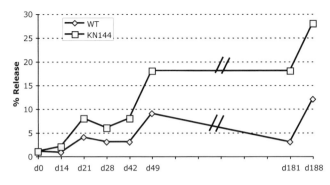

Figure 1. Histamine release assay for WT and chimeric IgE/IgG1 mice.

With our chimeric IgE/IgG1 "knock-in" mouse (KN 144) we could support our in vitro postulations. KN 144 showed elevated total and specific IgE titers after immunization, pointing out the influence of the chimeric antigen receptor. Total and specific serum IgE in KN 144 was elevated three to four times compared to WT mice. Furthermore, quantitative histamine release was elevated in the same range. Interestingly, as shown in Figure 1, the decrease of histamine release, reflecting the specific ph-Ox IgE antibodies, as observed in WT mice, was not detectable in KN 144. The previously described short-lived IgE response [7] seems to be reversed in KN 144, as a consequence of the chimeric IgE-IgG1 signaling. We hypothesize that during the germinal center reaction, the chimeric mIgE-IgG1 B cells preferable enter the differentiation pathway to long lived plasma cells. However, this has to be shown in future experiments.

Acknowledgments

Animal experiments were conducted in accordance with guidelines provided by the Austrian law on experimentation with live animals. The work was supported by the Austrian Science Foundation FWF (Hertha Firnberg fellowship T166-B12 and grant P-19017-B13) as well as the Austrian National Bank (OENB grant: 11710).

References

1. Haba S, Ovary Z, Nisonoff A: Clearance of IgE from serum of normal and hybridoma-bearing mice. J Immunol 1985; 134:3291–3297.
2. Yu P, Kosco-Vilbois M, Richards M, Kohler G, Lamers MC: Negative feedback regulation of IgE synthesis by murine CD23. Nature 1994; 369:753–756.
3. Achatz G, Lamers MC: The role of mIgE during thymus-dependent and thymus-independent immune responses. Allergy 1999; 54:1015–1021.
4. Oberndorfer I, Schmid D, Geisberger R, Crameri R, Achatz G: Indications for the existence of an IgE isotype specific signal transduction. Allergy Clin Immunol Int 2005; 2:15–18.
5. Achatz-Straussberger G, Karnowsky A, Lamers M, Achatz G: Studies on the regulation of IgE expression by the use of knock-in mice. Allergy Clin Immunol Int 2005; 2:18–22.
6. Karnowski A, Achatz-Straussberger G, Klockenbusch C, Achatz G, Lamers MC: Inefficient processing of mRNA transcripts for the membrane form of the IgE is a genetic mechanism to limit recruitment of IgE secreting cells. Eur J Immunol 2006 (in press).
7. Luger E, Lamers M, Achatz-Straussberger G, Geisberger R, Infuhr D, Breitenbach M, Crameri R, Achatz G: Somatic diversity of the immunoglobulin repertoire is controlled in an isotype-specific manner. Eur J Immunol 2001; 31:2319–2330.

Gernot Achatz

Department of Molecular Biology, Division Allergy and Immunology, Hellbrunnerstraße 34, A-5020 Salzburg, Austria, Tel +43 662 8044-5764, Fax +43 662 8044-183, E-mail gernot.achatz@sbg.ac.at

Mechanisms of Inhibition of Human Allergic Th2 Immune Responses

by Regulatory T-Cells Induced by Interleukin 10-Treated Dendritic Cells and Transforming Growth Factor β

I. Bellinghausen, B. König, I. Böttcher, J. Knop, and J. Saloga

Department of Dermatology, SFB 548, Johannes Gutenberg University, Mainz, Germany

Summary. *Background:* In grass pollen allergic individuals T-cell anergy can be induced by IL-10-treated dendritic cells (IL-10-DC) resulting in a decreased proliferation and Th1 as well as Th2 cytokine production. This study was set out to analyze whether such anergic T-cells are able to suppress the function of other T-cells and to analyze the role of TGF-β as potential inducer of regulatory T-cells (Treg) in the periphery in this system. *Methods:* Freshly isolated CD4$^+$ or CD4$^+$ CD25– T-cells from grass pollen allergic donors were stimulated with autologous mature monocyte-derived allergen-pulsed dendritic cells in the presence or absence of T-cells previously cultured with IL-10-DC- and/or TGF-β. *Results:* Anergic T-cells induced by allergen-pulsed IL-10-treated DC or allergen-pulsed DC and TGF-β alone enhanced IL-10 production and strongly inhibited IFN-γ production of fresh peripheral CD4$^+$ or CD4$^+$ CD25$^-$ T-cells while proliferation and Th2 cytokine production were only slightly reduced. The addition of TGF-β or the use of allergen-pulsed IL-10-treated DC and TGF-β had an additional effect leading to a much stronger suppression of Th2 cytokine production and proliferation. Suppression was not antigen-specific and was mainly mediated by cell-to-cell contact and by the molecule programmed death-1 (PD-1) and only partially by CTLA-4, TGF-β and IL-10. *Conclusions:* These data demonstrate that regulatory/suppressor T-cells that also suppress Th2 cytokine production are induced most efficiently by DC that had been pretreated with IL-10 and by TGF-β. This might be exploited for future therapeutic strategies for allergic diseases.

Keywords: allergy, dendritic cells, Th1/Th2, regulation

Immunological tolerance is achieved by several mechanisms including the thymic deletion of autoreactive T-cells and the induction of anergy in the periphery. Besides these passive mechanisms, active suppression occurs by a population of regulatory T-cells (Treg) that co-express CD4 and CD25, the IL-2 receptor α-chain. Many animal and human studies have demonstrated that CD4$^+$ CD25$^+$ naturally occurring Treg play a critical role in the prevention of tumor immunity, organ-specific autoimmunity and allograft rejection [1]. Concerning the role of CD4$^+$ CD25$^+$ FoxP3$^+$ Treg in allergic inflammation we and others have shown that they are functional in most atopic patients with allergic rhinitis and are able to inhibit proliferation and Th1 as well as Th2 cytokine production of CD4$^+$ CD25$^-$ responder T-cells [2–4]. In about 5–10% of the examined patients however, CD4$^+$ CD25$^+$ T-cells themselves proliferated well, produced high levels of IL-4 and IL-10 and showed no regulatory activity despite of the regulation of IFN-γ production. In later studies we demonstrated that the suppressive activity of Treg is dependent on the allergen concentration with different thresholds for different allergens and individuals. For example, Treg from grass-pollen allergic donors failed to inhibit proliferation of CD4$^+$ CD25$^-$ T-cells at high allergen doses while Treg from nonallergic donors did not fail at these allergen concentrations [5].

The immunologic mechanisms that regulate Th2-dominated allergic/atopic diseases, such as allergic rhinitis, bronchial asthma, and atopic dermatitis, have been addressed in several recent studies. It appears that besides CD4$^+$ CD25$^+$ naturally occurring Treg, IL-10-producing Tr1 cells are also involved in the prevention of human allergic immune responses [6–9]. Tr1-like anergic T-cells can be induced by dendritic cells (DC) pretreated with the anti-inflammatory cytokine IL-10 which was added during their maturation phase or by immature DC [10;11]. Additionally, we have shown that IL-10-treated DC inhibit Th1 and Th2 cytokine production of naive and memory T-cells from allergic patients while IL-10 production was enhanced [12].

The present study was set out to investigate a potential inhibitory function of these IL-10-DC-induced anergic T-cells on peripheral responder T-cells. As it has recently been shown that regulatory T-cells can also be induced in the periphery by TGF-β and that IL-10-and TGF-β-producing T-cells are increased during allergen-specific immunotherapy [13–15], we have additionally analyzed the role of TGF-β in our allergen-driven culture system. Therefore, we stimulated CD4$^+$ CD25$^-$ T-cells from grass pollen allergic donors with autologous mature monocyte-derived allergen-pulsed dendritic cells in the presence of TGF-β or with IL-10-treated DC and TGF-β for one week. The TGF-β-treated induced Treg (iTreg) were able to inhibit proliferation of fresh CD4$^+$ CD25$^-$ T-cells to the same extent as observed with CD4$^+$ CD25$^+$ naturally occurring Treg used as positive control. Addition of TGF-β and IL-10-DC-treated iTreg to fresh

CD4$^+$ CD25$^-$ T-cells did not further diminish their proliferative response. The same was observed for the Th1 cytokine IFN-γ. However, Th2 cytokine production of fresh CD4$^+$ CD25$^-$ T-cells were only significantly inhibited by TGF-β and IL-10-DC-treated iTreg compared to the inhibition by CD4$^+$ CD25$^+$ naturally occurring Treg and not by TGF-β-treated iTreg alone. Furthermore, TGF-β-treated iTreg and especially TGF-β and IL-10-DC-treated iTreg produced high levels of IL-10 and enhanced the IL-10 production by fresh CD4$^+$ CD25$^-$ T-cells.

In a second approach we analyzed whether IL-10-DC-treated anergic CD4$^+$ T-cells are able to suppress the function of other peripheral CD4$^+$ T-cells and again the role of TGF-β in this system. We stimulated freshly isolated CD4$^+$ T-cells from the same allergic donor with allergen-pulsed DC in the presence or absence of anergic T-cells which had been precultivated with IL-10-DC in the presence or absence of TGF-β. Proliferation of fresh CD4$^+$ T-cells was only significantly inhibited by anergic T-cells which had been precultivated with IL-10-DC and TGF-β. The same was observed for Th2 cytokine production while Th1 cytokine IFN-γ was already inhibited by T-cells which had been precultivated only with IL-10-DC. Here, the addition of TGF-β had a synergistic effect. The production of IL-10 itself was significantly enhanced by IL-10-DC-pretreated T-cells and especially after addition of TGF-β which also led to an enhanced IL-10 production of fresh CD4$^+$ T-cells.

Suppression was not antigen-specific as the use of another allergen during induction of iTreg led to the same inhibition of proliferation of fresh CD4$^+$ or CD4$^+$ D25$^-$ T-cells. Blocking experiments revealed that suppression was strongly mediated by cell-to-cell contact and by PD-1, while neutralization of IL-10, CTLA-4 and TGF-β had only marginal effects on proliferation and Th1 cytokine production. However, Th2 cytokine production could be restored by a combination of anti-IL-10, anti-TGF-β and anti-CTLA-4 indicating that Th2 suppression is not only more difficult to induce, but is also easier to abrogate than suppression of Th1 cells.

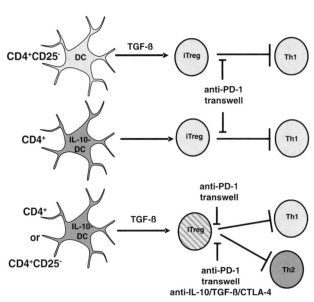

Figure 1. Inhibitory function of different induced regulatory T-cells (iTreg). Th2 immune responses are only suppressed by iTreg induced by IL-10-pretreated DC together with TGF-β while Th1 immune responses are already inhibited by iTreg induced by IL-10-treated DC or by TGF-β alone. All experiments were performed with autologous cells from sensitized atopic (allergic) donors.

To summarize, pretreatment of CD4⁺ T-cells with only IL-10-DC or CD4⁺ CD25⁻ T-cells with only TGF-β leads to the induction of regulatory T-cells which mainly inhibit Th1 immune responses. The further addition of TGF-β or IL-10-DC induces regulatory T-cells that also inhibit Th2 cytokine production (Figure 1). This might be exploited for future strategies for downregulation of allergic immune responses.

References

1. Piccirillo CA, Shevach EM: Naturally-occurring CD4⁺ CD25⁺ immunoregulatory T-cells: central players in the arena of peripheral tolerance. Semin Immunol 2004; 16:81–88.
2. Bellinghausen I, Klostermann B, Knop J, Saloga J: Human CD4⁺ CD25⁺ T-cells derived from the majority of atopic donors are able to suppress TH1 and TH2 cytokine production. J Allergy Clin Immunol 2003; 111:862–868.
3. Tiemessen MM, Van Hoffen E, Knulst AC, Van Der Zee JA, Knol EF, Taams LS: CD4 CD25 regulatory T-cells are not functionally impaired in adult patients with IgE-mediated cow's milk allergy. J Allergy Clin Immunol 2002; 110:934–936.
4. Ling EM, Smith T, Nguyen XD, Pridgeon C, Dallman M, Arbery J, Carr VA, Robinson DS: Relation of CD4⁺ CD25⁺ regulatory T-cell suppression of allergen-driven T-cell activation to atopic status and expression of allergic disease. Lancet 2004; 363:608–615.
5. Bellinghausen I, König B, Böttcher I, Knop J, Saloga J: Regulatory activity of human CD4⁺ CD25⁺ T-cells depends on allergen concentration, type of allergen and atopy status of the donor. Immunology 2005; 116:103–111.
6. Hawrylowicz CM, O'Garra A: Potential role of interleukin-10-secreting regulatory T-cells in allergy and asthma. Nat Rev Immunol 2005; 5:271–283.
7. Robinson DS, Larche M, Durham SR: Tregs and allergic disease. J Clin Invest 2004; 114:1389–1397.
8. Akdis M, Blaser K, Akdis CA: T regulatory cells in allergy: novel concepts in the pathogenesis, prevention, and treatment of allergic diseases. J Allergy Clin Immunol 2005; 116:961–968.
9. Foussat A, Cottrez F, Brun V, Fournier N, Breittmayer JP, Groux H: A comparative study between T regulatory type 1 and CD4⁺ CD25⁺ T-cells in the control of inflammation. J Immunol 2003; 171:5018–5026.
10. Steinbrink K, Graulich E, Kubsch S, Knop J, Enk AH: CD4(+) and CD8(+) anergic T-cells induced by interleukin-10-treated human dendritic cells display antigen-specific suppressor activity. Blood 2002; 99:2468–2476.
11. Jonuleit H, Schmitt E, Steinbrink K, Enk AH: Dendritic cells as a tool to induce anergic and regulatory T-cells. Trends Immunol 2001; 22:394–400.
12. Bellinghausen I, Brand U, Steinbrink K, Enk AH, Knop J, Saloga J: Inhibition of human aller-

gic T-cell responses by interleukin-10-treated dendritic cells: differences from hydrocortisone-treated dendritic cells. J Allergy Clin Immunol 2001; 108:242–249.

13. Zheng SG, Gray JD, Ohtsuka K, Yamagiwa S, Horwitz DA: Generation ex vivo of TGF-β-producing regulatory T-cells from CD4$^+$ CD25$^-$ precursors. J Immunol 2002; 169:4183–4189.

14. Jutel M, Akdis M, Budak F, Aebischer-Casaulta C, Wrzyszcz M, Blaser K, Akdis CA: IL-10 and TGF-β cooperate in the regulatory T-cell response to mucosal allergens in normal immunity and specific immunotherapy. Eur J Immunol 2003; 33:1205–1214.

15. Bellinghausen I, Knop J, Saloga J: The role of interleukin 10 in the regulation of allergic immune responses. Int Arch Allergy Immunol 2001; 126:97–101.

Iris Bellinghausen

Universitäts-Hautklinik, Langenbeckstraße 1, D-55131 Mainz, Germany, Tel.+ 49 6131 172298, Fax+ 49 6131 175505, E-mail bellinghausen@hautklinik.klinik.uni-mainz.de

Anaphylactic and Anaphylactoid Reactions to Paclitaxel, Carboplatin, and Doxorubicin: Treatment with Rapid Desensitization

N.M. Tennant, K. Keenan, U.A. Matulonis, and M.C. Castells

Brigham and Women's Hospital and Dana Farber Cancer Institute, Boston, MA, USA

Summary. We have generated a standardized protocol for rapid desensitization to chemotherapy and used it in patients who had presented IgE-mediated hypersensitivity reactions. Suboptimal doses were infused for 4–6 h until reaching the optimal dose, without the induction of anaphylaxis. *Objectives:* We wanted to provide evidence of efficacy and safety of a 3-solution, 12-step desensitization protocol for the treatment of IgE and non-IgE mediated hypersensitivity reactions to chemotherapy drugs. We also wanted to demonstrate the feasibility of chemotherapy desensitizations in the outpatient setting. *Methods:* Patients with ovarian, breast and other gynecological malignancies and anaphylactic/anaphylactoid reactions to paclitaxel, carboplatin and doxorubicin were evaluated for desensitization. Skin testing was done for carboplatin reactions. Desensitization was performed, starting at 1/100 the optimal dose and by doubling doses at 15 min intervals, until reaching the final dose. The first desensitization was performed in the MICU and then in the inpatient or outpatient oncology facilities. *Results:* A total of 322 desensitizations were done in 73 patients: 17 patients received 109 paclitaxel courses, 55 patients received 208 carboplatin courses and 3 patients received 5 doxorubicin courses. 90.8% of patients receiving carboplatin had a positive skin test. Mild side effects occurred in 38 patients (66 desensitizations), but no anaphylaxis or anaphylactoid reactions occurred. *Conclusions:* Patients with anaphylactic and anaphylactoid reactions to chemotherapy drugs can be safely treated by rapid desensitization using the three-solution, 12-step protocol in the outpatient setting, once the safety of the procedure has been established in the inpatient setting.

Keywords: anaphylaxis, anaphylactoid, paclitaxel, carboplatin, doxorubicin, desensitization, hypersensitivity reactions

Introduction

An acute need for rapid desensitizations to chemotherapy drugs has been apparent since more cancer survivors have been exposed to many chemotherapy cycles [1]. Of the patients treated with carboplatin, 27% develop IgE-mediated anaphylactic reactions after 6–8 cycles, preventing the use of an important drug, active against their cancer [2]. Although desensitizations remain empirical [3, 4] and pose high risk by reintroducing a potentially lethal medication into the allergic patient, *in vitro* data indicate that suboptimal antigen down regulates syk preventing mast cell and basophil activation at optimal doses, and that STAT6 is implicated [5].

Table 1. Standardized desensitization protocol for outpatient treatment of chemotherapy hypersensitivity reactions to paclitaxel, carboplatin, and doxorubicin

Carboplatin			
Full Dose	300.0 mg		total mg to be injected in each bottle
Solution 1	100 cc of	0.030 mg/ml	3.000
Solution 2	100 cc of	0.300 mg/ml	30.000
Solution 3	100 cc of	2.941 mg/ml	294.098

Note to pharmacy: the total mg injected is more than the final dose because solutions 1 and 2 are not completely infused

Step	Solution	Rate (cc/h)	Time (min)	Administered dose (mg)	Cumulative dose (mg)
1	1	2	15	0.0150	0.0150
2	1	5	15	0.0375	0.0525
3	1	10	15	0.0750	0.1275
4	1	20	15	0.1500	0.2775
5	2	5	15	0.3750	0.6525
6	2	10	15	0.7500	1.4025
7	2	20	15	1.5000	2.9025
8	2	40	15	3.0000	5.9025
9	3	10	15	7.3524	13.2549
10	3	20	15	14.7049	27.9598
11	3	40	15	29.4098	57.3696
12	3	75	66	242.6304	300.0000
	Total time =		231 minutes		

Methods

Patients with ovarian, breast and other gynecological malignancies and anaphylactic/anaphylactoid reactions to paclitaxel, carboplatin and doxorubicin were evaluated for desensitization. Skin testing was done for carboplatin reactions. Desensitization was performed, starting at 1/100 the optimal dose and by incremental administration of doubling suboptimal doses at 15 min intervals, until reaching the final dose. The initial desensitization occurred in the MICU, and subsequent desensitizations occurred in the outpatient oncology center for patients presenting no side effects during the first infusion. For patients presenting side effects, one desensitization with a modified protocol was performed in the inpatient setting before outpatient desensitization was permitted.

Results

A total of 323 desensitizations were performed in 73 patients: 17 patients received 109 paclitaxel courses, 55 patients received 208 carboplatin courses, and 3 patients received 5 doxorubicin courses. The majority of patients, 90.8%, receiving carboplatin had a positive skin test. Mild side effects occurred in 38 patients for a total of 66 desensitizations, but no anaphylaxis or anaphylactoid reactions occurred. Side effects consisted of flushing, warmth, tingling, pruritus, erythema, rash, hives, and pain at infusion site. Rarely nausea, vomiting, swelling, abdominal pain, nasal congestion, mild shortness of breath, chest tightness, and throat tightness were observed.

Discussion

Patients with anaphylactic and anaphylactoid reactions to chemotherapy drugs can be safely treated by rapid desensitization using this 3-solution, 12-step protocol in the outpatient setting, once the safety of the procedure has been established in the inpatient setting. The rapid desensitization protocol has proven to be safe and effective in the outpatient setting. This protocol has allowed appropriate patients with moderate to severe hypersensitivity reactions to continue on chemotherapy and should be considered in standard clinical practice. An IgE-mediated mechanism is supported in carboplatin hypersensitivity reactions by the prolonged period required for sensitization, by the symptoms consistent with mast cell activation, and by positive skin tests.

Acknowledgments

We would like to thank all nurses and personnel, and especially the patients from DFCI that participated in the Desensitization Program.

References

1. Feldweg AM, Lee C, Matulonis UA, Castells MC: Rapid desensitization for hypersensitivity reactions to paclitaxel and docetaxel: a new standard protocol used in 77 successful treatments. Gynecol Oncol 2005; 96:82409.
2. Markman M, Hsieh F, Zanotti K, Webster K, Peterson G, Kulp B et al.: Initial experience with a novel desensitization strategy for carboplatin-associated hypersensitivity reactions: carboplatin-hypersensitivity reactions. J Cancer Res Clin Oncol 2004; 130:25–28.
3. Lee CW, Matulonis UA, Castells MC: Carboplatin hypersensitivity: a 6-h 12-step protocol effective in 35 desensitizations in patients with gynecological malignancies and mast cell/IgE-mediated reactions. Gynecol Oncol 2004; 95:370–376.
4. Lee CW, Matulonis UA, Castells MC: Rapid inpatient/outpatient desensitization for chemotherapy hypersensitivity: Standard protocol effective in 57 patients for 255 courses. Gynecol Oncol 2005; 99:393–399.
5. Morales AR, Shah N, Castells MC: Antigen-IgE desensitization of mast cells by suboptimal antigen is abrogated in signal transducer and activator of transcription (STAT) 6 deficient mast cells. Ann Allergy Asthma Immunol 2005; 94:575–80.

Mariana Castells

One Jimmy Fund Way, Smith Building, Room 626D, Boston, MA 02115, USA, Tel. +1 617 525-1265, Fax +1 617 525-1310, E-mail mcastells@partners.org

Regulatory Natural Killer Cells Suppress Antigen-Specific T Cell Responses

G. Deniz[1,2], G. Erten[1,2], M. Akdis[2], C. Karagiannidis[2], E. Aktas[1,2], K. Blaser[2], and C.A. Akdis[2]

[1]Institute for Experimental Medical Research, Department of Immunology, Istanbul University, Turkey, [2]Swiss Institute of Allergy and Asthma Research (SIAF), Davos, Switzerland

Summary. The immune system has a variety of regulatory/suppressive processes, which define the equilibrium between healthy and allergic response to environmental antigens. Natural Killer (NK)1 and NK2 subsets have been demonstrated to display counter-regulatory and provocative roles in allergic immune responses, similar to Th1 and Th2 cells. Although T regulatory cells that suppress both Th1 and Th2 responses have been the focus of intensive research during the last decade, regulatory subsets of NK cells have not been reported so far. To investigate the existence of regulatory NK cells in humans, NK cell subsets were characterized according to their IL-10 secretion and IL-10-secreting and IL-10-nonsecreting NK cells were purified by magnet-activated cell sorting. IL-10-secreting NK cells expressed CD16 and CD56, activation markers CD25, CD69, CD49d, CD45RA, CD45RO, and killer activatory CD94, CD161 and killer inhibitory receptors, CD158a, NKAT2, NKB1 on their surface. NK cells showed up to forty-fold increase in IL-10 mRNA by PHA and IL-2 stimulation. In contrast, stimuli which were shown to stimulate IL-10 in T cells, such as dexamethasone and/or vitamin D3 induced 3 to 4 fold increased IL-10 mRNA in NK cells. Frequency of IL-10-secreting NK cells was significantly low (2–6%) compared to IFN-γ-secreting NK cells (61–89%). As previously observed in IFN-γ^+ and IFN-γ^- NK subsets, IL-10$^+$ and IL-10$^-$ NK cells did not show any difference in their natural cytotoxicity to K562 cells. The effect of IL-10$^+$ NK cells on antigen-specific T cell proliferation was examined in bee venom major allergen, phospholipase A$_2$- or purified protein derivative of *M. bovis*-induced T proliferation. IL-10$^+$ NK cells significantly suppressed both allergen/antigen-induced T cell proliferation, particularly due to secreted IL-10. For comparison IFN-γ-secreting NK cells did not show any suppression. These results demonstrate that a small fraction of NK cells display regulatory functions similar to T regulatory cells in humans.

Keywords: regulatory NK cells, KIR, KAR

Introduction

Natural Killer (NK) cells mediate the early, nonadaptive responses against virus-, intracellular bacteria-, and parasite-infected cells, and modulate the activity of other effector cells of the innate immune system. NK1 and NK2 subsets have been demonstrated to display counter-regulatory and provocative roles in allergic immune responses, similar to Th1 and Th2 cells. Although T regulatory cells suppressing both Th1 and Th2 responses have been the focus of intensive research during the last decade, regulatory subset of NK cells has not been reported so far. To investigate the existence of regulatory NK cells in humans, NK cell subsets were purified and characterized according to their IL-10 secretion property [1, 2].

Material and Methods

NK cells were purified by magnet-activated cell separation (MACS, Miltenyi USA). IFN-γ and IL-10-secreting and nonsecreting NK cells were isolated by MACS. PHA stimulated peripheral blood mononuclear cells (PBMCs) from healthy individuals were analyzed by using a dual-specific, anti-CD45/anti-IL-10 mAb followed by microbead-labeled anti-PE antibody. PBMC and NK cells were stained with FITC-conjugated anti-CD4, -CD8, -CD16, -CD25, -CD45RO, -CD49d, -CD56, -CD69, -CD94, -CD158a, -CD161, -NKAT2, -NKB1, and flow cytometric analysis was performed with EPICS XL. IFN-γ and IL-10-secreting NK cells were measured by ELIS-POT (R & D Systems). RNA was isolated using the RNeasy Mini Kit (Qiagen, Hamburg, Germany) according to the manufacturer's protocol. Reverse transcription was performed with TaqMan® reverse transcription reagents (Applied Biosystems, Rotkreuz, Switzerland) and quantitative-RT PCR was performed and relative mRNA expression was quantified compared to housekeeping (18s) mRNA expression. Antigen-specific T cell proliferative response was determined by stimulation of 2 × 10⁵ PBMC alone or together with freshly purified cytokine-secreting NK cells for 5 d with bee venom major allergen, phospholipase A2- or purified protein derivative of *M. bovis*. Cytotoxic activity of NK cell subsets was determined by using green fluorescent labeled K562 target cells (Orphagen Pharma, Heidelberg, Germany) (3, 4).

Results and Discussion

We first investigated the expression of IL-10 and co-expression of NK cell markers in human PBMC. Within the PBMCs population, the percentage of IL-10-secreting cells was approximately 3–4%. The percentage of both CD4⁺ and CD8⁺ IL-10-secreting T cells were in the range of 1.4–2.7%. Within the NK cell population, the percentage of CD16⁺ IL-10-secreting and CD56⁺ IL10-secreting NK cells was approximately 7% (6.9–7.5). The majori-

ty of these IL-10-secreting NK cells were CD45RO⁺ (4.5–5.1%). Almost all of the IL-10-secreting NK cells expressed CD49d, CD94, CD158a, CD161 and NKAT2. In contrast, NKB1 did not appear to be a marker of IL-10-secreting NK cells.

By using a microbead-labeled anti-PE antibody, PE-stained IL-10-secreting NK cells and IL-10-negative fraction were purified. After purification, the IL-10-secreting NK subset was enriched to more than 85%. Within the whole NK cell population, the frequency of IL-10-secreting NK cells was significantly low compared to IFN-γ-secreting NK cells (2–6% versus 61–89%). IL-10-secreting NK cells showed forty-fold increased IL-10 mRNA immediately after purification without any further stimulation compared to NK cells, which do not secret any IL-10. The regulation of IL-10 mRNA expression was investigated by stimulation of freshly purified NK cells with PHA with IL-2 and VitD3/Dex at 4 h. NK cells showed up to forty-fold increase in IL-10 mRNA by PHA and IL-2 stimulation. In contrast, stimuli which were shown to stimulate IL-10 in T cells, such as dexamethasone and/or vitamin D3 induced 3 to 4 fold increased IL-10 mRNA in NK cells. There was no significant difference between purified IL-10-secreting and IL-10-nonsecreting NK cells in natural cytotoxic activity.

As few as 4 × 10³ IL-10⁺ NK cells were able to induce antigen-specific suppression in PBMCs. IL-10-secreting NK cells significantly suppressed both PLA- & PPD -induced T cell proliferation, particularly due to secreted IL-10. However IFN-γ-secreting NK cells did not show any suppression. In comparison, IL-10- and IFN-γ-secreting NK cells did not exert any suppressive effect on anti-CD3 stimulation. Suppression of antigen-specific T cell proliferation by IL-10-secreting NK cells was inhibited by blocking of IL-10R. Neutralization of IL-10 activity significantly enhanced antigen-induced T cell proliferation.

Taken together, direct purification of IL-10-secreting and nonsecreting NK cell subsets from peripheral blood enabled to demonstrate the *in vivo* existence of a regulatory NK cell subset, which may play immune regulatory and suppressor roles.

References

1. Taylor A, Verhagen J, Blaser K, Akdis M, Akdis CA: Mechanisms of immune suppression by interleukin-10 and transforming growth factor-B: the role of T regulatory cells. Immunol 2006; 117:433–442.
2. Aktas E, Akdis M, Bilgic S, Disch R, Falk CS, Blaser K, Akdis C, Deniz G: Different natural killer (NK) receptor expression and immunoglobulin E (IgE) regulation by NK1 and NK2 cells. Clin Exp Immunol 2005; 140:301–309.
3. Deniz G, Christmas SE, Brew R, Johnson PM: Phenotypic and functional cellular differences between human CD3⁻ decidual and peripheral blood leukocytes. J Immunol 1994; 152:4255–4261.
4. Deniz G, Akdis M, Aktas E, Blaser K, Akdis CA: Human NK1 and NK2 subsets determined by purification of IFN-γ-secreting and IFN-γ-nonsecreting NK cells. Eur J Immunol 2002; 32:879–884.

Gunnur Deniz

Istanbul University, Institute for Experimental Medical Research (DETAE), Department of Immunology, Vakif Guraba Cad. 34280, Sehremini, Istanbul, Turkey, Tel. +90 212 414-2232, Fax +90 212 532-4171, E-mail gdeniz@istanbul.edu.tr

Environmental Prenatal Factors of Allergy in Lithuania

R. Dubakienë and D. Vaicekauskaite

Vilnius University, Lithuania

Summary. The relationship between ecological factors and allergy during pregnancy was analyzed and their influence on the health status of pregnant women in Lithuania was evaluated. A total of 205 pregnant women were interviewed with a questionnaire that included 235 questions about health status, housing conditions, socioeconomic status, environmental factors, smoking habits, family history of atopy, allergies, and other items. Of these, 121 (59.02%) were healthy, 58 (28.29%) were allergic, 26 (12.68%) were atopic, thus, 84 (40.88%) were allergic/atopic. The differences between healthy women and those who were allergic or atopic were significant in some cases: There was no significant difference for smoking in healthy and allergic/atopic women ($p = .1209/.8927$), but a great difference in family history of allergy ($p < .0001$), allergy history, pollinosis in the family, soft furniture at home, and a dry home environment. The father's smoking was a great risk factor for miscarriage ($p = .046$). The environmental factors influencing the health status of pregnant women were: heating by gas ($p = .038$) and dry home ($p = 0023$).

Keywords: pregnancy, allergy, environment

Introduction

Environmental factors have been discussed as critical influences in the development of allergic diseases in many publications all over the world. The aim of this study was to evaluate the role of environmental factors during pregnancy on allergic sensitization in newborns of Lithuanian women.

Materials and Methods

A total of 205 pregnant women were included in the study. One month before each predicted birth, informed consent and the questionnaire were collected. Each neonate's cord blood was collected immediately after birth. In the questionnaire, the pregnant women were asked about their age, number of live births, educa-tion level, self-reported environmental pollutants, history of atopic diseases (atopic dermatitis, allergic rhinitis, asthma) in their maternal and paternal families, and pets at home. Information about dampness of the house, carpets at home, as well as tobacco smoking before and during pregnancy was also included in the questionnaire.

Neonate health data at birth were also collected from the hospital records: head circumference, weight, height, and weeks of gestation. None of the women had any complications during pregnancy.

Statistical Analysis

Data analysis was done using statistical analysis of determinations of mean and standard error of numeric variables. Multivariate logistic regression analysis was done to detect associations between dependent and independent variables. The variables were included in the multivariate logistic regression analysis according to the data-missing percentage from low to high. The Pearson χ^2 test was used to determine the difference of frequency between two or more groups, p values were determined by a two-tailed test, and statistical significance was set at $p < .05$.

Results

A total of 205 pregnant women were included in the study. Of these, 121 (59.02%) were healthy, 58 (28.29%) were allergic, 26 (12.68%) were atopic, thus, 84 (40.88%) were allergic/atopic.

The characteristics of pregnancy in both allergic/atopic and healthy women, with calculations of odds ratios (OR) and 95% confidence interval (CI) are presented in Table 1.

The risk of preterm delivery was statistically significant in allergic women, while there were less inflammatory respiratory diseases.

The environmental influences are presented in Table 2.

The following environmental factors, evaluated by logistic regression, had no significant influence: illness of brothers, sisters; living in a town or in a village; the age of building and it's nature; number of living persons in a flat; number of rooms in a house; molds in a house; contact with animals, and others. There were significant associations of complications with level of education (unfinished university; OR 4.4) and father's smoking (OR 2.3), while a dry atmosphere seemed protective (OR 0.4). There was no significant difference between smoking habits in healthy and allergic/atopic women ($p = .1209/.8927$), but a great difference in family history of allergy ($p < .0001$).

The newborns of the women studied were followed up for symptoms of allergy. This group formed the first Lithuania birth cohort pilot study, in which the cord blood and maternal milk from healthy and from allergic women were studied for specific IgE to a mixed panel of 36 allergens (milk, egg, wheat, cat, dog, house dust mites *D. pteronyssinus* and *D. farinae*, mugwort, etc.) and were determined using multiple allergosorbent chemiluminescent assay (MAST CLA; Hitachi, USA) technique. Those data are under statistical evaluation now.

After 1.5 years, of the 205 mothers studied in the first Lithuanian birth cohort, the data reported by telephone conversation were as follows (see Figure 1):

Table 1. Characteristics of pregnancy and role of allergy during the course of pregnancy.

Women groups	Yes n (%)	No n (%)	OR and 95% CI	p
		Risk of preterm delivery		
Allergic	30 (35.71)	54 (64.29)	2.4 (1.26;4.56)	**.007**
Healthy	22 (18.8)	95 (81.2)	1(ref)	
		Inflammatory respiratory diseases		
Allergic	37 (44.05)	47 (55.95)	0.475 (0.268;0.839)	**.01**
Healthy	73 (62.39)	44 (37.61)	1(ref)	
		Anemia		
Allergic	10 (11.9)	74 (88.10)	1.84 (0.694; 4.884)	.22
Healthy	8 (6.84)	109 (93.16)	1(ref)	
		Risk of miscarriage		
Allergic	21 (25.00)	63 (75.00)	0.967 (0.507;1.843)	.92
Healthy	30 (25.64)	87 (74.36)	1(ref)	
		Miscarriage in history		
Allergic	13 (15.48)	71 (84.52)	0.89 (0.414;1.903)	.76
Healthy	20 (17.09)	97 (82.91)	1(ref)	

Table 2. Environmental and demographic influence on course of pregnancy.

		No n (%)	Yes n (%)	p	OR	CI_below	CI_above
Risk of preterm delivery							
Education	University	33 (84.6)	6 (15.4)		1 (ref)		
	Unfinished university	8 (57.1)	6 (42.9)	**.036**	**4.470**	**1.104**	**18.104**
	High school	38 (69.1)	17 (30.9)	.088	2.507	0.872	7.210
	Basic	63 (74.1)	22 (25.9)	.143	2.136	0.775	5.889
Father's smoking	Nonsmoker	45 (84.9)	8 (15.1)		1(ref)		
	Stopped smoking	22 (73.3)	8 (26.7)	.202	2.057	0.679	6.233
	Smoker	83 (70.3)	35 (29.7)	**.046**	**2.372**	**1.014**	**5.548**
Risk of miscarriage							
House heating	Central	97 (83.6)	19 (16.4)		1 (ref)		
	Gas	9 (60.00)	6 (40.00)	**.038**	**3.380**	**1.068**	**10.700**
	Electricity	3 (100.0)	0	–	–	–	–
	Wood	32 (86.5)	5 (13.5)	.675	0.796	0.275	2.307
	Mixed (centr. + wood)	27 (90.0)	3 (10.00)	.387	0.565	0.155	2.058
Father's smoking	Nonsmoker	51 (96.2)	2 (3.80)		1 (ref)		
	Stopped smoking	20 (66.7)	10 (33.3)	**.002**	**13.230**	**2.644**	**66.209**
	Smoker	97 (82.2)	21 (17.8)	**.024**	**5.533**	**1.247**	**24.551**
Dry home	No	66 (41.3)	94 (58.8)		1 (ref)		
	Yes	25(61.0)	16 (39.0)	**.023**	**0.435**	**0.213**	**0.890**

*The models of logistic regression were corrected based upon women's dependence to allergic or healthy group.

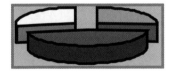

Figure 1. Newborns characteristics from the studied women.

- 53 allergic babies – 25.8% from all (205) delivered and 37.8% from all answered (149)
- 96 healthy, 56 (no data because of missing at home)

Conclusions

1. The course of pregnancy has an influence on child allergy: Preterm delivery was sig-nificantly higher in allergic versus healthy women (*p* = .007; OR of 2.4).
2. Inflammatory respiratory diseases were 2.1 times more common in healthy compared to allergic women.
3. The father's smoking implied a risk factor for miscarriage (OR 2.3).
4. Other environmental factors, such as heating by gas (OR 3.3) increased the risks, while a dry home seemed to be associated with a low risk of complications.
5. After 1.5 years, in a telephone conversation, 53 out of 205 babies delivered were report-ed to be allergic – 25.8%, i.e., 37.8% of those responding (149). Half of them were born to atopic mothers and a quarter to healthy and allergic mothers.

References

1. Jarvis D, Luczynska C, Chinn S, Burney P: The association of age, gender, and smoking with total IgE and specific IgE. Clin Exp Allergy 1995; 25:1083–1089.
2. Kulig M, Luck W, Lau S, Niggemann B, Bergmann R, Klettke U, Guggenmoos-Holzmann I, Wahn U: Effect of pre- and postnatal tobacco smoke exposure on specific sensitization to food and inhalant allergens during the first 3 years of life. Multicenter Allergy Study Group, Germany. Allergy 2001; 56:466–469.
3. Lin YC, Wen HJ, Lee YL, Guo YL: Are maternal psychosocial factors associated with cord immunoglobulin E in addition to family atopic history and mother immunoglobulin E? Clin Exp Allergy 2004; 34:548–554.
4. Lopez N, de Barros-Mazon S, Vilela MM, Silva CM, Ribeiro JD: Genetic and environmental influences on atopic immune response in early life. J Investig Allergol Clin Immunol 1999; 9:392–398.
5. Oldak E: Effect of smoking in the families of newborn infants on levels of immunoglobulin E in cord blood. Pediatr Pol 1995; 70:723–726.
6. Platts-Mills TA, Erwin EA, Allison AB, Blumenthal K, Barr M, Sredl D, Burge H, Gold D: The relevance of maternal immune responses to inhalant allergens to maternal symptoms, passive transfer to the infant, and development of antibodies in the first 2 years of life. J Allergy Clin Immunol 2003; 111:123–130.
7. Dubakiene R, Dautartiene A, Sliesoraityte I: Changes in house dust mite fauna in Lithuanian's dwellings and sensitization to Dpt among healthy young people. WHO Proceedings 2004; 255–258.

Ruta Dubakiene

Allergy Centre, Vilnius University, Antakalnio 124, Vilnius 10200, Lithuania, E-mail ruta.dubakiene@mf.vu.lt

Antibody Responses to Minor Allergen Bet v 2 During Allergen-Specific Immunotherapy in Birch Pollen-Allergic Patients

J.N. Larsen[1], U. Bødtger[2], L.K. Poulsen[2], M. Ferreras[1], and M. Svenson[2]

[1]*ALK-Abelló, Hørsholm,* [2]*National University Hospital, Copenhagen, both Denmark*

Summary. Antibodies to the major birch pollen allergen Bet v 1 and the minor allergen Bet v 2 were investigated in sera of SIT treated patients. All sera were positive for IgG and IgE against Bet v 1 before and after SIT. In contrast, 22% of non-treated patients were positive for IgE anti-Bet v 2 and 48% for IgG anti-Bet v 2. Prevalences were unchanged after 1.5 years of SIT, however, after 5 years of treatment the prevalence of IgG anti-Bet v 2 was 91% while the prevalence of IgE anti-Bet v 2 was unchanged. The relative binding activities of IgG compared to IgE were up to 30 times higher after SIT. Thus, whereas existing responses, i.e., to the major allergen, are increased early in SIT, increase in IgG responses to the minor allergen require prolonged treatment. No new IgE sensitivities were observed when analyzed by quantitative immunoassay; however, 3 sera became IgE anti Bet v 2 positive after 5 years of treatment when measured by immunoblotting. This result may possibly indicate differences in assay sensitivity with respect to denaturation insensitive epitopes.

Keywords: specific immunotherapy, antibody response, minor allergen, birch pollen

Background

Allergen specific immunotherapy (SIT) induces small changes in the level of specific IgE but most pronounced is a quantitative increase in allergen specific IgG. The effect on antibodies to minor as compared to major allergens is not clear. In this study antibodies toward Bet v 1 and Bet v 2 of *Betula verrucosa* were investigated in sera of SIT-treated patients.

Methods

Sera from 50 adult patients allergic to birch pollen, including 17 patients SIT treated for 30 weeks, 11 for 3 years, and 21 patients treated for 5 years, were used in the study [1, 2]. SIT was performed with Alutard SQ (ALK-Abelló, Hørsholm, Denmark) and according to international guidelines. All patients reported marked improvements in symptoms during and following SIT. Serum samples were collected outside the birch pollen season.

Specific antibodies were assayed by the binding of ^{125}I-labeled purified natural Bet v 2 and recombinant Bet v 1.2801. Specific IgE was assayed following binding to anti-IgE monoclonal antibody coupled to paramagnetic beads. IgE depleted serum was tested for specific IgG and following incubation with the labeled allergen, free and bound allergen were

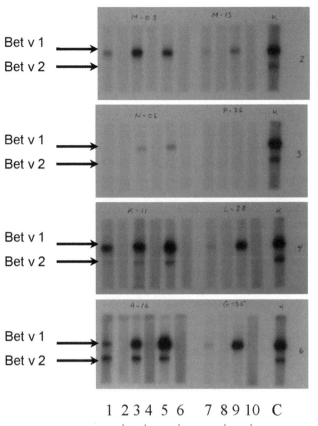

Figure 1. Autoradiograms of selected sera analyzed by immunoblotting. Autoradiograms of selected sera analyzed by immunoblotting with (+) or without (−) absorption using 1 mg birch pollen extract. Sera from study A [1] at 0 (lanes 1–2), 30 w (lanes 3–4), 5 years of SIT (lanes 5–6); sera from study B [2] at 0 (lanes 7–8) and 3 years (lanes 9–10) of SIT. Positive control serum (lane C).

Table 1. Activities and prevalences of IgG and IgE anti-Bet v 1 and anti-Bet v 2 during SIT. A: binding activities (ng$_{eq}$/ml). B: prevalence. For Bet v 1 this was 1 at all times (data not shown).

	Time 0, $N = 50$			Week 30, $N = 17$		
	Bet v 1	Bet v 2		Bet v 1	Bet v 2	
	A	A	B	A	A	B
IgG	61	2.5[1]	0.50[a]	180[1]	0[2]	0.41
	(0.1–310)	(0–1100)		(67–610)	(0–1900)	
IgE	2.8	0[1]	0.22[a,c]	2.9[1]	0	0.23
	(0.14–39)	(0–11)		(0.19–16)	(0–6.4)	
	Month 36, $N = 11$			Month 60, $N = 21$		
	Bet v 1	Bet v 2		Bet v 1	Bet v 2	
	A	A	B	A	A	B
IgG	270[1]	22[2]	0.73	315[1]	29[2]	0.90[b]
	(35–520)	(0–1900)		(132–1100)	(0–928)	
IgE	3.0[1]	0	0.36	1.2[1]	0	0.14[c]
	(0.22–8.0)	(0–2.1)		(0.20–6.5)	(0–4.6)	

[1] $p < .05$ compared to Bet v 1 at time 0, Wilcoxon's test for paired comparisons; [2] $p < .05$ compared to Bet v 2 at time 0, Wilcoxon's test for paired comparisons; [a] $p < .01$ compared to Bet v 1 at time 0 of the same patients, χ^2 test; [b] $p < .01$ compared to Bet v 2 at time 0 of the same patients, χ^2 test; [c] $p < .01$ compared to IgG anti-Bet v 2 of the same patients, χ^2 test.

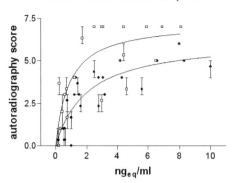

Immunoblot versus RIA, Bet v 1

□ SIT > 3 yrs
• pre - SIT

Figure 2. Relation between results obtained by immunoblotting (scored by 3 separate individuals) and results obtained by radio-immunoassay (RIA).

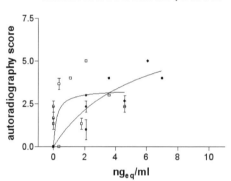

Immunoblot versus RIA, Bet v 2

□ SIT > 3 yrs
• pre - SIT

Table 2. Ratio of specific IgG/IgE for IgE positive individuals and the relative change of the ratio by SIT.

	IgG/IgE of non-SIT	Relative change of IgG/IgE after 3–5 years of SIT
IgE anti-		
Bet v 1	19 (0.1–100)[1] N = 50	9 (1–60) N = 32
Bet v 2	71 (4–1000)[2] N = 11	8 (1–22) N = 7

[1]median (range), [2]$p < .01$ compared to Bet v 1, Mann-Whitney test.

Table 3. Ratio of positive IgE reaction in immunoblotting for sera detected positive or negative in RIA for IgE against Bet v 1 or Bet v 2.

	Bet v 1		Bet v 2	
Time of SIT	RIA positive	RIA negative	RIA positive	RIA negative
0	0.81 (22/27)	0/0	1.0 (7/7)	0 (0/20)
30 weeks	1.0 (17/17)	0/0	1.0 (4/4)	0 (0/13)
3–5 years	0.95 (20/21)	0/0	0.86 (6/7)	0.21 (3/14)

Of the 27 patients tested at time 0, 6 were only retested at 30 weeks, 11 at all time points, and 10 were only retested at 3–5 years. Sera were judged positive for specific IgE by the following criteria: in immunoblot assay median score >= 1 (N = 3), and in the RIA assay bound cpm > 2 times background.

separated by protein G affinity chromatography. Serum IgE activity against Bet v 1 was also assayed by the Pharmacia CAP system. Sera were tested in immunoblotting using radio-labeled anti-IgE followed by autoradiography, with or without absorption using 1 mg birch pollen extract. 0.5 µg rBet v 1.2801 and 1.0 µg nBet v 2 were applied in each lane.

Results

Figure 1 shows representative examples of immunoblotting. In all cases IgE binding to rBet v 1 and nBet v 2 could be completely blocked using 1 mg/ml birch pollen extract. Figure 2 shows the relation between RIA and immunoblot measurements, before and after >3 years of SIT. Note, that compared to RIA, signals of immunoblot measurements were increased by SIT.

Table 1 shows binding activities and prevalences of IgG and IgE specific antibodies during SIT. All sera ($n = 50$) were positive for IgG and IgE against Bet v 1 before and after SIT. The relative binding activities of IgG compared to IgE were up to 30 times higher after SIT. In contrast, 22% of nontreated patients were positive for IgE anti-Bet v 2 and 50% for IgG anti-Bet v 2. At 1.5 years of SIT, the prevalence of IgG- and IgE-anti-Bet v 2 was unchanged (data not shown), however, after 5 years of treatment, the prevalence of IgG anti-Bet v 2 was 90% but the prevalence of IgE anti-Bet v 2 was unchanged when analyzed by quantitative radio-immunoassay (RIA).

Table 2 shows the ratio between allergen specific IgG and IgE before SIT as well as the increase in the ratio after 3–5 years of SIT. The ratio is increased by a factor of approx. 10 to both the major allergen, Bet v 1, and the minor allergen, Bet v 2. Table 3 shows the concordance between the two assays in terms of IgE positivity. Before SIT all 27 sera were positive to Bet v 1 in RIA, whereas 22 were positive by immuno-blotting indicating a difference in detection limit between the assays. For Bet v 2 there was complete concordance between the assays. After SIT 3 of 14 (21%) sera, which were negative in RIA, were positive in immuno-

blotting. This discordance is difficult to explain. A possible hypothesis could be a relative increase in the occurrence of IgE directed toward epitopes insensitive to denaturation. This hypothesis could also explain the relative increase in signal strength during SIT observed by immunoblotting as compared to RIA, see Figure 2.

Conclusions

The dominating binding activity against Bet v 1 and Bet v 2 in sera from birch pollen allergic patients, both before and after SIT, resides in the IgG fraction. Prolonged SIT treatment induces IgG against minor allergens in most individuals. New IgE reactivities to Bet v 2 were observed after SIT in 3 patients by immunoblotting, however, this result was not confirmed by quantitative immunoassay and may indicate differences in assay sensitivity with respect to the detection of IgE binding epitopes induced by denaturation.

Acknowledgments

The authors wish to thank Lotte Friberg and Gitte Nordskov Hansen for excellent technical work. Henrik Ipsen and Anne Ejrnaes are thanked for help with the immunoblotting experiments and fruitful discussions.

References

1) Bødtger U, Poulsen LK, Jacobi HH, Malling HJ: The safety and efficacy of subcutaneous birch pollen immunotherapy – a one-year, randomized, double-blind, placebo-controlled study. Allergy 2002; 57:297–305.
2) Svenson M, Jacobi HH, Bødtger U, Poulsen LK, Rieneck K, Bendtzen K: Vaccination for birch pollen allergy. Induction of affinity-matured or blocking IgG antibodies does not account for the reduced binding of IgE to Bet v 1. Mol Immunol 2003; 39:603–612.

Jørgen Nedergaard Larsen

ALK-Abelló, Bøge Allé 6–8, 2970 Hørsholm, Denmark, Tel. +45 4574 7445, fax +45 4574 8607, E-mail jnl@dk.alk-abello.com

Induction of "Regulatory" T-Cells by *Cynodon dactylon*-Specific Allergen Immunotherapy

S. Li[1], J.M. Rolland[1], G. Paukovics[2], J.A. Douglass[3], L. Baxter[3], K. Deckert[3], C. Suphioglu[4], J.M. Weiner[5], and R.E. O'Hehir[1,3]

[1]*Department of Immunology, Monash University, Melbourne,* [2]*Macfarlane Burnet Institute of Medical Research, Commercial Road, Melbourne, Victoria,* [3]*Department of Allergy, Immunology and Respiratory Medicine, Alfred Hospital and Monash University, Melbourne,* [4]*Australian Centre for Blood Diseases, Monash University, Melbourne,* [5]*Department of Respiratory Medicine, St Vincent's Hospital, Melbourne, all Australia*

Summary. *Background:* Efficacy of allergen-specific injection immunotherapy is associated with altered T-cell function but the exact mechanism for this change is controversial. Decreased production of IL-4 with expansion of IL-10-producing T-cells and CD4$^+$ CD25$^+$ T-cells has been reported. CD30 is a member of the TNF receptor family and has been suggested to govern Th1/Th2 balance. CD30-CD30L interaction may be involved in Treg cell function. In this study we investigated the induction of a CD25$^+$ CD30$^+$ T-cell population in conventional, effective aeroallergen injection immunotherapy. *Methods:* Ten subjects treated for Bermuda grass pollen allergy by subcutaneous immunotherapy were compared with nonimmunotherapy-treated allergic and nonatopic subjects. Basophil activation as assessed by surface CD63 expression and T-cell phenotype in seven-day allergen-stimulated PBMC were analyzed by flow cytometry. *Results:* Allergen-induced basophil activation analyzed by flow cytometry was decreased for treated subjects compared with a panel of untreated allergic subjects, confirming desensitization. Seven-day allergen-stimulated PBMC cultures for treated subjects showed decreased proportions of CD4$^+$ T-cells producing IL-4 and increased production of IL-10 and TGF-β compared with untreated allergic subjects. A CD25$^+$ lymphocyte subset coexpressing CD30 was also increased in treated subject cultures. These cells expressed CTLA-4 and TGF-β but not IFN-γ. *Conclusions*: Our results show that clinically-effective subcutaneous grass pollen immunotherapy is associated with expansion of CD25$^+$ CD30$^+$ T-cells expressing CTLA-4 and TGF-β. Levels of this T-cell subset may be useful for monitoring efficacious allergen-specific immunotherapy.

Keywords: grass pollen allergy, immunotherapy, T-cells, CD25, CD30, TGF-β, CTLA-4

Introduction

Bermuda grass (*Cynodon dactylon*) pollen is an important and increasingly recognized cause of seasonal asthma and allergic rhinitis in subtropical and temperate regions. Pharmacotherapy is effective but may offer insufficient relief to patients with moderate or severe allergy. Allergen specific immunotherapy (SIT) has been demonstrated unequivocally to be an effective treatment for allergic disease [1] but its precise mechanism of action is unclear. Efficacy of SIT can be attributed to T-cell anergy induction, immune deviation, increased apoptosis of allergen-specific T-cells, induction of blocking antibodies or a combination of these [2]. An increasing body of evidence suggests that SIT also causes the induction of regulatory T (Treg) cell populations (reviewed in [3]).

We and others have shown that SIT induces expansion of CD4$^+$ CD25$^+$ T-cells, with increased production of IL-10 and TGF-β as the suggested mechanisms for antigen-specific suppression [4, 5]. Whether these CD4$^+$ CD25$^+$ T-cells represent natural or induced Treg cells is unclear. There are data supporting a role for Type 1 regulatory cells (Tr1), defined by their production of high levels of IL-10 and variable levels of TGF-β early in the course of SIT [5, 6]. The exact phenotype of the Treg cells and mechanisms of suppression following SIT remain controversial and no robust laboratory assays have yet been identified to monitor efficacy of treatment.

Expression of the TNF receptor family member CD30 has been suggested to govern Th1/Th2 balance [7] and murine studies suggest that CD30-CD30L interaction may be involved in Treg cell control of allograft rejection and graft-versus-host disease [8]. In the current study we investigated the induction of a CD25$^+$ CD30$^+$ T-cell population in conventional, effective aeroallergen injection immunotherapy.

Materials and Methods

Subjects

BGP allergic patients ($N = 10$) were treated with conventional specific injection immunotherapy (SIT) using Alustal® (Stallergenes, Antony, France) standardized extract for at least one year, and all reported decreased symptoms and medication use following therapy. Control groups comprised age-matched non-SIT treated BGP allergic (No SIT) and nonatopic subjects. Allergy to BGP was determined by clinical history and evidence of sensitization to BGP by positive skin prick test (wheal > 5 mm) and/or CAP-FEIA (Pharmacia Diagnostics, Uppsala, Sweden) score ≥ 2 (> 0.7 kU/ml). The Alfred Hospital Ethics Committee approved the study.

Basophil Activation Assay

Whole blood was incubated with BGP (0.0001–10 µg/ml) for 20 min and cells analyzed for surface expression of CD63 by flow cytometry as described previously [9].

BGP Extract-Stimulated 7-Day Polyclonal T-Cell Cultures

PBMC were stimulated with 50 µg/ml BGP (Greer Laboratories Inc. Lenoir, NC, USA) for 7 days as described previously [10] and stained and analyzed by flow cytometry for surface and intracellular markers [4]. The results are presented either as the proportion of positively stained cells (with isotype control values subtracted) or as the net geometric mean fluorescence intensity (net GMFI = GMFI test – GMFI isotype control).

Statistical Analysis

Data were analyzed with the aid of the SPSS statistical package. Statistical significance of differences between groups was analyzed using a nonparametric Mann Whitney test. A p value of less than .05 was considered statistically significant.

Results

Allergen-Induced Basophil Activation Is Decreased by SIT

Basophil activation by BGP was decreased in the SIT group compared with the non-SIT treated allergic group, reaching statistical significance at 10 µg/ml BGP ($p < .05$).

SIT Decreases the Proportion of CD4$^+$ T Lymphocytes Producing IL-4

For PBMC cultures of SIT-treated patients and nonatopic controls, the percentage of CD4$^+$ T-cells that were IL-4 positive was significantly decreased compared with non-SIT treated BGP allergic subjects ($p < .05$ and $p = .001$, respectively; data not shown). Values for the

A

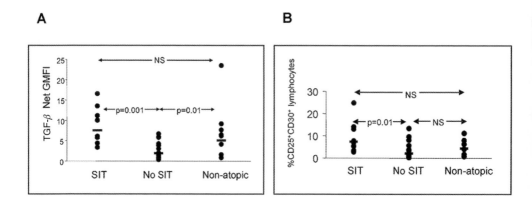

B

C

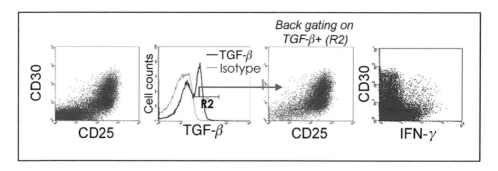

D

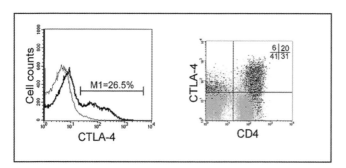

Figure 1. A. Increased production of TGF-β by lymphocytes following SIT. Net GMFI of TGF-β staining of lymphocytes in 7-day BGP-stimulated PBMC cultures for 9 SIT treated, 14 BGP allergic untreated and 8 nonatopic subjects. The bars indicate mean values. B. Increased proportion of CD25⁺ CD30⁺ lymphocytes following SIT. Summary of percentages of CD25⁺ CD30⁺ lymphocytes in 7-day BGP-stimulated PBMC cultures for 10 SIT treated, 16 BGP allergic untreated and 8 nonatopic subjects. The bars indicate geometric mean values. C. CD25⁺ CD30⁺ lymphocytes express TGF-β but not IFN-γ. The left-hand dot plot shows that CD30⁺ cells express high levels of CD25. By back gating, TGF-β⁺ lymphocytes (shown in histogram) were shown to largely colocalize to the CD25⁺ CD30⁺ lymphocytes. The CD30⁺ lymphocytes did not produce IFN-γ (right-hand dot plot). Representative data for 10 SIT-treated patients. D. SIT induces CTLA-4 expression by lymphocytes. Representative profile of CTLA-4 expression on lymphocytes in a BGP-stimulated culture for 10 SIT-treated subjects. The grey line in the histogram represents the isotype control. The dot plot shows that CTLA-4 is expressed mainly by CD4⁺ T-cells. Backgating for CD25⁺ CD30⁺ cells (black dots) shows that the majority (~ 80%) are CTLA-4 positive.

SIT group were not significantly different from the nonatopic group. In contrast, the proportions of CD4$^+$ T-cells producing IFN-γ were not significantly different between the SIT-treated and non-SIT treated allergic groups. Values for both allergic groups were greater than those in the nonatopic group ($p <$ .01 and $p =$ .001, respectively).

SIT Increases IL-10 and TGF-β Production

Low proportions of IL-10 positive cells were detected in PBMC cultures for all groups, but comparison of the net GMFI of positive cells showed that the SIT-treated subjects had significantly increased production of IL-10 compared with the nontreated allergic and nonatopic subjects ($p <$ .01 and $p <$ .05, respectively) [data not shown]. Similarly, small proportions of TGF-β-positive cells were present in the PBMC cultures, but the production of TGF-β was significantly greater for both the SIT-treated and nonatopic groups compared with the non-SIT treated group ($p =$ .001 and $p =$ .01 respectively; Figure 1A).

SIT Enhances the Proportion of CD25$^+$ CD30$^+$ Lymphocytes

The proportions of CD4$^+$ CD25$^+$ lymphocytes (data not shown) and CD25$^+$ CD30$^+$ lymphocytes (Figure 1B) were increased significantly in PBMC cultures for the SIT group compared to the non SIT treated group ($p <$ .05). IL-10 staining co-localized with CD4$^+$ CD25$^+$ cells. Further analysis of the CD30$^+$ subset in the SIT-treated subject cultures showed that these cells co-expressed high levels of CD25 (Figure 1C) and CD45RO but not CD69 [data not shown]. The CD25$^+$ CD30$^+$ lymphocytes produced TGF-β but not IFN-γ (Figure 1C). CD30 was not expressed on unstimulated PBMC T-cells [data not shown].

SIT Enhances the Proportion of Lymphocytes Expressing CTLA-4

The proportion of CTLA-4 positive lymphocytes was significantly higher in the SIT-treat-ed group compared with the non-SIT-treated group ($p <$ .01) [data not shown]. The majority of CTLA-4 positive cells were CD4$^+$ CD25$^+$ CD30$^+$ (Figure 1D).

Discussion

In agreement with our previous study of HDM SIT [4], we observed that following successful SIT for Bermuda grass pollen allergy, the proportions of CD4$^+$ CD25$^+$ lymphocytes and IL-10 production in BGP-stimulated PBMC cultures were greater than those for non-SIT treated allergic subjects, and IL-10 staining co-localized with CD4$^+$ CD25$^+$ cells. However, we noted a substantial subset of CD30$^+$ T-cells within the CD4$^+$ CD25$^+$ cell population. The CD25$^+$ CD30$^+$ cells produced the inhibitory cytokine TGF-β but no detectable IFN-γ. IFN-γ producing CD4$^+$ CD25$^+$ cells were CD30$^-$, possibly representing anergic T-cells as we have described previously [11]. The correlation between intracellular CTLA-4 and CD30 expression further supported an inhibitory phenotype of the CD25$^+$ CD30$^+$ cells.

Concurrent with reduced basophil reactivity to BGP, we detected a decreased proportion of IL-4 producing CD4$^+$ T-cells following SIT. Specific IgE was not monitored in this study as it is well established that clinical efficacy of SIT precedes decreased serum allergen-specific IgE. T-cell changes more closely correlate with clinical improvement on allergen encounter [12]. Taken together, our findings of decreased proportions of CD4$^+$ T-lymphocytes producing IL-4 and decreased allergen-induced basophil activation following SIT with a concomitant expansion of T-cells which respond to allergen by co-expressing CD25 and CD30 together with immunoregulatory CTLA-4 and TGF-β but not IFN-γ are consistent with Treg cell-mediated down-regulation of allergen-specific Th2-type responses. It further suggests a possible role for these cells as a monitorable marker of effective treatment of allergy.

Acknowledgments

This work was funded by the National Health and Medical Research Council, Australia, and the Cooperative Research Centre for Asthma, Sydney, Australia.

References

1. Abramson MJ, Puy RM, Weiner JM: Allergen immunotherapy for asthma. Cochrane Database Syst Rev 2003; CD001186.
2. Rolland JM, Drew AC, O'Hehir RE: Advances in development of hypoallergenic latex immunotherapy. Curr Opin Allergy Clin Immunol 2005; 5:544–551.
3. Taylor A, Verhagen J, Akdis CA, Akdis M: T regulatory cells in allergy and health: a question of allergen specificity and balance. Int Arch Allergy Immunol 2004; 135:73–82.
4. Gardner LM, Thien FC, Douglass JA, Rolland JM, O'Hehir RE: Induction of T "regulatory" cells by standardized house dust mite immunotherapy: an increase in CD4$^+$ CD25$^+$ interleukin-10 + T-cells expressing peripheral tissue trafficking markers. Clin Exp Allergy 2004; 34:1209–1219.
5. Jutel M, Akdis M, Budak F, Aebischer-Casaulta C, Wrzyszcz M, Blaser K, Akdis CA: IL-10 and TGF-β cooperate in the regulatory T-cell response to mucosal allergens in normal immunity and specific immunotherapy. Eur J Immunol 2003; 33:1205–1214.
6. Akdis M, Verhagen J, Taylor A, Karamloo F, Karagiannidis C, Crameri R, Thunberg S, Deniz G, Valenta R, Fiebig H, Kegel C, Disch R, Schmidt-Weber CB, Blaser K, Akdis CA: Immune responses in healthy and allergic individuals are characterized by a fine balance between allergen-specific Treg1 and Th2 cells. J Exp Med 2004; 199:1567–1575.
7. Pellegrini P, Berghella AM, Contasta I, Adorno D: CD30 antigen: not a physiological marker for TH2 cells but an important costimulator molecule in the regulation of the balance between Th1/Th2 response. Transpl Immunol 2003; 12:49–61.
8. Blazar BR, Levy RB, Mak TW, Panoskaltsis-Mortari A, Muta H, Jones M, Roskos M, Serody JS, Yagita H, Podack ER, Taylor PA: CD30/CD30 ligand (CD153) interaction regulates CD4$^+$ T-cell-mediated graft-versus-host disease. J Immunol 2004; 173:2933–2941.
9. Drew AC, Eusebius NP, Kenins L, de Silva HD, Suphioglu C, Rolland JM, O'Hehir RE: Hypoallergenic variants of the major latex allergen Hev b 6.01 retaining human T-lymphocyte reactivity. J Immunol 2004; 173:5872–5879.
10. Eusebius NP, Papalia L, Suphioglu C, McLellan SC, Varney M, Rolland JM, O'Hehir RE: Oligoclonal analysis of the atopic T-cell response to the group 1 allergen of Cynodon dactylon (bermuda grass) pollen: pre- and post-allergen-specific immunotherapy. Int Arch Allergy Immunol 2002; 127:234–244.
11. O'Hehir RE, Yssel H, Verma S, de Vries JE, Spits H, Lamb JR: Clonal analysis of differential lymphokine production in peptide and superantigen induced T-cell anergy. Int Immunol 1991; 3:819–826.
12. Jutel M, Pichler WJ, Skrbic D, Urwyler A, Dahinden C, Muller UR: Bee venom immunotherapy results in decrease of IL-4 and IL-5 and increase of IFN-γ secretion in specific allergen-stimulated T-cell cultures. J Immunol 1995; 154:4187–4194.

Robyn O'Hehir

Department of Allergy, Immunology, and Respiratory Medicine, The Alfred Hospital, Commercial Road, Melbourne, 3004, Victoria, Australia, Tel. +61 3 9076-2251, Fax +61 3 9076-8692, E-mail robyn.ohehir@med.monash.edu.au

α-Melanocyte Stimulating Hormone and Fragments: Potential Therapeutic Agents in Inflammation

Thomas A. Luger and Thomas Brzoska

Department of Dermatology and Boltzmann Institute for Cell- and Immunobiology of the Skin,
University of Münster, Germany

Summary. α-Melanocyte stimulating hormone (α-MSH) exerts numerous immunomodulatory and antiinflammatory activities, which are, at least partly, mediated through the melanocortin receptor 1 (MC-1R). Accordingly, α-MSH downregulates the production of proinflammatory cytokines and the expression of costimulatory molecules on antigen-presenting cells (APC) via inhibiting the activation of transcription factors such as NF-κB. Besides α-MSH, its C-terminal-tripeptide (KPV) and the IL-1β derived tripeptide KPT are capable of modulating APC functions. Using a mouse model of contact hypersensitivity (CHS), application of α-MSH, KPV, or KPT inhibited CHS induction and induced hapten-specific tolerance. Moreover, α-MSH treated DC-inhibited CHS and induced hapten-specific tolerance, via the induction of regulatory T-lymphocytes (T^{reg}). These findings further support the therapeutic potential of α-MSH related peptides for the treatment of inflammatory, autoimmune, and allergic diseases.

Keywords: inflammation, neuropeptide, melanocyte stimulating hormone, contact hypersensitivity

Introduction

The proopiomelanocortin (POMC) derived melanocortin α-MSH has recently been shown to exhibit antiinflammatory as well as immunomodulating activities [1]. In addition to their pituitary origin, POMC peptides also have been detected in several other organs and cells including the skin and immunocompetent cells [2]. POMC-peptides exert their various biological effects via binding to MCRs belonging to the group of G-protein coupled receptors with seven transmembrane domains. Among the five known melanocortin receptors α-MSH predominantly binds with high affinity to the MC-1R [3].

Effect of α-MSH on APCs

There is evidence from several studies that α-MSH is able to modulate the function of MC-1R expressing APCs. Accordingly, α-MSH upregulates the production of IL-10 but downregulates the synthesis of proinflammatory cytokines such as IL-1, IL-6, and TNFα, as well as nitric oxide in monocytes and macrophages [4, 5]. Furthermore, α-MSH significantly suppresses the expression of costimulatory molecules such as CD40 and CD86 on monocytes and dendritic cells [6]. There is further evidence that α-MSH exerts its antiinflammatory effects by generally inhibiting the activation of the transcription factor NFκB [7, 8].

Effect of α-MSH on CHS

The *in vitro* immunomodulating capacity of α-MSH was further supported by a murine model of contact hypersensitivity (CHS). Systemic or topical application of very low amounts of α-MSH (5 μg) prior to the sensitization with potent contact allergens such as dinitrochlorobenzene (DNCB) inhibited both the sensitization as well as the elicitation of CHS and induced hapten-specific tolerance. In addition, KPV and the IL-1β derived tripeptide KPT turned out to exhibit the same antiinflammatory activity [1, 9].

To further evaluate the effect of α-MSH on APC *in vivo,* bone marrow derived immature murine DC were generated (cultured for 6 days in the presence of GM-CSF and IL-4) and treated *in vitro* with the soluble antigen DNBS alone or in the presence of α-MSH (10^{-10} M). Subsequently cells were i.v.-injected into naive syngenic mice. Upon epicutaneous challenge with the same hapten (DNBC) the ear-swelling response was significantly reduced in mice treated with haptenized and α-MSH pulsed DC. These animals could not be resensitized after 2 weeks with the same hapten, suggesting the induction of immune tolerance. Furthermore, CHS inhibition and tolerance induction were also observed upon injection of T-cells, which were coincubated with haptenized and α-MSH treated DC *ex vivo,* suggesting the generation of a population of regulatory T-cells [10, 11].

Conclusion

The POMC-derived tridecapeptide α-MSH and fragments such as KPV as well as KPT turned out to exhibit a potent antiinflammatory potential. Using animal models, α-MSH was found to prevent sensitization with potent contact-allergens and to induce immune-tolerance (Figure 1). These immunomodulating effects of α-MSH appear to be predominantly mediated via its effect on MC-1R expressing APCs. Therefore, KPV and KPT, because of their smaller size and

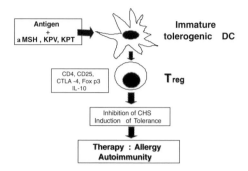

Figure 1. Possible role of αMSH in the treatment of allergic and autoimmune disease

lower antigenicity, appear to be suited to be developed as anti-inflammatory and immunomodulating compounds for the treatment of inflammatory, autoimmune, and allergic diseases.

References

1. Luger TA, Scholzen TE, Brzoska T, Bohm M: New insights into the functions of α-MSH and related peptides in the immune system. Ann N Y Acad Sci 2003; 994:133–140.
2. Luger TA, Scholzen T, Grabbe S: The role of α-melanocyte-stimulating hormone in cutaneous biology. J Investig Dermatol Symp Proc 1997; 2:87–93.
3. Abdel-Malek ZA: Melanocortin receptors: their functions and regulation by physiological agonists and antagonists. Cell Mol Life Sci 2001; 58:434–441.
4. Bhardwaj RS, Schwarz A, Becher E, Mahnke K, Riemann H, Aragane Y, Schwarz T, Luger TA: Pro-opiomelanocortin-derived peptides induce IL-10 production in human monocytes. J Immunol 1996; 156:2517–2521.
5. Lipton JM, Catania A: Antiinflammatory actions of the neuroimmunomodulator α-MSH. Immunol Today 1997; 18:140–145.
6. Becher E, Mahnke K, Brzoska T, Kalden DH, Grabbe S, Luger TA: Human peripheral blood-derived dendritic cells express functional melanocortin receptor MC-1R. Ann N Y Acad Sci 1999; 885:188–195.
7. Manna SK, Aggarwal BB: α-melanocyte-stimulating hormone inhibits the nuclear transcription factor NF-κ B activation induced by various inflammatory agents. J Immunol 1998; 161:2873–2880.

8. Kalden DH, Scholzen T, Brzoska T, Luger TA: Mechanisms of the antiinflammatory effects of α-MSH: Role of transcription factor NF-kB and adhesion molecule expression. Ann NY Acad Sci 1999; 885:254–261.

9. Grabbe S, Bhardwaj RS, Steinert M, Mahnke K, Simon MM, Schwarz T, Luger TA: α-melanocyte stimulating hormone induces hapten-specific tolerance in mice. J Immunol 1996; 156:473–478.

10. Brzoska T, Schwarz A, Moeller M, Altmann B, Kalden DH, Scholzen T, Schwarz T, Grabbe S, Luger TA: Treatment of murine BMDC with α-MSH results in the generation of T-suppressor cells. J Invest Dermatol 2001; 117:453.

11. Taylor A, Namba K: *In vitro* induction of CD25+ CD4+ regulatory T-cells by the neuropeptide α-melanocyte stimulating hormone (α-MSH). Immunol Cell Biol 2001; 79:358–367.

Thomas Luger

Department of Dermatology, University of Münster, Von-Es-march-Str. 58, D-48149 Münster, Germany, Tel. +49 251 835-6504, Fax +49 251 835-6522, E-mail luger@uni-muenster.de

Mechanisms of Immune Tolerance to High Dose Allergen Exposure in Healthy Individuals

J. Zumkehr[1], F. Meiler[1], M. Larche[2], K. Blaser[1], C.A. Akdis[1], and M. Akdis[1]

Swiss Institute of Allergy and Asthma Research (SIAF), Davos, Switzerland

Summary. *Background:* Natural ways for the induction and life span of T regulatory cells have been an essential question in this rapidly developing area. *Methods:* Mechanisms of allergen-specific T-cell tolerance in high dose venom exposure in healthy beekeepers, who were followed throughout several years was investigated and compared to aeroallergens. *Results:* As soon as they received multiple bee stings at the beginning of each bee-keeping season, beekeepers showed very significant T-cell tolerance within 3 to 7 days as determined by abolished proliferative response to the bee venom major allergen phospholipase A_2. The frequency of allergen-specific Tr1 cells significantly increased, Th1 and Th2 cells decreased within 7 days. In parallel, allergen-induced IL-10 secretion increased and IL-4, IL-13 and IFN-g secretion decreased. Peripheral T-cell tolerance lasts a few months after the bee stings and returns to initial levels out of the season every year. The analysis of suppressor factors revealed the roles of IL-10, CTLA-4, PD-1 and histamine receptor 2 (HR2) in Tr1 cells. These data were supported in a study of phospholipase A_2 peptide immunotherapy (PIT), which showed significantly increased histamine receptor 2 expression in allergen-specific T-cells. *Conclusion:* The rapid generation capacity of allergen-specific Tr1 cells rather than their long life span and use of multiple suppressor factors including IL-10, CTLA-4, PD-1 and histamine receptor 2 (HR2) represent decisive mechanisms of immune tolerance to high dose of allergens in healthy individuals.

Keywords: T regulatory cells, immunotherapy, tolerance, anergy, IgE, T-cells, histamine, G-protein-coupled receptors

The studies on T-cell unresponsiveness suggest that anergy, tolerance and active suppression are not entirely distinct, but rather, represent linked mechanisms possibly involving the same molecular events. It is still not understood why exposure to allergens leads to atopic disorders in some individuals, but not others. However, it is clear that a strong interaction of environmental and genetic factors is involved. The initial event responsible for the development of allergic diseases is the generation of allergen-specific CD4+ T helper cells [1, 2]. The current view is that under the influence of interleukin 4 (IL-4), naive T-cells activated by antigen-presenting cells (APC) differentiate into T helper (Th)2 cells. Once generated, effector Th2 cells produce IL-4, IL-5, and IL-13 and exert several regulatory and effector functions. These cytokines induce the production of allergen-specific IgE by B cells, the development and recruitment of eosinophils, the production of mucus and the contraction of smooth muscles. Furthermore, the degranulation of basophils and mast cells by IgE-mediated cross-linking of receptors is the key event in type I hypersensitivity, which may lead to chronic allergic inflammation. Importantly, although Th2 cells are responsible for the development of allergic diseases, Th1 cells may contribute to chronicity and effector phase in allergic diseases [3]. Distinct Th1 and Th2 subpopulations of T-cells counterregulate each other and play a role in distinct diseases. In addition, a further subtype of T-cells, with immunosuppressive function and cytokine profiles distinct from either Th1 and Th2 cells, termed regulatory/suppressor T-cells (Treg) has been described. In addition to Th1 cells, Treg cells are able to inhibit the development of allergic Th2 responses and play a major role in allergen-specific immunotherapy (SIT) [4].

The symptoms of IgE-mediated allergic reactions, such as rhinitis, conjunctivitis and asthma can be alleviated by temporary suppression of inflammatory mediators and immune cells (e.g., by antihistamines, antileukotrienes, β2 adrenergic receptor agonists and corticosteroids). However, the only long-term solution is allergen-specific immunotherapy, which specifically restores normal immunity to allergens [5]. Allergen-SIT is most efficiently used in allergy to insect venoms and allergic rhinitis. Increased allergen-blocking IgG antibodies particularly of the IgG4 class, which may block allergen and IgE-facilitated antigen presentation, and a reduction in the numbers of mast cells and eosinophils, including the release of inflammatory mediators were shown to be associated with successful allergen-SIT. Furthermore, allergen-SIT was found to be associated with a decrease in IL-4 and IL-5 production by CD4$^+$ T-cells. The induction of a tolerant state in peripheral T-cells represents the crucial step in allergen-SIT. Peripheral T-cell tolerance is characterized mainly by suppressed proliferative and cytokine responses against allergens and their isolated T-cell epitopes. T-cell tolerance is initiated by the autocrine action of IL-10, which is increasingly produced by allergen-specific T-cells. It seems, however, that the demonstration of the modulation of peripheral immune responses is pivotal for the effects of allergen-SIT [6]. Local tissue responses do not necessarily reflect peripheral tolerance and are dependent upon a number of mechanisms like cell apoptosis, migration, homing and survival

signals, which are highly dependent on natural allergen exposure and environmental factors [2, 7].

Investigation of immune response to bee venom represents a suitable model to analyse peripheral tolerance in high dose allergen exposure. As soon as they receive multiple bee stings at the beginning of each bee-keeping season, beekeepers show very significant T-cell tolerance within 3 to 7 days as determined by abolished proliferative response to the bee venom major allergen phospholipase A$_2$. Allergen-specific Tr1-cells significantly increased, Th1 and Th2 cells decreased within 7 days. In parallel, allergen-induced IL-10 secretion increased and IL-4, IL-13, and IFN-γ secretion decreased. Peripheral T-cell tolerance lasts a few months after the bee stings and returns to initial levels out of the season every year. The analysis of suppressor factors revealed the roles of IL-10, CTLA-4, PD-1, and histamine receptor 2 (HR2) in Tr1 cells. These data were supported in a study of phospholipase A$_2$ peptide immunotherapy, which showed significantly increased histamine receptor 2 expression in allergen-specific T-cells [8]. In this recent study, subjects receiving peptides showed a decrease in the magnitude of the late-phase cutaneous reaction to bee venom compared with controls in parallel to the decreased proliferation of venom-stimulated PBMCs. Peptide treatment reduced the production of IL-13 by PLA-stimulated PBMCs and IFN-γ, and increased the production of IL-10. Transcription of the suppressor of cytokine signaling (Socs)3 gene was significantly increased following therapy [8].

Interestingly, healthy and allergic individuals exhibit all three subsets of CD4$^+$ T-cells, but in different proportions [9]. In healthy individuals, type 1 regulatory (Tr1) cells represent the dominant subset for common environmental allergens, whereas a high frequency of allergen-specific IL-4 secreting (Th2) cells is found in allergic individuals. Hence, a change in the dominant subset may lead to either the development of allergy or recovery from the disease. Accordingly, allergen-specific peripheral T-cell suppression mediated by IL-10 and TGF-β and other suppressive factors, and a deviation toward a Treg cell response has been observed in normal immunity as a key event for the healthy immune response to allergens.

As a small molecular weight monoamine that binds to 4 different G-protein-coupled receptors, histamine has recently been demonstrated to regulate several essential events in the immune response [10]. Histamine receptor (HR) 2 is coupled to adenylate cyclase and studies in different species and several human cells demonstrated that inhibition of characteristic features of the cells by primarily cAMP formation dominates in HR2-dependent effects of histamine [11]. Histamine enhances Th1-type responses by triggering the histamine receptor HR1, whereas both Th1- and Th2-type responses are negatively regulated by HR2 [12]. Human Th1 cells predominantly express HR1 and Th2 cells mostly express HR2, which results in their differential regulation by histamine. Histamine induces the production of IL-10 by DC. In addition, histamine induces IL-10 production by Th2 cells, and enhances the suppressive activity of TGF-β on T-cells. All three of these effects are mediated via HR2, which is relatively highly expressed on Th2 cells and suppresses IL-4 and IL-13 production and T-cell proliferation [13]. Apparently, these recent findings suggest that HR2 may represent an essential receptor that participates in peripheral tolerance or active suppression of inflammatory/immune responses. Histamine also regulates antibody isotypes including IgE. High amount of allergen-specific IgE is induced in HR1-deleted mice. In contrast, deletion of HR2 leads to significantly lower amounts of allergen-specific IgE, probably due to direct effect on B cells and indirect effect via T-cells [12].

Conclusion

The role of peripheral T-cell tolerance in the healthy immune response development has been well documented in allergy, autoimmunity, transplantation, cancer and infection. Changes in the fine balance between allergen-specific Treg cells and Th2 and/or Th1 cells is crucial in the development and also in the treatment of allergic diseases. There is strong evidence supporting the role for Treg cells and/or immunosuppressive cytokines as a mechanism, by which allergen-SIT and healthy immune response to allergens is mediated. In addition to the treatment of established allergy, it is essential to consider prophylactic approaches before initial sensitization has taken place. Allergen-specific Treg cells may in turn dampen both the Th1 and Th2 cells and cytokines, ensuring a well-balanced immune response. Enhancement of the number and activity of Treg cells could be an obvious goal for the treatment of many diseases related to dysregulation of the immune response. Small molecular weight compounds that may generate Treg cells or increase their suppressive properties are an important target not only for the use in allergy and asthma, but also for transplantation and autoimmunity. Treg cells may not always be responsible for a healthy immune response, since several studies have shown that they may be responsible for the chronicity of infections and for tumor tolerance. The application of current knowledge of Treg cells and related mechanisms of peripheral tolerance, may lead to more rational and safer approaches to prevention and cure of allergic disease in the near future.

Acknowledgments

The authors' laboratories are supported by the Swiss National Foundation Grants: 32–105865, 32–112306 and Global Allergy and Asthma European Network (GA²LEN).

References

1. Akdis CA, Akdis M, Trautmann A, Blaser K: Immune regulation in atopic dermatitis. Curr Opin Immunol 2000; 12:641–646.
2. Akdis CA, Blaser K, Akdis M: Apoptosis in tissue inflammation and allergic disease. Curr Opin Immunol 2004; 16:717–723.
3. Trautmann A, Akdis M, Brocker EB, Blaser K, Akdis CA: New insights into the role of T-cells in atopic dermatitis and allergic contact dermatitis. Trends Immunol 2001; 22:530–532.

4. Akdis M, Blaser K, Akdis CA: T regulatory cells in allergy: novel concepts in the pathogenesis, prevention, and treatment of allergic diseases. J Allergy Clin Immunol 2005; 116:961–968, quiz 9.

5. Akdis CA, Blaser K, Akdis M: Genes of tolerance. Allergy 2004; 59:897–913.

6. Akdis CA, Blaser K: Bypassing IgE and targeting T-cells for specific immunotherapy of allergy. Trends Immunol 2001; 22:175–178.

7. Verhagen J, Akdis M, Traidl-Hoffmann C, Schmid-Grendelmeier P, Hijnen D, Knol EF, Behrendt H, Blaser K, Akdis CA: Absence of T-regulatory cell expression and function in atopic dermatitis skin. J Allergy Clin Immunol 2006; 117:176–183.

8. Tarzi M, Klunker S, Texier C, Verhoef A, Stapel SO, Akdis CA, Maillere B, Kay AB, Larche M: Induction of interleukin-10 and suppressor of cytokine signaling-3 gene expression following peptide immunotherapy. Clin Exp Allergy 2006; 36:465–474.

9. Akdis M, Verhagen J, Taylor A, Karamloo F, Karagiannidis C, Crameri R, Thunberg S, Deniz G, Valenta R, Fiebig H et al.: Immune Responses in Healthy and Allergic Individuals Are Characterized by a Fine Balance between Allergen-specific T Regulatory 1 and T Helper 2 Cells. J Exp Med 2004; 199:1567–1575.

10. Jutel M, Watanabe T, Akdis M, Blaser K, Akdis CA: Immune regulation by histamine. Curr Opin Immunol 2002; 14:735–740.

11. Del Valle J, Gantz I: Novel insights into histamine H2 receptor biology. Am J Physiol 1997; 273:G987–G996.

12. Jutel M, Watanabe T, Klunker S, Akdis M, Thomet OAR, Malolepszy J, Zak-Nejmark T, Koga R, Kobayashi T, Blaser K, et al.: Histamine regulates T-cell and antibody responses by differential expression of H1 and H2 receptors. Nature 2001; 413:420–425.

13. Akdis CA, Simons FE: Histamine receptors are hot in immunopharmacology. Eur J Pharmacol 2006; 533:69–76.

Mübeccel Akdis

Swiss Institute of Allergy and Asthma Research (SIAF), Obere Strasse 22, CH-7270 Davos, Switzerland, Tel. +41 81 4100848, Fax +41 81 4100840, E-mail akdism@siaf.unizh.ch

Clinical Improvement and Immunological Changes of Atopic Dermatitis

in Patients Undergoing Subcutaneous Immunotherapy with Depigmented Polymerized House Dust Mite Allergens

C. Bussmann[1], A.J. Hart[1], S. Vrtala[2], J.-P. Allam[1], K.-W. Chen[2], W.R. Thomas[4], A. Sager[5], R. Valenta[3], and N. Novak[1]

[1]*Department of Dermatology, University of Bonn, Germany,* [2]*Division of Immunopathology, Department of Pathophysiology and* [3]*Center for Physiology and Pathophysiology, Department of Pathophysiology, Medical University of Vienna, Austria,* [4]*Center for Child Health Research, University of Western Australia, Telethon Institute of Child Health Research, Perth, Australia,* [5]*Leti Pharma, Witten, Germany*

Summary. House dust mite (HDM) allergens are important perennial triggering factors for some patients with atopic dermatitis (AD). Subcutaneous specific immunotherapy (SCIT) is a well-accepted therapy for allergic rhinoconjunctivitis and mild allergic asthma and could represent a therapeutic option for AD patients, but studies on SIT in AD are rare. We performed a SIT with a house dust mite extract in 24 AD patients and measured the subjective and the objective SCORAD as well immunological parameters during the therapy. The subjective and objective symptoms decreased significantly already 4 weeks after the start of the therapy. IL-10 levels increased, while CCL17 and IL-16 decreased. Allergen-specific IgE decreased in parallel to increase of specific IgG4. Specific immunotherapy with a house dust mite extract led to a significant improvement of AD mirrored by a reduction of the SCORAD as well as immunological and serological changes.

Keywords: allergy, atopic dermatitis, house dust mite, allergen specific immunotherapy

House dust mites (HDM) such as *Dermatophagoides pteronyssinus (Der p)* and *Dermatophagoides farinae (Der f)* are one of the most important indoor allergen sources for patients with atopic dermatitis (AD). HDM allergens induce both, allergic reactions of the immediate-type as well as allergic reactions of the delayed-type, which contribute to flare-ups of eczema and impairment of the course of AD [8]. Since allergen-reduction achieved mainly by consequent encasing strategies does not always lead to improvement of the clinical symptoms, subcutaneous immunotherapy (SCIT) against HDM might represent an attractive therapeutic option for the long-time treatment of these patients [5, 7]. However, studies on the effectiveness of HDM SCIT in patients with AD have provided controversial clinical results [2, 9]. Therefore, HDM SCIT is currently not accepted as standard therapy for AD. To evaluate the therapeutic value and immunologic response of patients with AD under SCIT, we performed HDM SCIT with a depigmented polymerized HDM extract in a total of 24 adult AD patients with a mean age of 31.9 ± 18.2 years and moderate to severe chronic persisting AD [3]. The mean subjective SCORAD of the patients was 44.31, the mean objective SCORAD of the patients was 36.52. Sensitizations against *Der p* and *Der f* have been evaluated by positive CAP RAST >3, positive Prick Test and/or positive Atopy Patch Test to *Der p* and *Der f*. The build up phase had a duration of 4 weeks, followed by regular allergen-application every 4 weeks during the maintenance phase.

Subjective and objective SCORAD improved statistically significant already within 4 weeks of treatment in >80% of the patients ($p = .001$). A statistically and clinically significant reduction of the objective SCORAD of 48.6% ($p < .001$) and the subjective SCORAD of 52% ($p < .001$) was obtained after 6 months of treatment. In patients with a positive atopy patch test this effect was even more pronounced. The concomitant treatment predominantly consisting of emollients, topical immunomodulators and corticosteroids was reduced by 6–7% each after 6 months of treatment. Generally SCIT was well tolerated. 2 patients withdrew related to side effects: 1 patient due to worsening of AD and 1 patient due to bronchial obstruction. The amount of chemokines correlating with the disease severity such as TARC/CCL17, MDC/CCL22 and IL-16 in the sera of the patients decreased during SCIT. In addition, the level of allergen-specific IgE against HDM decreased, while the serum level of allergen-specific IgG4 against HDM significantly increased during treatment [4].

Taken together, SCIT with HDM extract leads to significant improvement of the subjective and objective SCORAD as well as immunological markers known to go along with the therapeutical effect of SCIT in patients suffering from moderate to severe AD sensitized against HDM.

References

1. Angelova-Fischer I, Hipler UC, Bauer A, Fluhr JW, Tsankow N, Fischer TW, Elsner P: Significance of interleukin-16, macrophage derived chemokine, eosinophil cationic protein, macrophage derived chemokine, eosinophil cationic protein and soluble E-selectin in reflecting disease activity of atopic dermatitis – from laboratory parameters to clinical scores. Br J Dermatol 2006; 154:1112–1117.
2. Bussmann C, Bockenhoff A, Henke H, Novak N: Does Allergen-specific immunotherapy represent a therapeutic option for patients with atopic dermatitis? J Allergy Clin Immunol 2006; 118: 1292–1298.
3. Bussmann C, Maintz L, Hart J, Allam JP, Vratala S, Chen KW, Bieber T, Thomas WR, Valenta R, Zuberbier T, Sager A, Novak N: Clinical an immunological changes in atopic dermatitis patients undergoing subcutaneous immunotherapy with a house dust mite allergoid. Clin Exp Allergy 2007; 37:1277–1285.
4. Einarsson R, Dreborg S, Hammarstorm L, Lofkvist T, Smith CI, Svensson G: Monitoring of mite *Dermatophagoides farinae* allergen-specific IgG and IgG subclass distribution in patients on immunotherapy. Allergy 1992; 47:76–82.
5. Gutgesell C, Heise S, Seubert S, Domhof S, Brunner F, Neumann C: Double-blind placebo-controlled house dust mite control measures in adult patients with atopic dermatitis. Br J Dermatol 2001; 145:70–74.
6. Jahnz-Rozyk K, Targowski T, Paluchowska E, Owczarek W, Kucharczyk A: Serum thymus and activation-regulated chemokine, macrophage derived chemokine and exotaxin as markers of the severity of atopic dermatitis. Allergy 2005; 60:685–688.
7. Larche M, Akdis CA, Valenta R: Immunological mechanisms of allergen specific immunotherapy. Nat Rev Immunol 2006; 6:761–771.
8. Tupker RA, De Monchy JG, Coenraads PJ, Homan A, van der Meer JB: Induction of atopic dermatitis by inhalation of house dust mite. J Allergy Clin immunol 1996; 97:1064–1070.
9. Werfel T, Breuer K, Rueff F, Przybilla B, Worm M, Grewe M, Ruzicka T, Brehler R, Wolf H, Schnitker J, Kapp A: Usefulness of specific immunotherapy in patients with atopic dermatitis and allergic sensitisation to house dust mites: a multi-centre randomised dose response study. Allergy 2006; 61:202–205.

Natalija Novak

Department of Dermatology, University of Bonn, Sigmund-Freud-Str. 25, D-53105 Bonn, Germany, Tel. +49 228 287-15542, Fax +49 228 287-14333, E-mail natalija.novak @ukb.uni-bonn.de

A Potent Adenosine A$_{2B}$ Receptor Antagonist

Attenuates Methacholine-Induced Bronchial Hyperresponsiveness, Mucus Production, and IgE Levels in an Allergic Mouse Model

M. Aparici[1], A. Nueda[1], J. Beleta[1], N. Prats[2], R. Fernández[2], and M. Miralpeix[1]

[1]*Biology Department and* [2]*Preclinical Development Division,*
Research Center, Almirall Prodesfarma, Barcelona, Spain

Summary. *Background and objective:* Substantial evidence highlights the importance of adenosine in the pathogenesis of asthma and COPD. The objective of our work was to study the effect of LAS 38096, a potent and selective adenosine A$_{2B}$ receptor antagonist, on methacholine-induced bronchoconstriction, lung inflammation, mucus production and IgE levels in an allergic mouse model. *Methods:* Female Balb/c mice were sensitized with two injections (i.p.) of ovalbumin (OVA, 10 µg) plus Alum (2 mg/ml) on days 1 and 10. Aerosol challenges were performed with 5% OVA for 20 min from day 19 to 24. LAS38096 was administered orally twice daily 1 h before – and 6 h after – each OVA challenge. 24 h after last OVA-challenge, methacholine-induced bronchial hyperresponsiveness (BHR) was measured using whole body plethysmography (Buxco). A bronchoalveolar lavage (BAL) was then performed for cellular infiltration determination, and lung tissue and blood samples were collected for histopathology and OVA-specific IgE level measurements, respectively. *Results and conclusions:* OVA-challenged mice treated with LAS38096 showed significantly less BHR, mucus production and OVA-specific IgE levels. Overall, these results suggest that blockade of the A2B receptor may provide clinical benefits in the treatment of chronic respiratory diseases.

Keywords: adenosine, A$_{2B}$, mouse model, IgE, mucus, hyperresponsiveness

Introduction

Adenosine causes dose-related bronchoconstriction in patients with asthma and COPD but not in healthy volunteers, and this response appears to be orchestrated by adenosine mediated activation of mast cells through one of the four described adenosine receptors (A$_1$, A$_{2A}$, A$_{2B}$, A$_3$) [1]. While the A$_{2B}$ receptor appears to be responsible for mast-cell degranulation in humans, in rodents, both A$_{2B}$ and A$_3$ receptors could be playing this role [2]. The A$_{2B}$ receptor mediates the release of proinflammatory cyto-kines and chemokines in mast cells, Th2 cells, lung fibroblasts and bronchial smooth muscle cells which overall may participate in the chronicity of airway inflammation and remodeling [3]. Recent evidence has shown that an adenosine A$_{2B}$ receptor antagonist (CVT-6883) prevents AMP-induced bronchoconstriction in an allergic mouse model [4] and attenuates pulmonary inflammation, fibrosis and alveolar airway enlargement in adenosine deaminase (ADA)-deficient mice [5].

Our objective was to study the effect of LAS 38096, a potent and selective adenosine

A_{2B} receptor antagonist over methacholine-induced bronchoconstriction, lung inflammation, mucus production and IgE levels in an allergic mouse model.

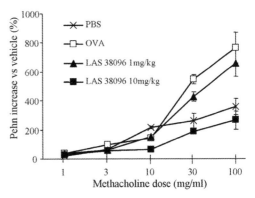

Methods

Functional and Radioligand Binding Assays

Rat colon whole organ functional assays were performed as previously described [6]. Binding with rat receptors: ^{3}H-CCPA, ^{3}H-CGS21680 and ^{125}I AB-MECA were used as ligands for A_1, A_{2A}, and A_3 binding assays respectively. All bindings assays were performed at CEREP, except rat A_3 assay which was performed at MDS.

Figure 1. LAS 38096 reverts methacholine induced airway hyperresponsiveness in conscious mice. Percentages of Penh increase *versus* vehicle were calculated for PBS, OVA and treated groups. Data represent the mean ± SEM of the percentage of Penh change *versus* vehicle for each group of animals in response to inhaled methacholine dose range. *$p <$ .05 *versus* OVA group for 30 and 100 mg/ml methacholine doses in the PBS and LAS 38096 10 mg/kg groups.

Compound Preparation

LAS 38096 (1, 3, and 10 mg/kg) was prepared as a suspension in 0.5% methylcellulose containing 0.1% Tween 80. The volume of administration was 10 ml/kg.

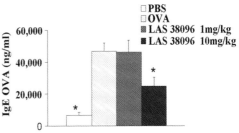

Statistics

Student's *t*-test was used to determine the significant difference between the OVA-challenged group and the other experimental groups.

Figure 3. LAS 38096 reduces OVA specific IgE levels in serum. OVA-specific IgE levels in serum were measured at 24 h after the last OVA challenge by a noncommercial sandwich ELISA (mouse IgE from Serotec; biotin rat antimouse IgE from Biosource International) . Data represent means ± *SEM* *$p <$ .05 versus OVA group.

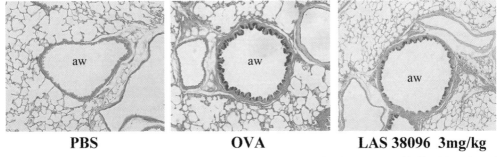

Figure 2. LAS 38096 decreases mucus accumulation in the lung. Lungs were fixed in 10% neutral-buffered formalin and cross-sections were obtained from the left and right lungs and embedded in paraffin. Sections were stained with periodic acid Schiff (PAS) for mucin detection in the airway epithelium of a first generation airway (aw).

Results and Discussion

LAS 38096 is a potent A_{2B} receptor antagonist ($pA_2 = 7.78$ for rat A_{2B} receptor) with good selectivity *versus* A_1, A_{2A} and A_3 adenosine receptors (60, 35, and >5000 fold selectivity *versus* rat receptors respectively).

Compared to PBS-challenged mice, untreated OVA–challenged mice showed a significant increase in bronchial hyperreactivity (BHR), eosinophil lung infiltration, BAL Th2 cytokines, plasma OVA-IgE levels, and airway mucus production. In contrast, OVA-challenged mice treated with LAS 38096 showed significantly less BHR (Figure 1), mucus production (Figure 2) and OVA-specific IgE levels (Figure 3) and a slight decrease in eosinophil infiltration and Th2 cytokine levels (not shown).

Overall, these results suggest that blockade of the A_{2B} receptor may provide clinical benefits in the treatment of chronic respiratory diseases.

References

1. Holgate ST: The Quintiles Prize Lecture 2004. The identification of the adenosine A2B receptor as a novel therapeutic target in asthma. Br J Pharmacol 2005; 145:1009–1015.
2. Fozard JR, Hannon JP: Species differences in adenosine receptor-mediated bronchoconstrictor responses. Clin Exp Allergy 2000; 30:1213–1220.
3. Mohsenin A, Blackburn MR: Adenosine signaling in asthma and chronic obstructive pulmonary disease. Curr Opin Pulm Med 2006; 12:54–59.
4. Fan M, Zeng D, Belardinelli L, Mustafa SJ: American Thoracic Society Meeting 2005; Poster H75.
5. Sun CX, Zhong H, Molina JG, Berlardinelli L, Zeng D, Balckburn MR: American Thoracic Society Meeting 2005; Poster C34.
6. Fozard JR, Baur F, Wolber C: Antagonist pharmacology of adenosine A_{2B} receptors from rat, guinea pig, and dog. Eur J Pharmacol 2003; 475:79–84.

Montse Miralpeix

Respiratory Therapeutic Group, Biology Department, Research Center, Almirall Prodesfarma, Laureà Miró 408–410, 08980 Sant Feliu de Llobregat, Barcelona, Spain, Tel. +34 93 291-3468, Fax +34 93 291-3420, E-mail mmiralpe@almirall.es

Differential Regulation of Different TLR Responses by IL-10 Derived from Different Cell Types

L. Siewe[1], M. Bollati-Fogolin[2], C. Wickenhauser[3], T. Krieg[1], W. Müller[2], and A. Roers[1]

[1]Department of Dermatology and [3]Department of Pathology, University of Cologne, [2]Department of Experimental Immunology, German Research Center for Biotechnology, Braunschweig, all Germany

Summary. *Background:* Interleukin-10 (IL-10) is an important regulator of immune responses secreted by different cell types. We have previously shown that mice with selective inactivation of the IL-10 gene in T-cells suffer from deregulated T-cell responses similar as observed in IL-10$^{-/-}$ animals. Unlike IL-10$^{-/-}$ mice, however, T-cell-specific mutants do not mount an enhanced innate response to LPS, which must, therefore, be subject to control by IL-10 from non-T-cells. *Methods:* Mice with cell type-specific inactivation of the IL-10 gene in macrophages and neutrophils were generated using the Cre-loxP recombination system. Inflammatory innate responses to subcutaneously injected TLR ligands were investigated by histology and quantification of serum cytokine levels and compared in wt, IL-10$^{-/-}$ and in T-cell- as well as macrophage/neutrophil-specific IL-10 mutant mice. *Results:* We show that subcutaneous injection of LPS, causing a moderate local inflammation in WT and T-cell-specific IL-10 mutant mice, resulted in an augmented inflammatory response in the macrophage/neutrophil-specific mutant mice. Correspondingly, serum levels of proinflammatory cytokines were increased in the macrophage/neutrophil-specific IL-10 mutants after i.p. administration of LPS when compared with WT mice. In contrast, the inflammatory response of these mutants to CpG oligodeoxynucleotides was not different from that of WT mice. *Conclusion:* These results show that different innate responses can be subject to control by IL-10 from different cellular sources.

Keywords: macrophages, neutrophils, knock out mice, inflammation, cytokines

The innate immune system senses microbial infection by receptors which detect conserved pathogen-associated molecular patterns and mediate inflammatory responses [1, 2]. TLR4 recognizes lipopolysaccharide (LPS) of Gram-negative bacteria and mediates secretion of proinflammatory cytokines, most notably, TNF-α, IL-12 and IFN-γ [3] TLR9 triggers an inflammatory response upon recognition of unmethylated CpG motifs in bacterial or viral DNA, which are less common in mammalian DNA [4].

IL-10 is an immunoregulatory cytokine, which limits immune responses and minimizes immunopathology [5]. The importance of IL-10 for the control of innate responses was demonstrated by an increased sensitivity of IL-10-deficient animals to lipopolysaccharide (LPS) [6].

We have previously shown that mice with a T-cell-specific inactivation of the *IL-10* gene reproduce the deregulated T-cell responses of completely IL-10-deficient animals but develop normal innate responses to LPS or skin irritation [7]. These innate responses must, therefore, be subject to control by IL-10 derived from non-T-cells.

As described in detail elsewhere [8], we have generated mice with a deficiency for IL-10 in macrophages and neutrophils by crossing *IL-10^{FL}* animals [7] *lysM-Cre* transgenic mice on a C57BL/6 background. LysM-Cre mice express the Cre recombinase in macrophages and neutrophilic granulocytes [9]. Efficiency and specificity of Cre-mediated deletion were verified by Southern blot analysis of DNA extracted from FACS-sorted cell populations. Complete deletion of the loxP-flanked fragment was found in F4/80+ macrophages from the peritoneal cavity and in Gr1+ neutrophilic granulocytes from the spleen of *IL-10^{FL/FL} lysM-Cre+* mice. In contrast, no or only insignificant deletion was observed in CD19+ splenic B cells, CD3+ T-cells, CD11c+ splenic dendritic cells or in tail biopsies from the same animals.

In order to test the importance of IL-10 derived from different cell types for the control of the local inflammatory response to TLR ligands, we first established regimens of repetitive s.c. administration of LPS or CpG oligonucleotides, which produced a clear difference between IL-10^{-/-} mice and wt animals with respect to the local inflammatory response. These treatments resulted in extensive tissue necrosis in IL-10 deficient, but only moderate inflammation in the wt animals as determined by histology and determination of serum cytokine levels (Table 1). Upon s.c. injection of LPS, macrophage/neutrophil-specific IL-10 mutant mice developed augmented inflammatory infiltration with extensive necrosis similar to the local response in mice with complete IL-10 deficiency while T-cell-specific IL-10 mutant mice [7] showed the same moderate local response as wt animals. Correspondingly, serum levels of proinflammatory cytokines were significantly elevated in macrophage/neutrophil-specific mutants as compared to wt mice. In order to characterize the local inflammatory response to TLR9 stimulation, CpG-oligodeoxynucleotides [4] were repetitively injected s.c., the injection site was excised and analyzed by histology. In WT or

Table 1. Overview of inflammatory local responses of wt and IL-10 mutant mice to LPS or CpG-DNA. While wt mice develop only moderate inflammation at the injection site and no or little immunopathology (ø), severe tissue necrosis (+++) is observed in IL-10^{-/-} mice upon subcutaneous injection of LPS or CpG. Mice with selective deficiency for IL-10 in macrophages and neutrophils (IL-10^{FL/FL} lysM-Cre+) show differential responses to the two stimuli.

	immunopathology in response to	
	LPS	CpG
wt	ø	ø
IL-10^{-/-}	+++	+++
IL-10^{FL/FL} lysM-Cre+	+++	ø

Cre− control animals, this treatment resulted in a moderate inflammatory infiltration as demonstrated by H&E stained paraffin sections. In marked contrast, the lesions of IL-10^{-/-} mice showed more massive infiltration by inflammatory cells and extensive necrosis of epidermis and dermis. The local response as well as the serum concentrations of proinflammatory cytokines after CpG s.c. in T-cell-specific but also macrophage/neutrophil-specific IL-10 mutant mice were as in WT mice. These results show that IL-10 secretion by different cell types serves distinct and nonredundant functions [8]. Different innate responses can be subject to control by IL-10 from different cellular sources.

References

1. Medzhitov R: Toll-like receptors and innate immunity. Nat Rev Immunol 2001; 1:135–145.
2. Akira S: Mammalian Toll-like receptors. Curr Opin Immunol 2003; 15:5–11.
3. Beutler B, Rietschel ET. Innate immune sensing and its roots: the story of endotoxin. Nat Rev Immunol 2003; 3:169.
4. Krieg AM: CpG motifs in bacterial DNA and their immune effects. Annu. Rev. Immunol. 2002; 20:709–760.
5. Moore KW, de Waal Malefyt R, Coffman RL, O'Garra A: Interleukin-10 and the interleukin-10 receptor. Annu Rev Immunol 2001; 19:683–765.
6. Berg DJ, Kuhn R, Rajewsky K, Muller W, Menon

S, Davidson N, Grunig G, Rennick D: Interleukin-10 is a central regulator of the response to LPS in murine models of endotoxic shock and the Shwartzman reaction but not endotoxin tolerance. J Clin Invest 1995; 96:2339–2347.

7. Roers A, Siewe L, Strittmatter E, Deckert M, Schlüter D, Stenzel W, Gruber AD, Krieg T, Rajewsky K, Müller W: T-cell-specific Inactivation of the interleukin-10 gene in mice results in enhanced T-cell responses but normal innate responses to lipopolysaccharide or skin irritation. J Exp Med 2004; 200:1289–1297.

8. Siewe L, Bollati-Fogolin M, Wickenhauser C, Krieg T, Muller W, Roers A: Interleukin-10 derived from macrophages and/or neutrophils regulates the inflammatory response to LPS but not the response to CpG DNA. Eur J Immunol 2006; 36:3248–3255

9. Clausen BE, Burkhardt C, Reith W, Renkawitz R, Förster I: Conditional gene targeting in macrophages and granulocytes using LysM-cre mice. Transgenic Research 1999; 8:265–277.

Axel Roers

Department of Dermatology, University of Cologne, Josef Stelzmann Str. 9, D-50931 Cologne, Tel. +49 221 478-3196 or -5554, E-mail axel.roers@uni-koeln.de

Pharmacodynamics of Latest Generation H$_1$-Antihistamines

Relevance of Drug Concentrations at Receptor Sites and of Affinity Values for H$_1$ Receptors

M. Strolin Benedetti[1], M. Gillard[2], N. Frossard[3], G. Pauli[3], A. Purohit[3], E. Baltes[4], and C. de Vos[5]

[1]*UCB, Drug Metabolism and Pharmacokinetics, Nanterre, France,* [2]*UCB, Cellular and Molecular Biology, Braine l'Alleud, Belgium,* [3]*EA3771, Faculté de Pharmacie, Université Louis Pasteur-Strasbourg I, Ilkirch, France,* [4]*UCB, Drug Metabolism and Pharmacokinetics, Braine l'Alleud, Belgium,* [5]*UCB, Global Medical Affairs, Brussels, Belgium*

Summary. *Introduction:* The percentage of receptor occupancy has been shown to correlate with the percentage of inhibition of histamine-induced wheal and flare by an H$_1$-antihistamine. The estimation of receptor occupancy requires the availability of both the drug concentration at receptor sites and affinity of the drug for the receptor. Classically, free plasma concentrations, calculated from plasma concentrations using plasma protein binding, are used as an approximation of the drug concentration at receptor sites. The purpose of this work is to estimate the drug concentration at receptor sites by an alternative approach, using the volume of distribution and the skin concentrations of the drug. *Methods and Results:* Skin concentrations were measured by validated methods in samples from 18 adult allergic volunteers 24 h after administration of 5 mg oral levocetirizine or desloratadine. Mean values were 40.7 and 56.3 ng/g, respectively). The volumes of distribution (V/F) of levocetirizine and desloratadine are 28 and 3430 L, respectively for a 70 kg man. Using the formula $V/F = V_p + \dfrac{f_{uP}}{f_{uT}} \cdot V_{TW}$, where F = absolute bioavailability (assumed to be 1), V$_P$ = volume of plasma (3.2 L for a 70 kg man), V$_{TW}$ = volume in which the drug is distributed outside plasma, f$_{uP}$ = fraction unbound in plasma and f$_{uT}$ = fraction unbound in tissue, it is possible to calculate f$_{uT}$ (0.14–0.052 for levocetirizine and 0.0017–0.0006 for desloratadine) and therefore the free tissue (skin) concentration by the relationship f$_{uT}$ • C$_T$, where C_T is the total tissue (skin) concentration. Based on these calculations, free skin concentrations ranged between 2.12–5.70 and 0.034–0.096 ng/g for levocetirizine and desloratadine, respectively. *Conclusion:* The estimated free skin concentration values are very similar to free plasma concentrations. Therefore, the free skin/plasma concentrations should be used to estimate the receptor occupancy by an H$_1$-antihistamine. High skin concentrations simply reflect an extensive distribution of a drug (skin ≈ 19% of body volume) and not necessarily the drug concentration at receptor sites, whereas high free skin concentrations are crucial for the efficiency of a drug given for skin allergic problems.

Keywords: wheal and flare inhibition, H$_1$ receptor occupancy

Introduction

Histamine is one of the many neurotransmitters that act via G-protein-coupled receptors. There are four major subtypes of histamine receptors, H$_1$ to H$_4$. The human H$_1$ receptor is a 487-amino acid G-coupled protein with seven transmembrane domains. H$_1$ receptors are widely distributed (e.g., in the skin). The percentage of receptor occupancy (RO) has been shown to correlate with the percentage of inhibition of histamine-induced wheal and flare as well as with the percentage of inhibition of allergen-induced wheal and flare by an H$_1$-antihistamine [1, 2]. The estimation of RO was calculated using:

$$RO = B_{max} (100\%) \times L/(L + K_i) \qquad (1)$$

where L = the "unbound" drug concentration at receptor sites
B$_{max}$ = the maximal number of binding sites (set to 100%)
K$_i$ = the equilibrium inhibition constant.

Values of Ki determined in conditions as near as possible to the physiopathological conditions were used [1–3]. Taking the classical approach, unbound plasma concentrations (C$_{uP}$) [calculated from total plasma concentrations (C$_P$) using the fraction unbound in plasma (f$_{uP}$):

$$C_{uP} = f_{uP} \times C_P \qquad (2)]$$

were used as an approximation of the drug concentration at receptor sites (L), as only unbound drug is capable of entering and leaving the plasma and tissue compartments (C$_{uP}$ = C$_{uT}$) (see Figure 1). However, this assumes the absence of an active transport mechanism (at least for the target tissues containing the H$_1$ receptors).

The purpose of this work was to estimate the drug concentration at receptor sites (L) by an alternative approach, i.e., by using the volume of distribution and the total skin concentrations of the drug. The data analyzed are those collected from a study investigating the inhibition of allergen-induced wheal and flare by levocetirizine and desloratadine administered as a single 5 mg oral dose to 18 adult allergic volunteers [2].

PLASMA   **TISSUE**

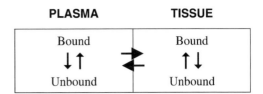

Figure 1. At equilibrium, the distribution of a drug within the body depends on binding to both plasma proteins and tissue components. In the model, only unbound drug is capable of entering and leaving the plasma and tissue compartments.

Methods

Skin and blood samples were obtained from the 18 allergic volunteers 24 h after administration of levocetirizine or desloratadine. Skin biopsies were performed on the internal surfaces of the arm using a 3 mm Accu Punch® device (depth = 7 mm). Total skin and plasma concentrations were measured by validated methods using Liquid Chromatography-Mass Spectrometry (LC-MS/MS) in the Turbo Ion Spray (TIS) positive mode (UCB data on file). The limit of quantitation (LOQ) in plasma was 0.200 ng/ml for levocetirizine 5 mg and 0.100 ng/ml for desloratadine 5 mg. The LOQ in skin was 25 ng/g for both drugs. As 5 subjects for each drug had skin concentrations < LOQ, it was decided to estimate the mean drug concentration at receptor sites by two ways, taking into account:

1. only subjects with skin concentration > LOQ (n = 13) (mean values = 48.92 and 69.08 ng/g for levocetirizine and desloratadine, respectively)
2. all subjects (n = 18) using extrapolated values for the 5 subjects with skin concentrations < LOQ (mean values = 40.73 and 56.33 ng/g, for levocetirizine and desloratadine, respectively).

Calculations have been made using the formula:

$$V/F = V_P + \frac{f_{uP}}{f_{uT}} \cdot V_{TW} \qquad (3)$$

where V = volume of distribution,
F = absolute bioavailability (assumed to be 1),
V$_P$ = volume of plasma (about 3.2 L for a 70 kg man [4, 5]),
V$_{TW}$ = volume in which the drug is distributed outside plasma,

Table 1. Total skin and plasma concentrations of levocetirizine (LCTZ) and desloratadine (DES) 24 h after administration of a single oral 5 mg dose.

Subject No.	LCTZ		DES	
	Total skin concentration (C$_T$) (ng/g)	Total plasma concentration (C$_P$) (ng/ml)	Total skin concentration (C$_T$, ng/g)	Total plasma concentration (C$_P$) (ng/ml)
1	41.52	27.26	114.14	0.42
2	62.42	22.74	(31.43)*	0.31
3	33.56	19.47	51.19	0.62
4	66.71	35.39	67.82	0.53
5	(5.83)*	(5.77)*	(30.83)*	0.26
6	31.43	18.79	28.52	0.48
7	52.06	22.84	76.91	0.84
8	78.09	31.41	30.26	0.66
9	45.85	18.52	242.84	0.49
10	(17.90)*	(7.98)*	(13.32)*	0.43
11	(17.10)*	(10.00)*	58.86	0.52
12	61.12	27.29	35.97	0.35
13	(21.70)*	(11.48)*	(14.69)*	0.34
14	37.77	27.99	27.52	0.41
15	31.04	16.40	30.47	0.18
16	47.24	20.87	25.24	0.34
17	47.12	21.84	(25.71)*	0.40
18	(34.60)*	(14.46)*	108.23	0.43
Mean (n = 13)	48.92 ± 14.62	23.91 ± 5.59	69.07 ± 60.30	0.48 ± 0.17
Mean (n = 18)	40.73 ± 18.99	20.03 ± 8.13	56.33 ± 55.06	0.44 ± 0.16

()* = subjects with skin concentrations < LOQ

f_{uP} = fraction unbound in plasma
f_{uT} = fraction unbound in tissue.

Using formula (3), it is possible to calculate f_{uT} for levocetirizine and for desloratadine. Therefore, the unbound tissue (skin) concentrations (C$_{uT}$) are calculated by the relationship $C_{uT} = f_{uT} \cdot C_T$ *(formula 4)*, where C$_T$ is the total tissue (skin) concentration.

The apparent volumes of distribution (V/F) of levocetirizine and desloratadine are 28 and 3430 L, respectively for a 70 kg man [6]. The fraction unbound in human plasma (f$_{uP}$) is 0.09 and 0.15 for levocetirizine and desloratadine, respectively [6, 7]. If the assumption is made that a drug is distributed either into the extracellular water or into the total body water, then V$_{TW}$ will be obtained by subtracting the plasma volume from the extracellular water or from

the total body water. For a normal young male adult of about 70 kg, average values for extracellular water and total body water are 17.5 and 42 L, respectively [4, 5].

Results

Individual and mean total plasma and skin concentrations of levocetirizine and desloratadine, measured 24 h after a single 5 mg dose, are presented in Table 1. Unbound skin concentrations (C$_{uT}$) for levocetirizine and desloratadine, calculated using the formulas (3) + (4), are presented in Table 2. These values are consistent with those found using the classical approach in which the aforementioned formula (2) has been used [2].

For levocetirizine, it would appear that data

Table 2. Unbound skin concentrations (C$_{uT}$) of levocetirizine (LCTZ) and desloratadine (DES) calculated by the alternative approach, assuming that the drugs are either distributed into the extracellular water or into the total body water (those obtained by the classical approach are given for comparison).

Parameter	Alternative approach [formulas (3) + (4)]				Classical approach [formula (2)]	
	Extracellular water		Total body water			
	V$_{TW}$ = 17.5–3.2 = 14.3L		V$_{TW}$ = 42–3.2 = 38.8L		C$_{uP}$ = f$_{uP}$ × C$_P$	
	LCTZ	DES	LCTZ	DES	LCTZ	DES
f$_{uT}$	0.052	0.0006	0.14	0.0017	–	–
C$_{uT}$ (ng/g)						
n = 13	2.54	0.041	6.85	0.117	2.152 ± 0.503	0.072 ± 0.025
n = 18	2.12	0.034	5.70	0.096	1.803 ± 0.730	0.067 ± 0.023

calculated by the formulas (3) + (4) are more consistent with the data calculated by the formula (2) (1.803 ng/g) when the assumption is made that the drug distributes only into the extracellular water (2.12 ng/g) rather than into the total body water (5.70 ng/g). For desloratadine, the data calculated by the classical approach (0.067 ng/g) are in between those calculated by the formulas (3) + (4) when it is assumed that the drug is either distributed only into the extracellular water (0.034 ng/g) or into the total body water (0.096 ng/g).

For a better comparison of the data obtained by the formulas (3) + (4) with those obtained by the classical approach, it would of course be necessary to know the absolute bioavailability F of the drug. For levocetirizine, F can be estimated as very high (> 0.77, as it is known that 77% of the drug is recovered unchanged in urine [6, 8]). Therefore, the assumption can be made that F − 1 for levocetirizine. For desloratadine, data to estimate absolute bioavailability F are unavailable in the scientific literature.

For comparison of the data obtained by the two approaches, it is also important that the fraction unbound in plasma (f$_{uP}$) be correctly and precisely evaluated. This is the case again for levocetirizine, for which the percentage binding reported to human plasma proteins has been estimated using equilibrium dialysis and is 91 ± 0.7% [7], whereas for desloratadine, the methodology used and the precision of the data reported in the literature are less clear [the percentage binding to human plasma proteins reported generally ranges between 82–87% [6,

9]. A mean value of 85%, i.e., a fraction unbound in plasma (f$_{uP}$) of 0.15, has been used for our calculations.

Conclusion

The two different approaches used to estimate the concentrations of levocetirizine and desloratadine at the receptor sites, i.e., the classical one and that based on the volume of distribution, give data in reasonable agreement. The estimated free skin concentration values are very low for desloratadine compared with levocetirizine, in spite of the similar or even higher total skin concentrations of desloratadine. The high skin concentrations of desloratadine simply reflect its extensive tissue distribution (skin is a tissue representing ≈ 19% of the body volume) and not necessarily its concentrations at receptor sites, whereas high unbound skin concentrations are crucial for getting a high receptor occupancy and a high inhibition of the allergen-induced wheal and flare [2].

Acknowledgment

The authors thank Dr. I. Poggesi for very useful discussions and Ms. M. Rovei for preparation of the manuscript.

References

1. Gillard M, Strolin Benedetti M, Chatelain P, Baltes E: Histamine H$_1$ receptor occupancy and phar-

macodynamics of second generation H_1-antihistamines. Inflamm Res 2005; 54:367–369.

2. Frossard N, Strolin Benedetti M, Purohit A, Pauli G: Evidence of a direct relationship between receptor occupancy and potency in the skin: the H1-antihistamines example. EADV Congress, Rhodes, October 2006.

3. Gillard M, Chatelain P: Changes in pH differently affect the binding properties of histamine H_1 receptor antagonists. Eur J Pharmacol 2006; 530:205–214.

4. Rowland M, Tozer TN: Distribution; in Clinical pharmacokinetics: concepts and applications (3rd edition), Philadelphia, Williams & Wilkins, 1995, pp. 137–155.

5. Wagner JG: Body water compartments and the distribution of drugs. In Biopharmaceutics and relevant pharmacokinetics (1st ed.). Illinois: Hamilton Press, Drug Intelligence Publications, 1971, pp. 260–265.

6. Molimard M, Diquet B, Strolin Benedetti M: Comparison of pharmacokinetics and metabolism of desloratadine, fexofenadine, levocetirizine and mizolastine in humans. Fund Clin Pharmacol 2004; 18:399–411.

7. Bree F, Thiault L, Gautiers G, Strolin Benedetti M, Baltes E, Rihoux JP, Tillement.JP: Blood distribution of levocetirizine, a new nonsedating histamine H_1-receptor antagonist, in humans. Fund Clin Pharmacol 2002; 16:471–487.

8. Strolin Benedetti M, Plisnier M, Kaise J, Maier L, Baltes E, Arendt C, McCraken N: Absorption, distribution, metabolism and excretion of [^{14}C]levocetirizine, the R enantiomer of cetirizine, in healthy volunteers, Eur J Clin Pharmacol 2001; 57:571–582.

9. Physician Desk Reference: Clarinex (desloratadine) tablets, Prescribing information as of 2002, Montvale, NJ, USA Medical Economics Company, Inc.: http://www.pdr.net.

Margherita Strolin Benedetti

UCB, Drug Metabolism and Pharmacokinetics, 21, rue de Neuilly, F-92003 Nanterre Cedex, France, Tel. +33 1 4729 4582, Fax +33 1 4729 4591, E-mail margherita.strolin@ucb-group.com

Conformational Change in the IgE-FcεRI Interaction as a Target for Inhibitor Design

A.J. Beavil, J. Hunt, R.L. Beavil, H.J. Gould, and B.J. Sutton

MRC & Asthma UK Centre in Allergic Mechanisms of Asthma, King's College London, UK

Summary. *Background:* The interaction between IgE and its high-affinity receptor FcεRI is a target for the design of inhibitors of the allergic response. The aim of this work is to understand the mechanism of this interaction at the atomic level to facilitate inhibitor design. *Methods:* X-ray crystallography and NMR were employed to determine the molecular structures; binding kinetics were determined by surface plasmon resonance analysis; analytical ultracentrifugation was used to determine binding stoichiometries and affinities. *Results:* The X-ray structure of IgE Fc revealed, unexpectedly, an asymmetrically and acutely bent conformation, with an extensive interface between Cε2 and Cε3 domains. The structure of the complex between a Cε3-Cε4 fragment and the soluble receptor (Fcε3–4/sFcεRIα) had earlier revealed both Cε3 domains engaged with receptor in the high-affinity complex, but in the bent IgE structure, only one of the two Cε3 domains is accessible for receptor binding. This implies substantial conformational change in both Cε2 and Cε3 upon receptor engagement, and NMR analysis of the Cε2:sFcεRIα interaction supported this hypothesis. In order to determine the effect of inhibiting this conformational change upon receptor binding, we generated a version of IgE Fc lacking the inter-heavy chain disulphide bridge. This modified Fcε3–4, which engages sFcεRIα through only a single Cε3 domain, displayed a 1000-fold lower affinity; this quantifies the potential effect of an inhibitor of the conformational change. *Conclusion:* Allosteric inhibition is an alternative and promising strategy, and fluorescently labeled IgE-based reagents have been produced to screen for small molecule inhibitors of the conformational change.

Keywords: IgE, FcεRI, X-ray structure, allostery, inhibition

Introduction

The binding of immunoglobulin E (IgE) to its high-affinity receptor (FcεRI) has long been seen as a potential target for therapeutic intervention in allergic disease [reviewed in 1], and the recently successful introduction into clinical use of an anti-IgE monoclonal antibody, Omalizumab [2], which competes with this interaction, provides support for this approach. We have been studying the three-dimensional structures of IgE and FcεRI and their interaction, and have discovered that substantial con-formational changes are involved in a biphasic binding event. Understanding the nature of these conformational changes opens up an alternative strategy for designing small molecules inhibitors, targeting the allosteric changes rather than direct, steric competition of the extensive protein-protein interface.

Materials and Methods

Production of the IgE Fc and sFcεRIα constructs has been described previously [3, 4 and

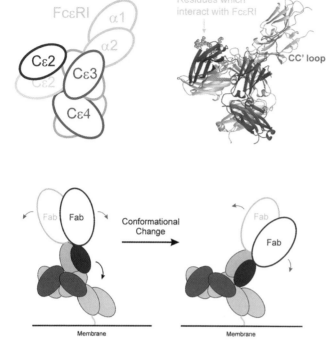

Figure 1. Upper panel: Model of the initial complex formed between the bent IgE Fc [9] and sFcεRIα based upon the contacts formed in the Fcεε3–4/sFcεRIα structure [8]. Cε2 residues shown in green are contacts for FcεRIα [7], and the CC' loop of the α2 domain of FcεRI is also indicated. Lower panel: schematic of the proposed conformational change in IgE ("unbending") upon receptor binding.

refs. therein]. The kinetics of binding of the IgE Fc variants to an IgG4-Fc(sFcεRIα)₂ fusion protein was measured by surface plasmon resonance (SPR) on BIAcore 1000, 2000, or 3000 instruments, and sedimentation equilibrium data were measured in an Optima XL-A analytical ultracentrifuge (Beckman Coulter Inc., Fullerton, CA, USA) [3].

Results

Analysis of the binding of IgE, IgE Fc (consisting of the dimer of Cε2, Cε3 and Cε4 domains) and a truncated version, IgE Fcε3–4 (lacking the Cε2 domains), to immobilized receptor by SPR indicated a biphasic interaction, with a fast initial contact followed by a slower phase [5, 6]. Furthermore, comparison between IgE Fc and Fcε3–4 revealed that in the absence of the Cε2 domains, both the on-rate and the off-rate was faster [5, 7]; thus the presence of the Cε2 domains is responsible in part for the characteristically slow dissociation rate of IgE from its high affinity receptor ($k_d \approx 10^{-4}$–10^{-5} s^{-1}). Evidence for a direct interaction

between Cε2 and FcεRI is provided by an NMR titration experiment using isotopically labelled Cε2 and unlabelled sFcεRIα [7].

The X-ray crystal structure of the complex between Fcε3–4 and sFcεRIα [8] revealed that both Cε3 domains make contact with the receptor. However, the structure of the uncomplexed but complete IgE Fc [9] showed that one of the Cε3 domains was inaccessible for receptor interaction, and also that the Cε2 domains were bent back onto the Cε3 domains and in no position to make contact with the receptor. This is shown in the top panel of Figure 1; on the right is a composite model of the bent IgE Fc structure and the sFcεRIα domains, the latter in the orientation adopted in the complex with Fcε3–4; the schematic on the left indicates the component domains. However, in this composite model, only one of the two Cε3 domains makes proper contact with the receptor, and the loop between the C and C' strands of the α2 domain of the receptor clashes with the other Cε3 domain. In order for the complete IgE Fc to engage with the receptor at both Cε3 domains, the Cε3 domains must move apart, which in turn requires movement of the Cε2 domains away

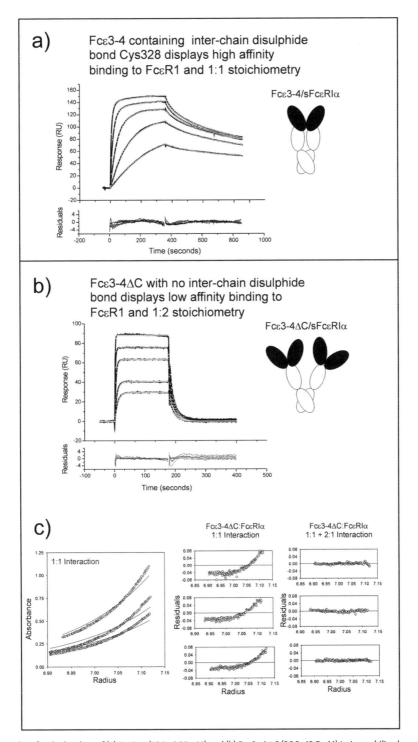

Figure 2. SPR data for the binding of (a) Fcε3–4 (100–6.25 nM) and (b) Fcε3–4ΔC (200–12.5 nM) to immobilized receptor, with the residuals for the curve-fitting. (c) Sedimentation data show that Fcε3–4ΔC forms a 1:2 complex with sFcεRIα (data collected at 11,000 rpm, with three loading ratios 1:1, 2:1, and 1:2), as indicated by the poor curve fits and residuals for 1:1 stoichiometry, and improved residuals for 1:2 binding model.

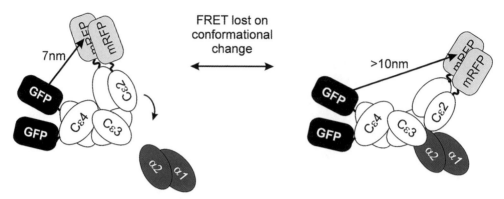

Figure 3. Schematic representation of an N- and C-terminally labelled IgE Fc derivative, constructed to monitor the conformational change in IgE Fc upon receptor binding.

from Cε3. The amino-acid residues that contact FcεRI in the complex, identified in the NMR analysis [7], are also shown in the top panel of Figure 1. We thus envisage a concerted set of conformational changes in which: (a) the Cε2 domains rotate away from Cε3 to make contact with the receptor, (b) the Cε3 domains move apart to engage the receptor at both sites, and (c) the CC' loop undergoes a rearrangement. This "unbending" of the IgE molecule is shown in a simplified schematic in the lower panel of Figure 1.

We propose that this structural model accounts for the biphasic interaction observed in the kinetic analysis. Initial, rapid and low-affinity contact at the one exposed Cε3 site in the bent IgE molecule leads to formation of the high-affinity complex (with contact at both Cε3 domains and also Cε2) after the slower conformational changes have taken place. If this conformational change could be prevented, what would be the affinity of IgE for FcεRI? Would it be sufficient to prevent mast cell or basophil activation, and long-term sensitization of these cells by IgE?

To answer the first of these questions, we generated a version of Fcε3–4 lacking the inter-heavy chain disulphide bridge at Cys328 (Fcε3–4ΔC) [4]. This molecule contained two fully-folded but unconstrained Cε3 domains. SPR analysis clearly indicated that the Fcε3–4ΔC displayed a markedly faster dissociation rate (Figure 2b) than the "native" Fcε3–4 (Figure 2a), and the sedimentation equilibrium data showed that Fcε3–4ΔC

bound two molecules of soluble receptor (Figure 2c), in contrast to the 1:1 stoichiometry of IgE, IgE-Fc and Fcε3–4. The affinity constants measured in solution from the sedimentation data for formation of the 1:1 and then the 2:1 complexes are respectively $K_{a1} = 1.8 \times 10^5 \, M^{-1}$ and $K_{a2} = 7.2 \times 10^5 \, M^{-1}$. Thus if the conformational change in IgE could be prevented, and interaction with the receptor restricted to only the one Cε3 domain that is accessible in the free (bent) molecule, then the affinity would be reduced 1000-fold at least (c.f. $K_a \approx 10^9$–$10^{10} \, M^{-1}$ for native IgE or IgE Fc).

In order to screen for small molecules that interfere with this conformational change, we have now generated derivatives of IgE Fc fluorescently labelled at their N- and C-termini with variants of GFP (Figure 3). The Fc crystal structures indicate that the change of conformation from "bent" to "open" upon receptor binding will lead to changes in distance between the fluorophores that can be detected by changes in the FRET (Förster Resonance Energy Transfer) signal.

Discussion

The structural, kinetic and equilibrium binding studies of IgE, FcεRI and their complex have led us to propose a model in which substantial, concerted conformational changes occur upon receptor engagement by IgE. This offers new target regions within the two molecules for allosteric inhibitor design, and provides an alternative to direct steric blocking of the interaction. This is important since it is difficult for a small molecule to compete with an extensive protein-protein interface [10]. We have now produced reagents that are sensitive to the conformational change in IgE, for screening small molecule libraries. The data presented here also indicate that if the conformational change can be blocked, then the affinity of IgE for FcεRI will be reduced at least 1000-fold, and preliminary studies (unpublished data) indicate that this is sufficient to have a significant inhibitory effect in both *in vitro* and *in vivo* functional assays.

Acknowledgments

We acknowledge the support of the Medical Research Council (UK), Asthma UK, the Biotechnology and Biological Sciences Research Council (UK) and The Wellcome Trust.

References

1. Gould HJ, Sutton BJ, Beavil AJ, Beavil RL, McCloskey N, Coker HA, Fear D, Smurthwaite L: The biology of IgE and the basis of allergic disease. Ann Rev Immunol 2003; 21:579–628.
2. Holgate S, Casale T, Wenzel S, Bousquet J, Deniz Y, Reisner C: The anti-inflammatory effects of omalizumab confirm the central role of IgE in allergic inflammation. J Allergy Clin Immunol 2005; 115:459–465.
3. Young RJ, Owens RJ, Mackay GA, Chan CMW, Shi J, Hide M, Francis DM, Henry AJ, Sutton BJ, Gould HJ: Secretion of recombinant human IgE-Fc by mammalian cells and biological activity of glycosylation site mutants. Protein Engineering 1995; 8:193–199.
4. Hunt J, Beavil RL, Calvert RA, Gould HJ, Sutton BJ, Beavil AJ: Disulphide linkage controls the affinity and stoichiometry of IgE Fcε3–4 binding to FcεRI. J Biol Chem 2005; 280:16808–16814.
5. Henry AJ, Cook JPD, McDonnell JM, Mackay GA, Shi J, Sutton BJ, Gould HJ: Participation of the N-terminal region of Cε3 in the binding of human IgE to its high affinity receptor FcεRI. Biochem 1997; 36:15568–15578.
6. Cook JPD, Henry AJ, McDonnell JM, Owens RJ, Sutton, BJ, Gould HJ: Identification of contact residues in the IgE binding site of human FcεRIα. Biochem 1997; 36:15579–15588.
7. McDonnell JM, Calvert R, Beavil RL, Beavil AJ, Henry AJ, Sutton BJ, Gould HJ, Cowburn, D: The structure of the IgE Cε2 domain and its role in stabilizing the complex with its high-affinity receptor FcεRI. Nature Struct Biol 2001; 8:437–441.
8. Garman SC, Wurzburg BA, Tarchevskaya SS, Kinet J-P, Jardetzky: Structure of the Fc fragment of human IgE bound to its high affinity receptor FcεRIα. Nature 2000; 406:259–266.
9. Wan T, Beavil RL, Fabiane SM, Beavil AJ, Sohi MK, Keown M, Young RJ, Henry AJ, Owens RJ, Gould HJ, Sutton BJ: The crystal structure of IgE Fc reveals an asymmetrically bent conformation. Nature Immunol 2002; 3:681–686.
10. Whitty A, Kumaravel G: Between a rock and a hard place? Nature Chem Biol 2006; 2:112–118.

Brian J. Sutton

MRC & Asthma UK Centre in Allergic Mechanisms of Asthma, Randall Division of Cell & Molecular Biophysics, King's College London, New Hunt's House, Guy's Campus, London SE1 1UL, UK, Tel. +44 20 7 848 6423, Fax +44 20 7 848 6410, E-mail brian.sutton@kcl.ac.uk

Protective Effects of CORM-3, a Water-Soluble Carbon-Monoxide-Releasing Molecule, in a Model of Vascular Inflammation

A. Vannacci[1], P. Failli[1], L. Giannini[1], F. Fabrizi[1], C. Uliva[1], L. Mazzetti[1], S. Franchi-Micheli[1], E. Masini[1], R. Motterlini[2], and P.F. Mannaioni[1]

[1]*Department of Preclinical and Clinical Pharmacology, University of Florence, Italy*
[2]*Vascular Biology Unit, Department of Surgical Research, Northwick Park Institute for Medical Research, Middlesex, UK*

Summary. *Background:* Induction of heme-oxygenase (HO-1) downregulates the response to antigen in guinea-pig mast cells, in human basophils and the anaphylactic reaction in isolated guinea-pig heart. The effects could be due to the end-products of HO-1 activity, carbon monoxide (CO), biliverdin and Fe^{2+}. CO-releasing molecules (CORMs) clarify whether the effects of HO-1 induction are attributable to CO. In previous experiments, a water insoluble CORM (CORM-2) decreases the immunological responses of guinea pig mast cells and of human basophils. Here we study the effects of a water-soluble CORM (CORM-3) in experimental models of vascular inflammation. *Methods:* Experiments were performed in isolated rat aorta, and in a bicellular model of rat coronary endothelial cells (EC) with human neutrophils (PMN). The tension of the aortic strip was evaluated with a transducer. In aortic homogenates cGMP were assessed through EIA kit. The adhesion molecules CD54 and CD11b were assayed through flow cytometric analysis on EC, and on PMN, respectively. *Results:* CORM-3 relaxes the precontracted aorta in a way which is blocked by ODQ and by charybdotoxin, and raises cGMP levels in aorta homogenates. EC coincubated with primed PMN overexpress CD54, and PMN overexpress CD11b in response to a chemotactic stimulus; these effects were blunted by CORM-3 and by superoxide-dismutase (SOD). *Conclusions:* The water soluble CORM-3 relaxes rat aorta through activation of the guanylyl cyclase/cGMP system, and the modulation of K^+ channels. CORM-3 reduced the expression of adhesion molecules by EC and PMN through a superoxide-dependent mechanism.

Keywords: carbon monoxide, neutrophils, endothelial cells

Introduction

Nitric oxide (NO), carbon monoxide (CO) and hydrogen sulphide (H_2S), once considered as toxic wastes and atmospheric pollutants, have been shown to modulate relevant biological processes. CO is endowed with anti-inflammatory activity [1] and downregulates the im-
mune system. These effects have been studied with the induction/over-expression of HO-1, or using CO as a gas [2, 3]. Previous experiments suggest a role for CO as a modulator of the allergic response. Both induction of HO-1 and administration of CO as a gas reduce the immunological response of guinea pig mast cells and of human basophils, and the anaphy-

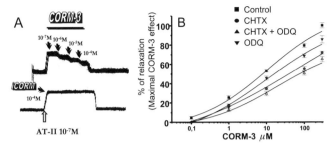

Figure 1. CORM-3 (10 mM–100 μM) induced the relaxation of angiotensin II (10^{-7} M) precontracted preparations. The angiotensin I induced contraction of the aortic strips was left unchanged by iCORM-3 (A). The relaxant effect was decreased by the guanylyl cyclase blocker ODQ, and by the K$^+$ channels blocker charybdotoxin (B).

lactic reaction in isolated guinea pig hearts [2, 3]. The introduction by Motterlini of the CO releasing molecules (CORMs) represents a tool to circumvent the criticism of the administration of CO [4]. In fact, to assert that the effects of HO-1 induction are attributable to CO is questionable, since HO-1 generates also biliverdin and Fe^{2+}, whose final products, bilirubin and ferritin, possess anti-inflammatory actions. A water-insoluble-CORM (CORM-2) abates the immunological response or guinea pig mast cells and or human basophils [5]. Our aim is to study the effects of tricarbonyl-chloro-glycinated-ruthenium (CORM-3), which was selected due to the solubility in water and to the kinetic of release of CO, in models of vascular inflammation.

Materials and Methods

Rat thoracic aorta strips were isolated and pre-contracted with angiotensin II, 10–7M according to Franchi-Micheli et al. [6]. The relaxation by CORM-3 was expressed as a decrease in the contractile force from the maximal contraction. In homogenates of rat aortic strip, the production of cGMP was assessed through the EIA kit.

Rat coronary endothelial cells (EC) were cultured in a a Petri dish at the density of 8,000–10,000 cells/cm^2. About 50,000 human polymorphonucleated neutrophilic granulocytes (PMN), isolated from healthy donors, were suspended in the supernatant of the EC cultures. PMN were then activated by the chemotactic peptide formyl-methionyl-leucyl-phenylalanine (fMLP) 10^{-8} M, in the presence or in the absence of CORM-3 (10 nM–100 μM). In some experiments, superoxide dismutase (300 IU/ml,

SOD) was used to assess the involvement of superoxide anion in the PMN-induced activation of EC. The activation of PMN was assessed through flow cytometric evaluation of CD11b expression, while EC activation was measured by the expression of the activation marker CD54.

The release of CO by CORM-3 was measured through direct reaction via headspace gas-analysis using a reductor gas detector (RGA-3 Trace Analytical Inc., Milan, Italy). The exact amount of CO released was measured in comparison with a CO standard curve.

When CORM-3 is incubated under air for 18 h in Krebs-Henseleit buffer a CO deprived, inactive CORM-3 was obtained (iCORM-3), suitable for use as internal control.

Results

CORM-3 in physiological solution (data not shown) under air released CO according to the concentrations.

In rat aorta strips, CORM-3 (10 mM–100 μM) induced the relaxation of angiotensin II (10–7 M) precontracted preparations in a concentration dependent fashion. The Angiotensin II (AT-II) induced contraction of the aortic strips was left unchanged by iCORM-3 (Figure 1a).

The relaxant effect was decreased by [1H-[1,2,4]oxadiazolo-[4, 3-a]quinoxalin-1-one] (ODQ) a blocker of guanylyl cyclase, and by charybdotoxin, a blocker of Ca^{2+} activated K$^+$ channels (Figure 1b). In rat aortic homogenates, CORM-3 increases cGMP levels, left unchanged by iCORM-3 (data not shown).

Quiescent EC express a small amount of CD54. The expression of CD54 was signifi-

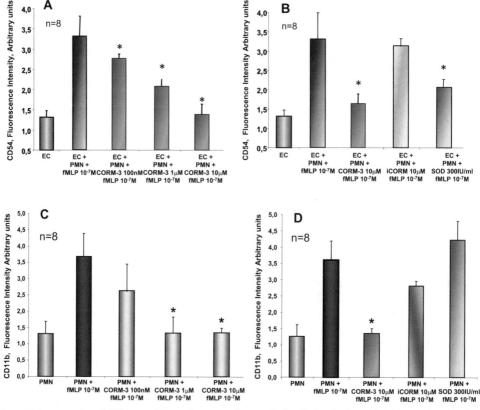

Figure 2. The expression of CD54 upon EC membrane was increased after the incubation with PMN stimulated by fMLP. CORM-3 was able to reduce the activation of EC (A), while the inactivated form of the drug (iCORM), unable to release CO, was ineffective (B). The treatment of the cells with SOD mimicked the effects of CORM-3 (B). CORM-3 reduced the activation of human PMN, assessed as membrane expression of CD11b (C). The inactivated form of CORM-3 (iCORM) and SOD were ineffective (D).

cantly increased by coincubation with PMN, and raised further when PMN were stimulated with increasing concentrations of fMLP. The maximal expression of CD54 by EC was abated by CORM-3 in a concentration dependent manner. The inhibitory effect of CORM-3 was shared by SOD; iCORM was ineffective. PMN express a small amount of CD11b which was increased by fMLP, and decreased by CORM-3. iCORM-3 and SOD did not modify the response of PMN to fMLP (Figure 2).

Discussion

CORM-3 releases CO, and the relaxant effect of CORM-3 on angiotensin–precontracted rat aorta is due to CO, since iCORM, incapable to

liberate CO, is inactive. The relaxation is attributable to the activation of the guanylyl cyclase/cGMP system, as shown by the increase in cGMP levels, and by the decrease of the relaxation by the inhibitor of guanylyl cyclase, ODQ. The relaxant effect is also attributable to modulation of K^+ channels, since a blocker of K^+ channels partially inhibits the relaxation.

The expression of adhesion molecules on the surface of EC and PMN is an essential step in inflammation. The inhibition by CORM-3 of the increase in ICAM-1 (CD54) expression on EC coincubated with fMLP-primed PMN, represents an antiinflammatory event, as well as the increase in the surface integrin CD11b expression in fMLP-stimulated PMN. We hypothesize that fMLP activates PMN to generate superoxide anion (O_2^-) and contextually to overexpress CD11b. Superoxide anion would in turn stimulate EC to express CD54. CO released by CORM-3 would block the generation of $O_2^-\cdot$ by the fMLP primed-PMN and the subsequent generation of CD54 by EC. Our preliminary data have shown that CORM-3 nullifies the release of $O_2^-\cdot$ by fMLP-stimulated PMN.

Through the dismutation of $O_2^-\cdot$ generated by the fMLP-stimulated PMN, SOD inhibits the CD54 expression by EC, in a similar fashion as CORM-3. SOD is ineffective on the CD11b expression by PMN, which does not depend upon O_2^- generation.

In conclusion, in view of the effects on the vessel tone and on the expression of adhesion molecules on cells which are relevant in the inflammatory process, CORM-3 would deserve further investigation as a anti-inflammatory drugs.

References

1. Sawle P, Foresti R, Mann BE, Johnson TR, Green CJ, Motterlini R: Carbon monoxide-releasing molecules (CO-RMs) attenuate the inflammatory response elicited by lipopolysaccharide in RAW264.7 murine macrophages. Br J Pharmacol 2005; 145:800–810.
2. Vannacci A, Baronti R, Zagli G, Marzocca C, Pierpaoli S, Bani D, Passani MB, Mannaioni PF, Masini E: Carbon monoxide modulates the response of human basophils to FcɛRI stimulation through the heme oxygenase pathway. Eur J Pharmacol 2003; 465:289–297.
3. Ndisang JF, Gai P, Berni L, Mirabella C, Baronti R, Mannaioni PF, Masini E: Modulation of the immunological response of guinea pig mast cells by carbon monoxide. Immunopharmacology 1999; 43:65–73.
4. Johnson TR, Mann BE, Clark JE, Foresti R, Green CJ, Motterlini R: Metal carbonyls: a new class of pharmaceuticals? Angew Chem Int Ed Engl 2003; 42:3722–3729.
5. Vannacci A, Di FA, Giannini L, Marzocca C, Pierpaolo S, Zagli G, Masini E, Mannaioni PF: The effect of a carbon monoxide-releasing molecule on the immunological activation of guinea-pig mast cells and human basophils. Inflamm Res 2004; 53 Suppl 1:S9–S10.
6. Franchi-Micheli S, Failli P, Mazzetti L, Bani D, Ciuffi M, Zilletti L: Mechanical stretch reveals different components of endothelial-mediated vascular tone in rat aortic strips. Br J Pharmacol 2000; 131:1355–1362.

P.F. Mannaioni

Department of Preclinical and Clinical Pharmacology, University of Florence, Viale G. Pieraccini 6, I-50139 Florence, Italy, Tel. +39 055 4271271, Fax +39 055 4271280, E-mail pierfrancesco.mannaioni@unifi.it

Insufficient T Regulatory Cell Expression and Function in Atopic Dermatitis Skin

J. Verhagen[1,2], A. Taylor[1,3], M. Akdis[1], K. Blaser[1], and C.A. Akdis[1]

[1]*Swiss Institute of Allergy and Asthma Research (SIAF), Davos, Switzerland,* [2]*Department of Cellular and Molecular Medicine, School of Medical Sciences, University Walk, Bristol, UK,* [3]*School of Chemical Sciences and Pharmacy, University of East Anglia, Norwich, UK*

Summary. *Background:* Although the role of T regulatory (Treg) cells in the control of allergic disease has been investigated intensively, it remains unclear where and how Treg cells exert their suppressive effect. *Methods:* Regulatory cytokines IL-10 and TGF-b as well as Treg cell-specific transcription factor FoxP3 were stained in situ in AD skin. T-cell cultures, cocultures with keratinocytes were performed. siRNA for SHP-1, transduced T-cells overexpressing dominant negative SHP-1 and SHP-1$^{-/-}$ mice T-cells were used. *Results:* We detected the presence of IL-10-secreting type-1 regulatory cells, but not FoxP3$^+$ CD4$^+$ CD25$^+$ Treg cells in the skin of AD patients. However, neither subtype of Treg cells could directly inhibit the T-cell-induced apoptosis of keratinocytes. IL-10 suppresses T-cells by blocking CD28 and ICOS costimulatory signals, but not the T-cell receptor signal in a rapid signal transduction cascade. IL-10 receptor-associated Tyk2 acts as a constitutive reservoir for SHP-1 and then tyrosine phosphorylates SHP-1 upon activation. SHP-1 rapidly binds to CD28 and ICOS costimulatory receptors and dephosphorylates them within minutes. In consequence, the binding of phosphatidylinositol 3-kinase and downstream signaling is inhibited. *Conclusions:* Treg cells cannot directly suppress keratinocyte apoptosis, the key tissue injury event in AD. IL-10, the major regulatory cytokine, exerts its effect through SHP-1 mediated suppression of costimulatory receptors. In the AD skin, effector T-cells are preactivated or reactivated in the presence of large amounts of superantigen and do not depend on costimulation. Therefore, IL-10-secreting regulatory T-cells cannot exert a suppressive effect.

Keywords: T regulatory cells, SHP-1, costimulation, allergy

T regulatory (Treg) cells have been shown to play an essential role in the control of allergy and autoimmune disease. Allergic patients have been demonstrated to have less IL-10-secreting type 1 regulatory (Tr1) cells in response to an encounter with allergen they are sensitized to, compared to healthy individuals. Conversely, they show higher levels of allergen-specific Th2 cells [1, 2]. Specifically altering this imbalance in the immune response has become the major target of immunotherapy.

Although the importance of allergen- or autoantigen-specific Treg cells has been shown repeatedly in several models, it remains unclear at which stage of inflammation and by which means Treg cells can exert their suppressive effect.

The four stages of allergic inflammation can be classified as activation, selective migration to diseased organs, prolonged survival and re-activation in the subepithelial tissue and effector functions [3]. Most of the studies on the role of Treg cells focus on their ability to prevent the activation of naïve/resting T-cells. In order to extend our understanding of the role of Treg cells, we first investigated second step of allergic inflammation, the infiltration of Treg cells in the skin of atopic dermatitis (AD) patients [4]. Interestingly, we demonstrated the presence of IL-10-secreting T-cells, but not CD4+ CD25+ FoxP3+ Treg cells in early lesions of AD skin and atopy patchy tests. Same findings were observed in psoriasis lesions. This might suggest that an impaired skin migration of CD4+ CD25+ FoxP3+ Treg cells is responsible for the observed lack of suppression of local inflammation. Previously, a dysfunction in FoxP3+ expression has been shown to lead to the development of immune dysregulation, polyendocropathy, enteropathy, X-linked (IPEX) syndrome, which is often associated with atopic dermatitis [5]. In co-culture experiments we demonstrated however, that CD4+ CD25+ FoxP3+ Treg cells, just like Tr1 cells, are unable to directly suppress keratinocyte apoptosis induced by effector T-cells. CD4+ CD25+ FoxP3+ Treg cells therefore seem unable to control the effector phase of inflammation that characterizes AD. It has previously been shown that superantigens, present in the skin of over 90% of all AD patients, downregulate the suppressive of CD4+ CD25+ FoxP3+ Treg cells [6]. We found significant numbers of IL-10-secreting cells in the infiltrate in AD skin. In order to explain the absence of regulation by these cells, we investigated how IL-10 suppresses the reactivation and effector functions of skin-infiltrating T-cells, stages 3 and 4 of allergic inflammation.

For any effector T-cell to be activated, it needs to receive both a primary signal through the T-cell receptor (TCR) as well as co-stimulatory signals from receptors such as CD28. Ligation of the IL-10 receptor has previously been demonstrated to result in the dephosphorylation of the immune tyrosine based activation motif (ITAM) in the cytoplasmic tail of CD28, thereby inhibition the binding of phosphatidylinositol-3-kinase (PI3K) and subsequent further intracellular signaling [7]. In a further investigation, we demonstrate that IL-10 has a similar inhibitory effect of signaling via the CD28 family member inducible co-stimulator (ICOS) [8]. In contrast, a strong TCR signal induced with anti-CD3 mAb or SEB is not inhibited by IL-10. In order to explain this differential effect, we sought for the link responsible for IL-10-mediated inhibition of the CD28- or ICOS-induced activation. The IL-10 receptor associated tyrosine kinase Tyk2 acts as a constitutive reservoir for the tyrosine phosphatase SHP-1. Within minutes of stimulating resting T-cells with CD28 or ICOS mAbs in the presence of IL-10, SHP-1 interacts with the PI3K binding site of these receptors and dephosphorylates them. In consequence, the binding of PI3K no longer occurs and downstream signaling is inhibited. In accordance with these data, CD4+ splenocytes of SHP-1 deficient mice showed increased proliferation to stimulation through CD28 and ICOS in comparison to wild-type mice, and this proliferation was not suppressed by IL-10. The generation of human T-cells overexpressing a dominant negative form of SHP-1 or silencing SHP-1 mRNA by transfection with specific siRNA also abolished the suppressive effect of IL-10. SHP-1 has no inhibitory effect on TCR signaling, confirming that only T-cell activation that requires co-stimulatory signals can be inhibited by IL-10.

In conclusion, the major factor responsible for a lack of T-cell regulation in chronically inflamed AD skin does not seem to be a defect in the migration of Treg cells into the skin, but rather the insensitivity of effector T-cells to IL-10-mediated suppression. One reason for this could be that skin-infiltrating T effector cells have been preactivated before migration and therefore require a lower level of costimulation that resting T-cells to exert their effect. The second reason could be high concentrations of SEB in the skin of most AD patients. Reactivation of SEB-responsive T-cells (which form the larger part of T-cells present in the skin of AD patients) does not require costimulation. In either case, the reduced requirement for costimulation in the reactivation of effector T-cells in the organs seems responsible for the absent regulation by the major suppressive cytokine, IL-10.

References

1. Akdis CA, Blesken T, Akdis M, Wüthrich B, Blaser K: Role of IL-10 in specific immunotherapy. J Clin Invest 1998; 102:98–106.
2. Akdis M, Verhagen J, Taylor A, Karamloo F, Karagiannidis C, Crameri R, Thunberg S, Deniz G, Valenta R, Fiebig H et al.: Immune responses in healthy and allergic individuals are characterized by a fine balance between allergen-specific T regulatory 1 and Th2 cells. J Exp Med 2004; 199:1567–1575.
3. Akdis CA, Akdis M, Trautmann A, Blaser K: Immune regulation in atopic dermatitis. Curr Opin Immunol 2000; 12:641–646.
4. Verhagen J, Akdis M, Traidl-Hoffmann C, Schmid-Grendelmeier P, Hijnen D, Knol EF, Behrendt H, Blaser K, Akdis CA: Absence of T-regulatory cell expression and function in atopic dermatitis skin. J Allergy Clin Immunol 2006; 117:176–183.
5. Chatila TA: Role of regulatory T-cells in human diseases. J Allergy Clin Immunol 2005; 116:949–959
6. Ou LS, Goleva E, Hall C, Leung DY: T regulatory cells in atopic dermatitis and subversion of their activity by superantigens. J Allergy Clin Immunol 2004; 113:756–763.
7. Akdis CA, Joss A, Akdis M, Faith A, Blaser K: A molecular basis for T-cell suppression by IL-10: CD28-associated IL-10 receptor inhibits CD28 tyrosine phosphorylation and phosphatidylinositol 3-kinase binding. Faseb J 2000; 14:1666–9.
8. Taylor A, Akdis M, Joss A, Akkoc T, Wenig R, Colonna M, Daigle I, Flory E, Blaser K, Akdis CA: IL-10 inhibits CD28 and ICOS co-stimulations in T-cells via SHP-1. Faseb J 2006; in press.

Cezmi A. Akdis

Swiss Institute of Allergy and Asthma Research (SIAF), Obere Strasse 22, CH-7270 Davos Platz, Switzerland, Tel. +41 81 4100-848, Fax +41 81 4100-840, E-mail akdisac@siaf.uzh.ch

Hymenoptera Venom Allergy: A New Ultra-Rush Immunotherapy

V. Patella[1], G. Florio[1], and G. Spadaro[2]

[1]Unit of Allergy and Clinical Immunology, Department of Medicine, Community Hospital of Agropoli of ASL SA/3, Salerno, [2]Division of Clinical Immunology and Allergy and Center for Basic and Clinical Immunology Research (CISI), University of Naples Federico II, Naples, all Italy

Summary. *Background:* Various protocols are currently used for hymenoptera venom immunotherapy (VIT). The primary objective of this study was to compare the tolerability and safety of a new ultra-rush protocol with those of other established protocols used for VIT. *Methods:* Seventy-five patients allergic to hymenoptera (51 M, 24 F, aged 16–76 years) underwent VIT with a standardized, purified venom preparation (ALK-Abelló) according to three different regimens. During the incremental phase, patients in Group A (n = 27; 18 allergic to *Vespula species* and 9 allergic to *Apis mellifera*) or Group B (n = 25; *Vespula species*: 16; *Apis mellifera*: 9) received an aqueous preparation with ultra-rush protocol in 3 h and with rush protocol in 3 days, respectively. Patients in Group C (n = 23; *Vespula species*: 16; *Apis mellifera*: 7) were treated with conventional VIT (15 weeks) using an aluminum-adsorbed depot preparation. Maintenance dose (100 micrograms) of aluminum-adsorbed depot was administered to all groups 15 days after the end of the incremental dose and, thereafter, once a month. *Results:* Treatment with the ultra-rush protocol evoked local and systemic reactions (SARs) less frequently than rush and conventional protocol during the incremental phase; Group A: 7/351 injections (1.9%), Group B: 14/375 injections (3.7%), Group C: 13/362 injections (3.5%); $p < .05$. No difference among groups was observed in the incidence of adverse reactions during the maintenance phase. A comparable number of patients in the three groups were accidentally restung by hymenoptera. Patients treated with the ultra-rush protocol (Group A) had only local reactions whereas patients in Groups B and C referred both large local as well as systemic reactions. *Conclusions:* The incremental phase of VIT can be significantly reduced using an ultra-rush protocol lasting 3 h without a significance increase in the incidence of side effects. The ultra-rush protocol has a therapeutic efficacy similar to that of currently used conventional and rush protocols.

Keywords: hymenoptera anaphylaxis, IgE, tolerability, safety, venom immunotherapy

In recent years a large number of protocols for VIT have been used; most of them with the aim of reducing the number of injections and, consequently, the number of visits. Previous studies also suggest that short (rush) VIT protocols carry a lower risk of systemic reactions [1, 2]. These findings stimulated interest in the development and application of alternative strategies to desensitize patients allergic to hymenoptera venom. It has been reported that ultra-rush therapy is better tolerated as compared to cluster or conventional therapy in children, adolescents, and adults [1, 3, 4]. In this study we compared different strategies for VIT in a cohort of patients with hymenoptera hypersensitivity (to *Apis mellifera* or *Vespula* species) to verify whether an ultra-rush protocol, with low cumulative doses, carries a lower risk of side effects and has comparable efficacy to other conventional protocols. During the incremental phase, patients were randomized in different groups: Group A (n = 27) and B

Table 1. Protocol of initial treatment for ultrarush, rush and conventional protocol immunotherapy.

Group A (aqueous preparation)		Group B (aqueous preparation)			Group C (depot preparation)	
Dose (USQ)	Min	Dose (USQ)	Day	Hour	Dose (USQ)	Week
1	0	20	1	0	20	1
10	15	40		2	40	2
40	30	80		4	80	3
50	45	200		6	200	4
100	60	400	2	0	400	5
400	75	800		2	800	6
500	90	2,000		4	2,000	7
1,000	105	4,000	3	0	4,000	8
4,000	120	8,000		2	8,000	9
5,000	135	10,000		4	10,000	10
10,000	150	20,000	4	0	20,000	11
40,000	165	40,000		2	40,000	12
50,000	180	60,000		4	60,000	13
–	–	80,000	5	0	80,000	14
–	–	100,000		2	100,000	15

($n = 25$) received an aqueous preparation according to ultra-rush (Group A) and rush protocols (Group B), while patients in Group C ($n = 23$) were treated with conventional immunotherapy using an adsorbed aluminium-hydroxide depot preparation (Table 1).

All patients in Group A received a cumulative dose of 111.101 µg (111,101 USQ) of hymenoptera venom (*Vespula spp.* or *Apis m.*) in 180 min (Table 1). Subsequently, these patients received two booster injections of 50 µg of an aluminium-adsorbed depot preparation on Day 15. The patients of Group B received an aqueous preparation according to a daily conventional rush therapy as reported in Table 1. Subsequently, these patients received two booster injections of 50 µg of an aluminium-adsorbed depot preparation on Day 15. Patients in Group C were treated with weekly conventional immunotherapy using a aluminium-adsorbed depot preparation as reported in Table 1 [5]. The maintenance dose (100,000 USQ/100 µg) was administered once a month in all groups as a depot preparation, according to information provided by the manufacturer (ALK-Abellò) that a dose of 100 µg of aqueous

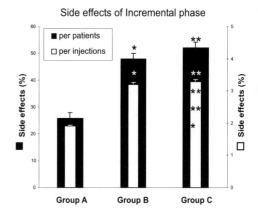

Figure 1. Frequency of local side effects in subjects of different groups. Results are shown per patients (■) or per injections (□). Each bar represents the mean ± SEM. *$p < .05$ vs. the corresponding group A. **$p < .001$ vs. the corresponding group A.

preparations corresponds to 100,000 USQ of Alutard™ preparations.

During the incremental phase of VIT, large local reactions (LLR) were reported in some patients. In Group A, during 351 injections of VIT, there were seven LLRs: 7/351 (1.99%); whereas in Group B there were 12 LLRs on 375 injections (3.7%) and in Group

C there were 13 LLRs on 362 injections (3.5%) (Figure 1). A number of severe allergic reactions (SAR), grade I, II, III and IV of anaphylaxis according to Mueller [6], occurred only in patients in Group B [2/375 (0.5%) *per* injections; 2/25 (8%) *per* patients] and in group C [1/362 (0.27%) *per* injections; 1/23 (4.3%) *per* patients]. No SAR occurred in patients in group A. During the maintenance phase, during a total period of 18 months (18 injections of maintenance dose), the incidence of side effects in group A, B and C was similar [group A: 1 LLRs and 1 SARs; group B: 2 LLRs and 1 SARs; group C: 2 LLRs and 1 SARs] . A comparable number of patients in the three groups were accidentally restung by hymenoptera. Patients treated with the ultra-rush protocol (group A) had only local reactions whereas patients in group B and C referred both large local as well as systemic reactions.

In conclusion, we report that the incremental phase of VIT can be reduced to 3 h (180 min), without a significance increase in side effects. The ultra-rush protocol has a therapeutic efficacy similar to that of conventional and rush protocols.

References

1. Birnbaum J, Ramadour M, Magnan A, Vervloet D: Hymenoptera ultra-rush venom immunotherapy (210 min): a safety study and risk factors. Clin Exp Allergy 2003; 33:58–64.
2. Cirillo A, Patella V, Ciccarelli A, Gallo L: Asthma in allergic patients to venom of Hymenoptera. In XVII International Congress of Allergology and Clinical Immunology, Sydney, Australia, October 15–20, 2000 International Association of Allergy & Clinical Immunology (Ed.). Seattle, Hogrefe & Huber, 2000, Special issue for Sydney 2000 ACI International, Supplement No. 2, 2000 p. 367.
3. Schiavino D, Nucera E, Pollastrini E, De Pasquale T, Buonomo A, Bartolozzi F, Lombardo C, Roncallo C, Patriarca G. Specific ultrarush desensitization in Hymenoptera venom-allergic patients. Ann Allergy Asthma Immunol 2004; 92:409–413.
4. Sturm G, Kranke B, Rudolph C, Aberer W. Rush Hymenoptera venom immunotherapy: a safe and practical protocol for high-risk patients. J Allergy Clin Immunol. 2002; 110:928–933.
5. Birnbaum J, Charpin D, Vervloet D: Rapid Hymenoptera venom immunotherapy: comparative safety of three protocols. Clin Exp Allergy. 1993; 23:226–230.
6. Mueller HL: Diagnosis and treatment of insect sensitivity. J Asthma Res. 1966; 3:331–333.

Vincenzo Patella, MD

Viale della Repubblica 54/b, I-84040 Capaccio-Paestum (Salerno), Italy, Tel. +39 0974 8275794, Fax +39 0974 8275793, E-mail info@allergiesalerno3.it

Anti-IgE Treatment

Overcomes Intolerability of Honeybee-Venom Ultra-Rush Immunotherapy in Indolent Systemic Mastocytosis

B. Wedi, D. Wieczorek, U. Raap, and A. Kapp

Department of Dermatology and Allergology, Hannover Medical University, Germany

Summary. Patients with elevated serum tryptase/mastocytosis are at risk for severe and fatal reactions following hymenoptera stings and can be unable to undergo venom immunotherapy because of intolerable side effects. We report the first case of a patient with indolent systemic mastocytosis and recurrent severe anaphylaxis to field stings and to venom immunotherapy, in whom a single dose of 150 mg omalizumab enabled ultra-rush honey bee venom immunotherapy.

Keywords: anti-IgE, mastocytosis, venom allergy, immunotherapy, ultra rush

Immunotherapy (IT) with hymenoptera venom reduces the risk of anaphylaxis with subsequent stings and is recommended in patients with systemic reactions and evidence of venom-specific IgE. Treatment with honey bee venom (HBV) induces anaphylactic reactions more frequently than yellow jacket venom [1]. Patients with elevated basal serum tryptase levels/mastocytosis are at risk for more-severe and even fatal reactions following stings and may be unable to undergo venom IT [2, 3].

We report the first case of a patient with indolent systemic mastocytosis and recurrent severe anaphylaxis to field stings and venom IT, in whom a single dose of omalizumab enabled ultra-rush IT within two days [4] with a total dose of 351.11 mg HBV (ALK SQ, Abello, Horsholm, DK). Thereafter, ten maintenance doses of HBV (100 mg) were tolerated.

In July 2003 the nonatopic 66-year old man developed severe anaphylaxis immediately after a honey bee sting. HBV allergy was diagnosed by specific IgE (sIgE), by ImmunoCAP (Pharmacia Diagnostics, Uppsala, Sweden), Immulite 2000 (Diagnostic Products Corporation, Los Angeles, CA, USA.), by basophil allergen stimulation test (CD63

surface expression, BasoTest, Orpegen Pharma, Heidelberg, Germany), and by cysteinyl leukotriene production (CAST2000, Bühlmann Laboratories, Allschwil, Switzerland). 3, 7, and 11 years ago severe anaphylactic shocks occurred immediately after yellow jacket stings. However, yellow-jacket sIgE was not found and titrated skin testing was negative. Total serum tryptase concentration (Pharmacia, Uppsala, Sweden) demonstrated 60 mg/l (normal < 11.4 mg/l). Mastocytosis was indolent (no skin lesions, organomegaly or mediator-related symptoms).

Ultra-rush HBV specific IT (ALK SQ Abello, Horsholm, DK) was initiated in november 2003. During initiation with aqueous extract the patient developed moderate reactions paralleled by an increase of serum tryptase (121 mg/l) and required systemic antiallergic treatment, but epinephrine was not needed. Thereafter the 4-weekly maintenance dose with depot HBV (100 mg) was well tolerated.

After 10 monthly injections of the maintenance dose the man was stung by a yellow jacket and developed severe anaphylaxis. Therefore, the maintenance dose of HBV was reduced to 80 mg by the allergologist and well tolerated. Four weeks later the dose was increased to 100 mg and within 5 min severe epinephrine resistant anaphylaxis followed.

Several weeks later he was submitted to hospital to reintroduce IT. Our initial aim was to increase the maintenance dose with bee venom. However, flushing and nausea occurred after 40 mg aqueous HBV and severe epinephrine resistant anaphylaxis after 80 mg (tryptase increased to 161 mg/l). We did not find potential triggering factors. Again, sIgE to yellow jacket was not detectable and skin testing was negative. Re-introduction of HBV IT was tried some weeks later but again severe flushing, nausea and hypotension developed after a concentration of 40 mg. Therefore, we gave omalizumab 150 mg s.c. and discharged the patient. One week later we restarted ultra-rush venom IT that then was tolerated.

Two weeks after omalizumab serum total IgE increased 2.8-fold and HBV sIgE 4.4-fold (CAP), 5.3-fold (Immulite) because of formation of omalizumab-IgE complexes, as has been described. This total IgE and sIgE increase remained stable for about 10 weeks and then decreased. Tryptase levels remained stable (49.1 ± 4.0 mg/l) during the following visits. Within one to three weeks after omalizumab cysteinyl leukotriene production and CD63 expression decreased and remained stable for over 17 weeks for leukotrienes whereas CD63 expression increased after 7 weeks above original values. Interestingly, the CD63 response to N formyl Met Leu Phe (fMLP) decreased significantly although no effect of omalizumab on fMLP-induced basophil histamine release has been demonstrated after a 3 months treatment with omalizumab [5].

Within the 20-week follow-up the patient tolerated 10 maintenance doses. He has now reached the regular 4-week intervals and we are planning to initiate yellow jacket venom IT. Furthermore, a sting challenge test will be performed within several months to clarify whether the maintenance dose of 100 mg HBV is protective.

This case demonstrates several important facts: (1) skin testing with HBV remained positive (similar threshold) two weeks after oma-

lizumab, (2) basophil CD63 expression to anti-FcεRIα mAb, fMLP, and HBV decreased with a maximum after three to five weeks after the single dose of omalizumab and thereafter increased above original levels, (3) cysteinyl leukotriene production to HBV decreased with a maximum two weeks after omalizumab and stayed on this low level for at least 17 weeks.

Taken together this case nicely demonstrates the overwhelming problems in the diagnosis and management of hymenoptera venom allergies in patients with elevated tryptase/mastocytosis and shows for the first time that a single injection of omalizumab enables ultra-rush HBV IT in risk patients with elevated tryptase levels.

References

1. Rueff F, Przybilla B: Venom immunotherapy: adverse reactions and treatment failure. Curr Opin Allergy Clin Immunol 2004; 4:307–311.
2. Dubois AE: Mastocytosis and Hymenoptera allergy. Curr Opin Allergy Clin Immunol 2004; 4:291–295.
3. Haeberli G, Brönnimann M, Hunziker T, Müller U: Elevated basal serum tryptase and hymenoptera venom allergy: relation to severity of sting reactions and to safety and efficacy of venom immunotherapy. Clin Exp Allergy 2003; 33:1216–1220.
4. Brehler R, Wolf H, Kutting B, Schnitker J, Luger T: Safety of a two-day ultrarush insect venom immunotherapy protocol in comparison with protocols of longer duration and involving a larger number of injections. Journal of Allergy and Clinical Immunology 2000; 105:1231–1235.
5. MacGlashan D, Jr., Bochner BS, Adelman DC, Jardieu PM, Togias A, McKenzie-White J, Sterbinsky SA, Hamilton R, Lichtenstein LM: Down-regulation of FcεRI expression on human basophils during in vivo treatment of atopic patients with anti-IgE antibody. J Immunol 1997; 158:1438–1445.

Bettina Wedi

Department of Dermatology and Allergology, Hannover Medical University, Ricklinger Str. 5, D-30449 Hannover, Germany, Tel. +49 511 9246-237, Fax +49 511 9246-309, E-mail wedi.bettina@mh-hannover.de

Immunomodulatory Effects of Viral Toll-Like Receptor Ligands

An Experimental Approach to the Hygiene Hypothesis

M. Wegmann[1], S. Sel[1], S. Sel[1], S. Bauer[2], H. Renz[1], and H. Garn[1]

[1]*Department of Clinical Chemistry and Molecular Diagnostics,* [2]*Institute of Immunology, Biomedical Research Center (BMFZ), Hospital of the Philipps University, Marburg, Germany*

Summary. Several viruses are known to lead to an exacerbation of already established asthma, whereas repeated infections in early life may prevent from the development of allergic asthma as suggested by the hygiene hypothesis. Toll-like receptors (TLRs) are key regulators of both innate and adaptive immune responses. We therefore hypothesized that activation of TLRs by virus-derived double or single stranded RNA may have an influence on initiation or progression of allergic asthma. To test this hypothesis we investigated the effects of synthetic TLR-3 and TLR-7 ligands, polyinosinic-poly-cytidylic acid (poly (I:C)) and R-848, respectively, in different mouse models of experimental asthma. Systemic application of viral TLR-ligands during the sensitization phase prevented allergic sensitization to OVA and consequently from development of experimental asthma. In animals with already established experimental asthma systemic application of viral TLR-ligands resulted in marked reduction of the phenotype involving improved airway reactivity to metacholine, lessened allergic airway inflammation and decreased mucus production in the airways. In conclusion, these data indicate that systemic exposure to viral TLR-ligands seems to have protective effects on the development of allergic diseases such as asthma.

Keywords: TLR, dsRNA, ssRNA, allergy, T-cells

Allergic bronchial asthma represents a major and increasing health care problem especially in industrialized countries. A complex interaction between genetic, environmental and developmental factors has a great impact on the pathogenesis of the disease. Epidemiological data support the concept that viral infections contribute to the pathogenesis of allergic asthma in opposite ways. In patients with already established disease, viral infections particularly of the upper respiratory tract play a major role in triggering acute asthma exacerbations [1]. In addition, infections with respiratory syncytial virus (RSV) in early childhood have been shown to represent a high risk factor for the development of asthma in susceptible individuals [2, 3]. However, the currently observed increase in asthma prevalence and incidence is inversely linked to repeated respiratory viral infections particularly in early childhood. This concept is reflected in parts by the "hygiene hypothesis." Although epidemiological and clinical data clearly support this concept, it still remains unclear why certain viral infections may exert such opposite effects on allergic conditions in the respiratory tract [4, 5]. Since toll-like receptors (TLRs) are known to be key regulators of both, innate

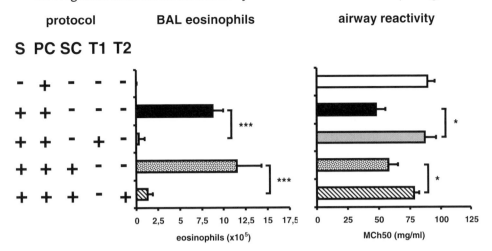

Figure 1. Effects of TLR-3 activation on experimental asthma. BALB/c mice were sensitized to ovalbumin by three intra-peri-toneal injections of ovalbumin (OVA) in the presence of Al(OH)₃ (S). Experimental allergic asthma was induced by primary allergen-challenge (PC) or secondary allergen-challenge with aerosolized OVA (SC). Treatment with poly (I:C) was performed either during the sensitization phase (T1) or during secondary allergen-challenge (T2). Absolute numbers of eosinophils in broncho-alveolar lavage fluid (BAL) were determined by light-microscopy of cytospins using standard morphological criteria. Airway reactivity was assessed by head-out body-pletysmography and expressed as concentration of methacholine that induces 50%-reduction baseline midexpiratory airflows (MCh50). All analyses were performed 24 h after the last allergen-challenge. Means ± SEM are represented. Statistical significance: $^*p < .05$, $^{***}p < .01$.

as well as adaptive immune responses, we hypothesized that viral TLR-3 or TLR-7 ligands such as double stranded RNA (dsRNA) or single stranded RNA (ssRNA) may contribute to asthma development and/or exacerbation.

We tested this hypothesis in two different mouse models of experimental asthma. For this purpose BALB/c mice were sensitized to and challenged with ovalbumin (OVA). During sensitization polyinosinic-polycytidylic acid (poly (I:C)) as a synthetic TLR-3 ligand was applied intra-peritoneally (i.p.). In contrast to untreated OVA-sensitized animals that developed a significant OVA-specific antibody response these animals showed only negligible titers of allergen-specific IgE or IgG1. Furthermore, inhalational OVA provocation did not result in the development of asthma pathology as indicated by infiltration of eosinophils into the airways and increased airway reactivity to methacholine (MCh) as assessed by head-out body-plethysmography (6) (Figure 1).

We further investigated the effects of viral TLR-activation on secondary allergic immune responses. Therefore, systemic application of

TLR-3 was performed during OVA rechallenge in OVA-sensitized BALB/c mice with already established experimental asthma. Whereas asthma pathology in untreated animals was characterized by marked influx of eosinophils into the airways together with increased mucus production and high IL-5 levels in broncho-alveolar lavage (BAL) fluids, TLR-ligand treated animals revealed only mild allergic airway inflammation with few eosinophils in BAL fluids or airway tissue. Furthermore, IL-5 levels in BAL fluids were markedly reduced and airway hyperresponsiveness (AHR) that was pronounced in untreated OVA-sensitized animals was nearly normalized in TLR-ligand treated mice (Figure 1). In addition serum titers of OVA-specific IgE and IgG1 were markedly reduced whereas serum titers of OVA-specific IgG2a appeared to be significantly increased. Similar effects were observed in animals receiving the synthetic TLR-7 ligand R-848 [data not shown].

In conclusion, we demonstrated that systemic application of viral TLR-ligands during the sensitization phase prevent from allergic sensitization and subsequently from development of experimental asthma. Furthermore, inhibitory effects of systemic TLR-3 and TLR-7 activation were also observed in already established experimental allergic airway inflammation. It still remains to be elucidated how systemic viral TLR-activation works in this model. Increased production of allergen-specific IgG2a together with decreased production of allergen-specific IgE and IgG1 may indicate the induction of a counter regulating TH1-driven immune-response. This would require production of interleukin-12 (IL-12) by TLR-activated antigen-presenting cells as it is described for other microbial products such as LPS or bacterial DNA containing unmethylated CpG-motifs [7]. Another mode of action could be the induction of regulatory T-cells producing IL-10 as it is reported for TLR-2 activation by candida albicans (8). Taken together, virus-induced TLR-activation may explain protective effects of viral infections on allergic immune-responses but may not account for exacerbation of already existing allergic asthma.

References

1. John AE, Berlin AA, Lukacs NW: Respiratory syncytial virus-induced CCL5/RANTES contributes to exacerbation of allergic airway inflammation. Eur J Immunol 2003; 33:1677–1685
2. Sigurs N, Bjarnason R, Sigurbergsson F, Kjellman B: Respiratory syncytial virus bronchiolitis in infancy is an important risk factor for asthma and allergy at age 7. Am J Respir Crit Care Med 2000; 161:1501–1507
3. Wright AL, Holberg CJ, Martinez FD, Morgan WJ, Taussig LM: Breast feeding and lower respiratory tract illness in the first year of life. Group Health Medical Associates. BMJ 1989; 299: 946–949.
4. Lemanske RF: Viral infections and asthma inception J Allergy Clin Immunol 2004; 114:1023–1026.
5. Message SD, Johnston SL: Viruses in asthma. Brit Med Bull 2002; 61: 29–43.
6. Wegmann M, Fehrenbach H, Fehrenbach A, Held T, Schramm C, Garn H, Renz H: Involvement of distal airways in a chronic model of experimental asthma. Clin Exp Allergy 2005; 35:1263–1271.
7. Robson NC, Beacock-Sharp H, Donachie AM, Mowat AM: The role of antigen-presenting cells and interleukin-12 in the priming of antigen-specific CD4+ T-cells by immune stimulating complexes. Immunology 2003; 110:95–104.
8. Netea MG, Sutmuller R, Hermann C, Van der Graaf CA, Van der Meer JW, van Krieken JH, Hartung T, Adema G, Kullberg BJ: Toll-like receptor 2 suppresses immunity against *Candida albicans* through induction of IL-10 and regulatory T-cells. J Immunol 2004; 172:3712–3718.

Michael Wegmann

Biomedizinisches Forschungszentrum (BMFZ), Abteilung für Klinische Chemie und Molekulare Diagnostik, Hans-Meerwein-Strasse 3, D-35033 Marburg, Germany, Tel. +49 6421 286-6035, Fax +49 6421 286-6086, E-mail wegmann@med.uni-marburg.de

Development of a Mucosal Polyvalent Allergy Vaccine for Primary Prevention of Multisensitization

U. Wiedermann[1], C. Wild[1], K. Hufnagl[1], K. Hoffmann-Sommergruber[2], H. Breiteneder[2], O. Scheiner[2], M. Wallner[3], and F. Ferreira[3]

[1]Department of Specific Prophylaxis and Tropical Medicine, Center for Physiology and Pathophysiology, Medical University of Vienna, [2]Department of Pathophysiology, Center for Physiology and Pathophysiology, Medical University of Vienna, [3]Department of Allergy and Immunology, Institute of Molecular Biology, University of Salzburg, all Austria

Summary. *Background:* Since many allergic patients become cosensitized to several allergens and are then difficult to treat by conventional immunotherapy, our research has focused on the development of novel treatment strategies against allergic polysensitization based on mucosal tolerance induction. *Methods:* A mouse model of polysensitization to the major birch and grass pollen allergens Bet v 1, Phl p 1, and Phl p 5 was established to evaluate if mucosal tolerance to several allergens can be induced simultaneously. Mucosal pretreatment was either induced with polypeptides, covering the immuno-dominant T-cell epitopes of the three allergens, or with a recombinant allergen chimer, consisting of the whole Bet v 1 molecule anchoring the immunodominant peptides of Phl p 1 and Phl p 5. The effectiveness, as well as the underlying mechanisms, were compared between polypeptide- and chimer-induced polytolerance. *Results:* Mucosal pretreatment with both polypeptides and allergen chimer prevented allergic polysensitization to all three aeroallergens. The underlying mechanisms of polytolerance, however, differed depending on the conformation of the molecules: While polypeptide-induced tolerance was mediated by cytokine independent mechanisms, intranasal tolerance induction with the chimer was associated with IL-10 and TGF-β-dependent regulatory mechanisms. *Conclusions:* The data indicate that mucosal tolerance induction with polypeptides or allergen chimers could provide a new treatment approach for preventive allergy vaccination against polysensitization. Both polypeptides and allergen chimers exhibit many advantages over conventional immunotherapy, but will need further investigation with respect to long-term efficacy and individual applicability.

Keywords: animal model, type I allergy, polysensitization, mucosal tolerance, allergen chimer, hybrid-peptides, T regulatory cells

Introduction

There is increasing clinical evidence that many monosensitized patients become cosensitized to several allergens with increasing age [1]. Conventional immunotherapy is less effective in these patients and is not even recommended for polysensitized patients because of the increased risk of anaphylactic side reactions [2].

Therefore, our current research has focused on the development of novel treatment strategies against multisensitivities based on mucosal tolerance induction.

In previous studies we demonstrated that allergic monosensitization can be prevented or treated by mucosal application of the major birch pollen allergen Bet v 1 [3]. Recently, a mouse model of polysensitization with the

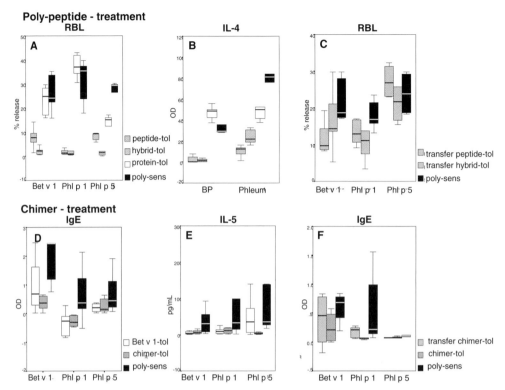

Figure 1. Intranasal tolerance induction. A, B: mucosal tolerance induction with polypeptides; C: adoptive cell transfer with splenocytes from polypeptide/hybrid-peptide tolerized mice; D, E: mucosal tolerance induction with the allergen chimer; F: adoptive cell transfer with splenocytes from chimer tolerized mice. *$p < .05$ pretreated versus polysensitized as determined by Mann-Whitney U test. RBL: rat basophil leukemia cell mediator release assay; BP: birch pollen.

major birch and grass pollen allergens Bet v 1, Phl p 1, and Phl p 5 was established in order to test whether mucosal tolerance can also be established against several allergens [4].

Based on the fact that tolerance could not be induced with a mixture of these protein allergens [4], only the immunodominant peptides of Bet v 1, Phl p 1, and Phl p 5, either as a mixture or as a hybrid-peptide, were used for mucosal application. As our previous studies demonstrated that Bet v 1 acts as a very strong tolerogen inducing a regulatory immune mechanism [5], another construct was produced for polytolerance induction, which used the complete Bet v 1 molecule as the backbone for linkage of the immunodominant peptides of Phl p 1 and Phl p 5. This new allergen chimer was also used for mucosal treatment prior to polysensitization with the birch and grass pollen allergens.

Material and Methods

Identification of the immunodominant peptides of Bet v 1, Phl p 1, and Phl p 5 was performed by epitope mapping experiments [4]. Subsequently, the respective peptides, as well as a hybrid-peptide, consisting of the immunodominant regions of all three allergens, were synthesized [4, 6].

For recombinant production of a birch-grass-chimer, Bet v 1 served as a scaffold for N- and C- terminal linkage of the immunodominant peptides of Phl p 1 and Phl p 5. The new construct was expressed in *E. coli*, purified by single step purification and characterized by biochemical and immunological analyses [7].

For intranasal tolerance induction, BALB/c mice were intranasally pretreated with either the peptide-mixture, the hybrid-peptide, or the birch-grass-chimer (three times in weekly intervals) prior to polysensitization with Bet v 1, Phl p 1, and Phl p 5. Sensitized controls were sham-pretreated with sodium chloride prior to polysensitization [4]. At sacrifice, serum samples and splenocytes were used for evaluation of allergen-specific humoral and cellular immune responses. For studies on underlying mechanisms, adoptive cell transfer experiments with splenocytes from polytolerized mice were performed.

Results

Intranasal pretreatment with the peptide mixture, the hybrid, as well as the allergen chimer, led to significantly reduced IgE-mediated basophil degranulation and serum IgE levels (Figure 1A, 1D). Similarly, IL-4 or IL-5 levels were significantly reduced by the polypeptide or chimer pretreatment compared to the polysensitized controls (Figure 1B, 1E). In contrast, IgG2a and IFN-g levels were markedly enhanced in chimer-, but not in polypeptide-, pretreated mice [data not shown].

Other than the immunological parameters, the mechanistic pathways of immunosuppression seemed to differ depending on the constructs being used: Polytolerance induced with the polypeptides was not transferable with splenocytes (Figure 1C) and IL-10 and TGF-β levels remained unchanged compared to polysensitized controls (data not shown). In contrast, splenocytes from chimer-tolerized mice could transfer polytolerance (Figure 1F), which was associated with an upregulation of the above mentioned regulatory cytokines.

Discussion

In the present study we demonstrated that it is possible to prevent the development of multisensitivities to birch and grass pollen allergens by intranasal application of the immunodominant peptides of Bet v 1, Phl p 1, and Phl p 5 (Figure 1A and 1B), or an allergen chimer consisting of the whole Bet v 1 and the immunodominant grass pollen peptides (Figure 1D and

PROs (+) and CONs (−)	
Polypeptide treatment	Chimer treatment
+ Easy, rapid and cheap production	+ No HLA and T-cell receptor restriction
+ No anaphylactic side reactions because of the lack of IgE epitopes (in case of secondary prevention)	+ Induction of regulatory mechanisms with long-lasting tolerance
− HLA and T-cell receptor restriction → individual design of peptide vaccine necessary	+ Standardized construction of the vaccine for general use
	− Laborious and time consuming production of the chimer
	− Correct folding and maintenance of conformation of chimer as prerequisite for treatment efficacy

Figure 2. Advantages and limitations of the different treatment regimes

1E). These results indicate that immunosuppression can equally well be established using different lengths of peptides or conformational allergen chimers. However, with respect to the underlying regulatory mechanisms, the conformation of the tolerogens seems important, since polypeptide pretreatment led to cytokine-independent immunosuppression [4] (Figure 1C) while the allergen chimer induced regulatory mechanisms (Figure 1F) [7]. These results are in line with our previous findings in monotolerized mice, showing that Bet v 1, but not Bet v 1 peptides, induced the formation of TGF β and IL-10 producing regulatory T-cells [5]. As we also demonstrated that long-term efficacy of the treatment was only achieved with the whole Bet v 1 molecule [5], one might speculate that polypeptide- and chimer-induced tolerance might also differ in the duration of immunosuppression.

There seem to be advantages, as well certain disadvantages, to using either polypeptides or chimers for polytolerance induction (Figure 2): Peptides are rapidly and easily produced and, since they lack IgE epitopes, anaphylactic side effects can be diminished. Nevertheless, the limitation of peptide treatment in humans lies in their HLA and T-cell receptor restriction, which implies the necessity of vaccine designs tailored to individual patients [8]. The use of allergen chimers, maintaining the conformation of a core allergen, might overcome these limitations, even though production of chimer-constructs in correct folding and stable conformation poses a challenging task (Figure 2).

Taken as a whole, we conclude that mucosal tolerance induction with polypeptides or allergen chimers represents a new strategy of primary and secondary prevention for atopic patients at risk for or with developed multisensitivities.

Acknowledgments

This work was supported by a grant from the Austrian Science Fund (SFB F01814 "Mucosal tolerance induction: A strategy for prevention and therapy of type I allergy").

References

1. Silvestri M, Rossi GA, Cozzani S, Pulvirenti G, Fasce L: Age-dependent tendency to become sensitized to other classes of aeroallergens in atopic asthmatic children. Ann Allergy Asthma Immunol 1999; 83:335–340.
2. Bousquet J, Van Cauwenberge P, Khaltaev N. ARIA Workshop Group, World Health Organization: Allergic rhinitis and its impact on asthma. J Allergy Clin Immunol 2001; 108:S147–334.
3. Wiedermann U: Prophylaxis and therapy of allergy by mucosal tolerance induction with recombinant allergen or allergen constructs. Curr Drug Targets Inflamm Allergy 2005; 4: 577–583.
4. Hufnagl K, Winkler B, Focke M, Valenta R, Scheiner O, Renz H, Wiedermann U: Intranasal tolerance induction with polypeptides derived from 3 noncross-reactive major aeroallergens prevents allergic polysensitization in mice. J Allergy Clin Immunol 2005; 116:370–376.
5. Winkler B, Hufnagl K, Spittler A, Ploder M, Kallay E, Vrtala S, Valenta R, Kundi M, Renz H, Wiedermann U: The role of Foxp3+ T-cells in long-term efficacy of prophylactic and therapeutic mucosal tolerance induction in mice. Allergy 2006; 61:173–180.
6. Focke M, Mahler V, Ball T, Sperr WR, Majlesi Y, Valent P, Kraft D, Valenta R: Nonanaphylactic synthetic peptides derived from B cell epitopes of the major grass pollen allergen, Phl p 1, for allergy vaccination. Faseb J 2001; 15:2042–2044.
7. Wild C, Wallner M, Hufnagl K, Fuchs H, Hoffmann-Sommergruber K, Breiteneder H, Scheiner O, Ferreine F, Wiedermann U: A recombinant allergen chimer as novel mucosal vaccine candidate for prevention of multi-sensitivities. Allergy 2007; 62:33–41.
8. Smith TR, Larche M: Investigating T-cell activation and tolerance *in vivo*: peptide challenge in allergic asthmatics. Cytokine 2004; 28:49–54.

Ursula Wiedermann

Department of Specific Prophylaxis and Tropical Medicine, Center for Physiology and Pathophysiology, Medical University of Vienna, Kinderspitalgasse 15, A-1090 Vienna, Austria, Tel. +43 1 40490 64890, Fax +43 1 40490 64899, E-mail ursula.wiedermann@meduniwien.ac.at

The Role of Advanced Glycation End Products in Asthma and Chronic Obstructive Pulmonary Disease

S.J. Wilson[1], C. Lai[1], C. Williams[1], P.H. Howarth[2], S.T. Holgate[2], and J.A. Warner[2]

[1]*Histochemistry Research Unit and* [2]*Allergy and Inflammation Research, Infection, Inflammation and Repair, School of Medicine, University of Southampton, UK*

Summary. *Background:* Advanced glycation end products (AGE) form on long-lived connective tissue and matrix components by a process of nonenzymatic glycosylation. AGE accumulation is a normal aging process; however it is accelerated in several pathological conditions, for example diabetes mellitus and pulmonary fibrosis. AGE have a number of chemical and biological properties that are potentially pathogenic, including induction of cytokine and growth factor synthesis, increase in vascular permeability, enhancement of cell proliferation and extracellular matrix production. This process may therefore play a role in the remodelling responses observed in asthma and COPD. *Methods:* To investigate this we have immunohistochemically stained bronchial biopsies from mild asthmatics and normal controls, and bronchial and parenchymal tissue from subjects with and without COPD for AGE. Immunoreactivity was assessed with the assistance of computerized image analysis in inflammatory cells, the extra-cellular matrix (ECM) and the bronchial epithelium. *Results:* Expression was increased in the bronchial epithelium of the asthmatics compared to normal control subjects, 2.64% vs 0.445% (*p* = .002). No differences were observed in the expression of AGE by inflammatory cells or in the ECM. In the bronchial tissue of subjects with and without COPD there was no difference in expression of AGE in the epithelium or the number of AGE immunoreactive inflammatory cells. We also did not observe any disease related difference in the AGE expression in the lung parenchyma. *Conclusion:* Advance glycation pathways may have a role in the pathophysiology of asthma but not COPD.

Keywords: advanced glycation end product, asthma, COPD, bronchial epithelium, remodelling

Advanced glycation end products (AGE) form on long-lived connective tissue and matrix components by the process of nonenzymatic glycosylation. Initially, the process is reversible, glucose chemically attaching to the amino group of proteins, forming Schiff bases, which then form the more stable Amadori-like products. These early glycation products then slowly undergo irreversible glycosylation forming AGE [1, 2]. This is a process that accompanies normal aging but is accelerated in several pathological conditions such as diabetes and lung fibrosis [3, 4].

AGEs have a number of chemical and biological properties that are potentially pathogenic including induction of cytokine and growth factor synthesis, increase in vascular permeability, enhancement of cell proliferation and extracellular matrix production [5, 6]. Of particular interest, is that AGEs are able to interact with AGE-specific receptors on the surface of fibroblasts leading to cell activation, proliferation and increased matrix synthesis. AGE-stimulated extracellular matrix production may therefore play a role in the basement membrane thickening that is commonly seen in DM tissues [5]. In the bronchi of subjects with DM thickening of the *lamina reticularis* is observed and this is morphologically similar to that that is characteristic of asthma [7].

Given the role that AGE in driving ECM accumulation we wished to investigate if they may contribute to the remodelling responses that are observed in the lungs of subjects with asthma and chronic obstructive pulmonary disease.

Materials and Methods

We have undertaken two studies to investigate the expression of AGE in subjects with asthma and COPD.

Study 1

Bronchial biopsies have been collected from mild asthmatics ($n = 10$), with a mean age of 30.1 years (19–40), and FEV1 of 76.1% predicted (71–109), and from normal controls ($n = 10$), mean age of 24 years (18–35) and FEV1% predicted 104.1% (89–112).

Study 2

Bronchial biopsies were collected by bronchoscopy and subsequently parenchymal tissue from surgical lung resections from subjects with COPD ($n = 15$) and without COPD ($n = 10$). The COPD subjects has a mean age of 66.2 years (48–77) and FEV1 of 63% predicted (32–75), and those without had a mean age of 62.8 years (51–75) and FEV1 of 96.4% predicted (82–112).

For both studies the tissue samples were processed into glycol methacrylate resin, as previously described [8]. Two micron sections were cut and stained immunohistochemically with a monoclonal antibody to carboxy methyl lysine-AGE (gift Roche Diagnostics, Penzberg, Ger-

many) using the strept-avidin biotin-peroxidase technique. The number of immunoreactive nucleated cells were counted within the bronchial and parenchymal tissue, area measured and positive cells per millimeter calculated. The percentage staining in the epithelium, the extracellular matrix of the bronchial tissue and in the parenchyma was assessed with the assistance of computerized image analysis based on red/blue/green colour balance as previously described [9]. Data were analyzed using nonparametric statistics.

Results

A diffuse staining pattern for AGE was observed in the basolateral area of the columnar within the bronchial epithelium, on the matrix components within the lamina propia of the bronchial tissue and in the parenchymal tissue. Some scattered immunoreactive cells within the bronchial mucosa were also seen. When comparing asthmatics to normal controls (Study 1) a significant increase ($p = .002$) in AGE immunoreactivity was observed in the bronchial epithelium, 2.64% versus 0.445%. No differences were seen in the expression of AGE by inflammatory cells (2.77 vs 1.09 mm^{-2}) or in the extracellular matrix (0.31% vs 0.74%). When comparing those subjects with COPD to those without (Study 2) no differences were observed in the number of inflammatory cells staining for AGE (14.1 vs 21.5 mm^{-2}), or in AGE expression in the bronchial epithelial (16.5% vs 10%) or the parenchyma (34.9% vs 28.9%).

Discussion

The studies presented here have shown the expression of AGE is increased in the bronchial epithelium in asthma, but not COPD. This suggests that AGE mediated pathways may be involved in the pathophysiology of asthma. As one of the effects of AGEs is enhanced extracellular matrix deposition and as discussed earlier increased thickness of the *lamina reticularis* is observed in diabetics, it is tempting to speculate that AGEs may be contributing to the mechanisms that drive the thickening of the *lamina reticularis* that is a hallmark of asthma. The role that AGEs may have in the remodelling response in asthma therefore warrants further investigation.

Acknowledgments

The authors would like to thank Professor H Magnussen and Dr. O Holz from Hospital Grosshansdorf, Germany, for providing the tissue samples for Study 2 (COPD vs. non-COPD).

References

1. Brownlee M, Cerami A, Vlassara H: Advanced glycosylation end products in tissue and the biochemical basis of diabetic complications. N Engl J Med 1988; 318:1315–1321.
2. Brownlee, M Advanced protein glycosylation in diabetes and aging. Annu Rev Med 1995; 46:223–234.
3. Monnier VM, Vishwanath V, Frank KE, Elmets CA, Dauchot P, Kohn RR: Relation between complications of type I diabetes mellitus and collagen- linked fluorescence. N Engl J Med 1986; 314:403–408.
4. Monnier VM, Kohn RR, Cerami A: Accelerated age-related browning of human collagen in diabetes mellitus. Proc Natl Acad Sci 1984; 81:583–587.
5. Vlassara H, Bucala R, Striker L: Pathogenic effects of advanced glycosylation: biochemical, biologic, and clinical implications for diabetes and aging. Lab Invest 1994; 70:138–151.
6. Brownlee, M: The pathological implications of protein glycation. Clin Invest Med 1995; 18:275–281.
7. Watanabe K, Senju S, Toyoshima H, Yoshida M: Thickness of the basement membrane of bronchial epithelial cells in lung diseases as determined by transbronchial biopsy. Respir Med 1997; 91:406–410.
8. Britten KM, Howarth PH, Roche WR: Immunohistochemistry on resin sections: a comparison of resin embedding techniques for small mucosal biopsies. Biotechnic Histochem 1993; 68:271–280.
9. Puddicombe SM, Polosa R, Richter A, Krishna MT, Howarth PH, Holgate ST, Davies DE: Involvement of the epidermal growth factor receptor in epithelial repair in asthma. FASEB J 200; 14:1362–1374.

Susan J. Wilson

Histochemistry Research Unit, Mailpoint 894, Level B, South Block, Southampton General Hospital, Tremona Road, Southampton SO16 6YD, UK, E-mail s.j.wilson@soton.ac.uk

Allergenicity and Immuno-genicity of Commercially Available Allergoid Products for Birch Pollen Immunotherapy

H. Wolf[1], L. Lund[2], P.A. Würtzen[2], G. Lund[2], H. Henmar[2], and J.N. Larsen[2]

[2]*Clinical Development, ALK-SCHERAX, Hamburg, Germany*
[1]*ALK-Abelló A/S, Research Department, Hørsholm, Denmark*

Abstract. The rationale for chemically modifying allergens (allergoids) is to reduce allergenicity and maintain immunogenicity. A statistical evaluation of adverse events reported to the German health authority over a 10 year period, however, did not indicate higher safety of allergoids compared with intact allergens. Four commercially available allergoids were compared to the intact allergen product Alutard SQ® by solid phase IgE inhibition assays and histamine release assays to investigate allergenicity, and immunogenicity by human T-cell proliferation and measurement of IgG titers following mouse immunizations. The SIT products were normalized with respect to the manufacturers recommended maintenance dose. Two of four allergoids tested did not show reduced IgE binding in the solid phase IgE inhibition analyses compared with the intact allergen product; different slopes of the inhibition curves for the allergoids indicate structural changes of the epitope composition. One of the four allergoid products did not show reduced histamine release compared to the intact allergen extract, patient-to-patient variation in histamine release assays was very large. All allergoids showed a reduced response in standard T-cell stimulation assays compared to Alutard SQ® regardless of the cell type used for antigen presentation (PBL or DC). All allergoids showed reduced capacity to induce allergen-specific IgG responses in mice. Commercial allergoid preparations do not fulfil the allergoid concept, since all allergoids showed reduced immunogenicity, and one allergoid did not show reduced allergenicity.

Keywords: immunotherapy, intact allergens, allergoids, Birch pollen, histamine release, IgE, T-cell proliferation

Introduction

Specific immunotherapy with intact allergens is a well documented treatment for IgE mediated allergic disorders. In an attempt to eliminate the small but significant risk of inducing systemic allergic reactions Marsh and co-workers in the seventies proposed the "allergoid" concept to reduce allergenicity and maintain immunogenicity by chemically modifying the allergen extract [1]. It has been claimed that allergoids are better tolerated than the native intact allergen extract and may provide an improved alternative for specific immunotherapy in terms of improved safety and efficacy [2]. However, data from German health authorities based on adverse events reporting over a 10-year period did not indicate increased safety of allergoids compared to intact allergens [3].

The objective of this study was to compare allergenicity in terms of histamine release and IgE inhibition and immunogenicity in terms of T-cell stimulation and mouse immunization of an intact allergen vaccine and four commercial allergoid products for birch pollen immunotherapy.

Materials and Methods

Intact allergen vaccine (Alutard SQ birch) and four commercially available allergoid products (A, B, C, and D) for birch pollen immunotherapy were investigated. The vaccines were analyzed in concentrations normalized on the basis of the recommended maximal therapy dose. Allergenicity was investigated by IgE inhibition analyses performed on an Advia Centaur system (Bayer Diagnostics,

Tarrytown, NY, USA) and by histamine release assays performed with freshly drawn blood from 10 birch allergic patients. Immunogenicity was investigated by measuring Bet v 1 specific IgG antibodies from mice im-

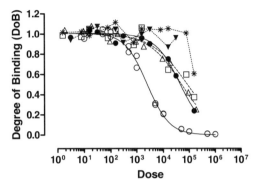

Figure 1. IgE Inhibition curves. Binding of biotinylated Bet v to solid phase bound IgE inhibited by: Bet v aqueous extract (○), Alutard SQ (●), Allergoid A (△), Allergoid B (▼), allergoid C (□) and Allergoid D (*).

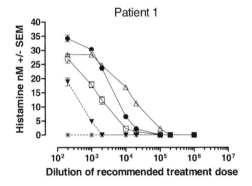

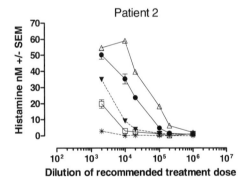

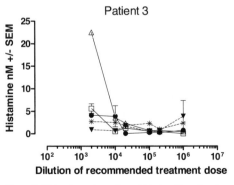

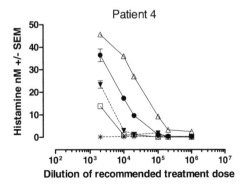

Figure 2. Histamine release from 4 birch pollen allergic patients. Alutard SQ (●), Allergoid A (△), Allergoid B (▼), Allergoid C (□) and Allergoid D (*).

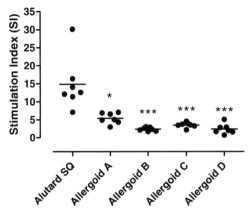

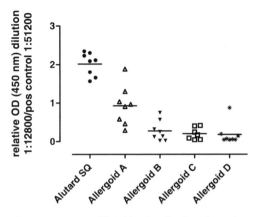

Figure 3. Reduced T-cell activation of Bet v 1-specific T-cell lines by Allergoid A, B, C and D compared to Alutard SQ. T-cell lines from seven allergic patients were tested. SI = Stimulation index, * = $p < .05$, *** = $p < .001$.

Figure 4A: Bet v 1 specific IgG in mice after three immunizations.

munized with the different products and by human T-cell proliferation using lines from 7 birch allergic individuals. Both PBMC and dendritic cells (DC) cells were investigated as antigen presenting cells.

Results

The IgE inhibition curves are shown in Figure 1. The data sets obtained for allergoid B and D vaccine products did not produce meaningful inhibition curves. The inhibition curves of the allergoid products A and C, although mutually parallel, were significantly nonparallel ($p = .0030$) to the birch pollen extract (Bet v) inhibition curve, indicating a difference in the IgE epitope composition. Figure 2 shows the histamine release results from the analysis of Alutard SQ and four allergoid products (four out of ten different birch pollen allergic patients shown). Three of four tested allergoid products showed reduced histamine release compared to the intact allergen vaccine and one allergoid product showed equal or higher release. Allergoid D caused low or no histamine release in all experiments. This was shown not to be due to toxicity of the product. The seven T-cell lines from seven birch pollen allergic patients exhibited strong proliferation when stimulated with Alutard SQ. In contrast, the

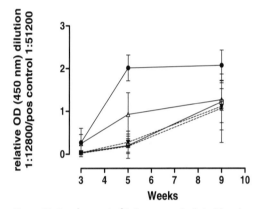

Figure 4B: Development of IgG response to Bet v1 in mice immunized with Alutard SQ (●), Allergoid A (△), Allergoid B (▼), Allergoid C (□) and Allergoid D (*). Error bars indicate standard deviation.

allergoid products induced significantly reduced or completely abrogated T-cell activation in all lines (Figure 3).

Comparison of T-cell activation using dendritic cells (DC) or peripheral blood lymphocytes (PBL) as antigen presenting cells (APC) were performed in nine experiments with T-cell lines from five patients. In general, comparable responses to the individual allergen preparations were obtained whether presented by DC or PBL (data not shown).

The Bet v 1 specific IgG antibody response in mice was already observed after two immunizations with Alutard SQ and allergoid A. After three immunizations specific IgG was significantly higher ($p < .001$) with Alutard SQ compared to allergoid A, B, C, and D (Figure 4A). Mice immunized with intact allergen vaccine developed IgG responses with an earlier onset than all tested allergoids and reached the maximum level after three immunizations (Figure 4B).

Discussion

The IgE inhibition experiments indicate that the IgE epitope composition is different comparing intact allergen extract with allergoids. Histamine release showed reduced allergenicity in three out of four allergoid products. However, although the allergenicity of most allergoid products was reduced the main finding was that the reduction in allergenicity was accompanied by a reduction in immunogenicity. This was shown by a generally reduced or even completely abrogated capacity to activate human Bet v 1-specific T-cell lines, which is in agreement with previously published data [4, 5]. In contrast, a study by Kahlert et al. [6] showed full responsiveness to an allergoid when stimulated with DC cells as APC. In our experiments we observed similar reactivity of Bet v 1-specific T-cell lines whether stimulated with PBMC or DC as APC. The capacity to induce Bet v 1-specific IgG antibodies in mice, were reduced for all allergoid products.

In conclusion, while some allergoids were associated with reduced allergenicity a clear reduction in immunogenicity was observed for all allergoid products compared to the intact allergen vaccine, and therefore the commercial allergoid products tested do not fulfil the allergoid concept. Furthermore, because of the change in epitope composition, clinical documentation from immunotherapy with intact allergen extracts cannot be used as documentation of modified allergen extracts.

Acknowledgments

The authors wish to thank Stina B. Thorup, Annette Giselsson, Lotte Heerfordt, Gitte Grauert, Gitte Koed, and Jette Skovsgaard for excellent technical work. Henrik Ipsen and Jens Holm are thanked for help with the IgE inhibition assays and histamine analyses, respectively.

References

1. Marsh DG, Lichtenstein LM, Campbell DH: Studies on "allergoids" prepared from naturally occurring allergens. I. Assay of allergenicity and antigenicity of formalinized rye group I component. Immunology 1970; 18:705–722.
2. Casanovas M, Fernandez-Caldas E, Alamar R, Basomba A: Comparative study of tolerance between unmodified and high doses of chemically modified allergen vaccines of *Dermatophagoides pteronyssinus*. Int Arch Allergy Immunol 2005; 137:211–218.
3. Lüderitz-Stanislawski B, Haustein D: Neubewertung des Risikos von Test- und Therapieallergenen – Eine Analyse der UWA-Meldungen von 1991 bis 2000. Bundesgesundheitsbl-Gesundheitforsch-Gesundheitsschutz 2001; 44:709–718.
4. Dormann D, Ebner C, Jarman ER, Montermann E, Kraft D, Reske-Kunz AB: Responses of human birch pollen allergen-reactive T-cells to chemically modified allergens (allergoids). Clin Exp Allergy 1998; 28:1374–1383.
5. Kalinski P, Lebre MC, Kramer D, De Jong EC, Van Schijndel JW, Kapsenberg ML: Analysiş of the CD4⁺ T-cell responses to house dust mite allergoid. Allergy 2003; 58:648–656.
6. Kahlert H, Grage-Griebenow E, Stuwe HT, Cromwell O, Fiebig H: T-cell reactivity with allergoids: influence of the type of APC. The Journal of Immunology 2000; 165:1807–1815.

Hendrik Wolf

ALK-SCHERAX Arzneimittel GmbH, Feldstraße 170, 22880 Wedel, Germany, Tel. +49 4103 7017-342, Fax +49 4103 7017-742. E-mail hendrik.wolf@alk-scherax.de

Human Antichimeric Antibodies to Infliximab and Infusion-Related Allergic Reactions in Patients with Rheumatoid Arthritis

D. Wouters[1], S. Stapel[3], M. Vis[2], H. de Vrieze[3], A.E. Voskuyl[2], W.F. Lems[2], M. Nurmohamed[2,4] L.A. Aarden[1], B.A.C. Dijkmans[2], R.C. Aalberse[1], and G.J. Wolbink[1,4]

[1]Department of Immunopathology, Sanquin Research at CLB, Amsterdam, [2]Department of Rheumatology, VU Medical Center, [3]Department Of Allergy, Sanquin Diagnostics, [4]Jan van Breemen Institute, Amsterdam, all The Netherlands.

Summary. *Background:* Infliximab-treated RA patients may develop antibodies to infliximab (HACAs; Human antichimeric antibodies), which is associated with reduced clinical response and infusion related allergic reactions. Recently, we found that infusion reactions are associated with formation of larger immune complexes. Since infusion reactions were not observed in all patients with HACAs, we investigated whether the occurrence of infusion reactions is influenced by the relative contribution of IgG4 to the HACA response, knowing that IgG4 cannot form large immune complexes. *Methods:* Out of 200 RA patients receiving infliximab we identified 19 patients with infusion reactions. Total IgG and IgG4 levels against infliximab were determined in sera collected prior to the reaction. As internal control, IgG and IgG4 were determined in sera collected prior to a previous infusion that did not cause clinical problems. Furthermore, results were compared with sera from patients with HACAs but without infusion reactions. *Results:* Infusion reactions in these 19 RA patients were mild. HACA levels were significantly higher in sera collected prior to the infusion reaction (median: 7.9 μg/ml; range: 0.46–1917) compared to internal controls (median: 0.24 μg/ml; range: 0.13–225). The median relative contribution of IgG4 to HACA levels is 29% (range: 1–100%). This is similar to the internal control (median: 33%; range: 1–100%) and to patients without infusion reaction (median 32%; range: 7–60%). *Conclusions:* Infusion reactions to infliximab are associated with increased HACA levels, however not all patients with HACAs show infusion reactions. This discrepancy cannot be explained by a difference in relative contribution of IgG4 to HACAs.

Keywords: rheumatoid arthritis, infliximab, antichimeric antibodies, allergic reaction

Introduction

Almost half of RA patients treated with infliximab develop antibodies to infliximab, (HACAs; Human antichimeric antibodies). Development of HACAs is related to a reduced clinical response to treatment and the occurrence of infusion related allergic reactions [1]. Recently, we found that infusion reactions are associated with the formation of larger immune complexes (unpublished data). Since infusion reactions were not observed in all patients that

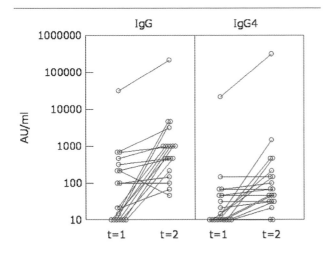

Figure 1. Both total IgG and IgG4 levels are significantly higher at infusion reaction (t = 2) compared to the internal control (t = 1).

develop HACAs, we investigated whether the occurrence of infusion reactions is influenced by the relative contribution of IgG4 to the HACA response knowing that IgG4 is unable to form large immune complexes and has been described to be protective against immune complex induced disease [2].

Material and Methods

From a cohort of 200 RA patients receiving infliximab every 8 weeks, we identified 19 patients with an infusion reaction. Infusion reactions consisted of erythema, dyspnea, fever and an increased heart rate, only few patients had a significant drop of blood pressure. All patients recovered within a few hours. Total IgG and IgG4 levels specific for infliximab were measured by an antigen binding assay [1, 3], in which the patients' IgG or IgG4 is trapped on a solid phase (Sepharose-coupled protein A or anti-IgG4, respectively) and specific anti-infliximab antibodies are detected by radiolabeled F(ab)₂ fragments of infliximab. Total IgG and IgG4 levels against infliximab were determined in sera collected prior to the infusion reaction (t = 2). Samples from the same patients prior to an infusion that did not result in an infusion reaction were used as internal control (t = 1). Results were also compared to matched controls, which had comparable anti-infliximab levels but no infusion related allergic reaction.

Results

All patients with infusion related allergic reactions had detectable antibodies against infliximab prior to the infusion that induced the allergic reaction. HACA levels were significantly higher at infusion reaction (t = 2) (median: 7.9 µg/ml; range: 0.46–19717) as compared to the internal control (t = 1) (median: 0.24 µg/ml; range: 0.13–225) (Figure 1). However, since IgG4 levels were also significantly higher at t = 2 compared to t = 1, we observed no difference in the relative contribution of gG4 to the HACA levels. Sera from 10 other RA patients, without allergic reaction, but with comparable total IgG anti-infliximab levels were used as matched controls. We also found no difference in the relative contribution of IgG4 to HACA levels between patients with allergic reaction and patients without allergic reaction (data not shown).

Discussion

We selected 19 infliximab treated RA patients that showed infusion related allergic reactions at some point during treatment. These patients all had detectable HACAs, and HACA levels were significantly increased at time of the allergic reaction as compared to an earlier infusion. Therefore we conclude that infusion related allergic reactions to infliximab are associated with increased HACA levels. However, not all patients with HACAs show infusion reactions. This discrepancy cannot be explained by a difference in the relative contribution of IgG4 to HACAs, since total IgG and IgG4 increased at the same rate. Further research is necessary to find out what causes infusion related allergic reactions.

References:

1. Wolbink GJ, Vis M, Lems W, Voskuyl AE, de Groot E, Nurmohamed MT, Stapel S, Tak PP, Aarden L, Dijkmans B: Development of anti-infliximab antibodies and relationship to clinical response in patients with rheumatoid arthritis. Arthritis Rheum 2006; 54:711–715.

2. Van der Zee JS, van Swieten P, Aalberse RC: Serologic aspects of IgG4 antibodies. II IgG4 antibodies form small, nonprecipitating immune complexes due to monovalency. J Immunol 1986; 137:3566–3571.

3. Aalberse RC, van der Gaag R, van Leeuwen J: Serologic aspects of IgG4 antibodies. J Immunol 1983; 130:722.

D. Wouters

Department of Immunopathology, Sanquin, Plesmanlaan 125, NL-1066 CX Amsterdam, The Netherlands, Tel. +31 20 512-3853, Fax +31 20 512-3170, E-mail d.wouters@sanquin.nl

LAS 36674, A New Generation of H1 Antihistamines: From Bench to Bedside and Back

M. Miralpeix[1], X. Cabarrocas[3], A. Cárdenas[2], I. Herrero[3], E. García[3], X. Luria[3], H. Ryder[1], and J. Beleta[1]

[1]Drug Discovery, [2]Development and [3]Medical Division, Research Center, Almirall Prodesfarma, Barcelona, Spain

Summary. *Background:* The objective of our work was to develop potent, selective and long lasting H_1 antihistamines devoid of cardiotoxicity, sedative effects and drug-drug interactions that may be favorably differentiated with respect to the second-generation antihistamines. In this study, we describe the profile of two new H_1 antihistamines named LAS 32928 and LAS 36674. *Methods and Results:* LAS 32928, an indolylpiperidinyl benzoic acid derivative, with a favorable preclinical profile, was initially selected for clinical development. In healthy male volunteers, LAS 32928 (10, 25, and 50 mg administered as an oral suspension during 5 consecutive days) showed a promising efficacy and safety profile, but its development was discontinued due to its short duration of action and elimination half-life. In order to improve the duration of action and pharmacokinetic profile of LAS 32928 new indolylpiperidinyl derivatives were synthesized. LAS 36674 was selected as a candidate for development based on its potent and long lasting antihistamine activity in rats, low brain penetration in mice and rats, lack of cardiotoxicity, no significant interaction with CYP450 isoforms and long elimination half-life in rats. *Conclusions:* LAS 36674 showed an improved preclinical pharmacological and ADME profile compared to its predecessor LAS 32928. LAS 36674 demonstrated a higher efficacy/safety ratio than second-generation antihistamines in preclinical models, suggesting the potential for a superior benefit/risk profile in humans.

Keywords: H_1 antihistamines, allergic rhinitis, indolylpiperidinyl benzoic acid derivatives, QT interval prolongation, sedative effects, drug-drug interactions, antihistamine activity in healthy volunteers

Introduction

H_1 antihistamines are still the first-line medication for patients with allergic rhinitis [1]. After several decades of research in the field of H_1 antihistamines there is still the opportunity to obtain a new class of antihistamines with improved and differentiated profiles with regard to the second-generation antihistamines. The "Consensus Group on New-Generation Antihistamines" concluded that three "prerequisites" will be necessary as pri-mary components of a new class of antihistamines: (1) lack of cardiotoxicity, (2) lack of drug-drug interactions, and (3) lack of central nervous system effects [2]. Moreover, there may be different kinds of new antihistamines, such as H_1 blockers with an additional effect (s) or H_1 blockers offering a special feature (e.g., being neutral antagonists). In this study, we describe the profile of two new H_1 antihistamines, indolylpiperidinyl benzoic acid derivatives, named LAS 32928 and LAS 36674.

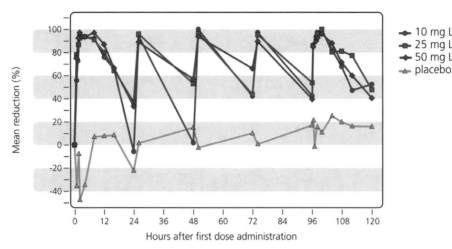

Figure 1. Mean percentage reduction of the wheal surface area following the treatment with 10, 25, 50 mg of LAS 32928 or placebo during 5 consecutive days. The percentage reduction of the histamine-induced wheal was measured at 15 minutes after histamine administration in the presence of LAS 32928 or placebo, as compared to the wheal area at predose (baseline). The intracutaneous histamine challenge (0.05 mL of a 100 µg/mL solution) was performed at predose, 30, 60, 90 minutes and 2, 4, 8, 12, 16, and 24 h postdose on days 1 and 5, and predose and 2 h postdose on days 2, 3, and 4.

Methods and Results

Twenty healthy male volunteers were randomized to receive LAS 32928 as oral suspension (10, 25, or 50 mg) and placebo in a ratio 2:1, in order to assess its antihistamine activity, tolerability, cardiovascular safety and pharmacokinetics. The administration regimen was once daily for 5 consecutive days for three study periods (one treatment per study period) with a wash out period of at least 7 days between each period. At all doses tested, LAS 32928 was safe and well-tolerated. Some somnolence episodes were reported at 50 mg whereas at lower doses not. No QTc interval prolongation was observed after administration of either the first or the last doses of LAS 32928 compared to time-matched values after placebo administration. Figure 1 shows that LAS 32928 was very effective reducing histamine-induced wheal healthy male volunteers at all doses tested, but with short duration of action and elimination half-life ($t_{1/2}$ 3 h) that compromised a once daily administration in humans. Thus, the development of LAS 32928 was discontinued and we went back to synthesize new indolyl-piperidinyl derivatives. LAS 36674 was selected as a new candidate for development based on its sustained duration of action in the histamine-induced cutaneous vascular permeability model in rat (Table 1) and longer elimination half-life in rat compared to its predecessor LAS 32928 (3.9 h *versus* 1.1 h), that together suggests a once daily administration in humans. Moreover, LAS 36674 had low potential of drug-drug interaction (not metabolize by P450 cytochrome and did not inhibit the 3A4, 2D6 and 2C9 isoforms of CYP450). LAS 36674 was devoid of cardiovascular side effects in the following preclinical models: (1)

	Binding H₁ IC₅₀ (nM)	Vascular Cutaneous Permeability ED₅₀ (mg/kg, p.o.)		
		1h	4h	8h
LAS 36674	460	0.03	0.05	0.14
LAS 32928	62	0.02	0.1	0.22
Loratadine	360	0.75	0.45	0.99
Cetirizine	226	0.51	4	9
Fexofenadine	214	8	30	>30

Table 1. Binding affinity for H₁ receptor, potency and duration of action in the histamine-induced cutaneous vascular permeability model in rat (1, 4, and 8 h after oral administration of the test compounds). Binding of [³H]-mepyramine to histamine-H1 receptors was performed in guinea pig cerebellum membranes.

blockage of K$^+$ hERG channel (IC$_{50}$ > 10 µM); (2) Action Potential Duration in piglet Purkinje fibers (no effect at 30 µM); and (3) QTc interval prolongation in anesthetized guinea-pig (no effect at 30 mg/kg). Finally, LAS 36674 showed low brain penetration in the H₁ *ex-vivo* binding assay in mouse and in the spontaneous motor activity model in rat.

Conclusions

LAS 32928 showed a promising efficacy and safety profile in healthy male volunteers, but its development was discontinued due to its short duration of action and elimination half-life. The new selected candidate for development, LAS 36674, showed an improved preclinical ADME profile that together with its low potential of cardiotoxicity, sedative effects and drug-drug interaction may it distinguish from the second-generation antihistamines. Thus, LAS 36674 may belong to a new class of H₁ antihistamines.

References

1. Simons FER: Advances in H1- Antihistamines. N Eng J Med 2004; 351:2202–2217.
2. Holgate ST, Canonica GW, Simons FER, Taglialatela M, Tharp M, Timmerman H, Yanai K: Consensus group on new-generation antihistamines (CONGA): present status and recommendations. Clin Exp Allerg 2003; 33:1305–1324.

Montse Miralpeix

Respiratory Therapeutic Group, Biology Department, Research Center, Almirall Prodesfarma, Laureà Miró 408-410, E-08980 Sant Feliu de Llobregat, Barcelona, Spain, Tel. +34 93 291-3468, Fax +34 93 291-3420, E-mail mmiralpe@almirall.es

B-Cell Development

From Bone Marrow to Peripheral Tissue in Allergy

A. Bossios and J. Lötvall

Lung Pharmacology Group, Department of Internal Medicine/Respiratory Medicine and Allergology, The Sahlgrenska Academy, Göteborg University, Sweden

Summary. B-cells generate the humoral immune response essential for antibody production. Their role in allergic inflammation is indispensable by the production of IgE. However these cells also share other roles in allergic inflammation, including activity as antigen presenting cells. After birth, B-cells develop originally within bone marrow from pluripotent haematopoietic stem cells, followed by further maturation in peripheral tissue. This composite process includes several stages and is under tight control. This mini-review summarizes the different stages of B cell development from the earliest B-cell precursors in the bone marrow until their development in functional plasma and memory B cells.

Keywords: B-cells, progenitors, bone marrow, maturation, differentiation

B-cells generate humoral immune response, protecting us from infections. Nevertheless deficient B-cell function can lead to severe disease such as hyper-immunoglobulin M syndromes [1]. Overproduction of specific IgE represents a major pathway in allergic inflammation, although other roles of B-cells in allergy, such as antigen presentation or potentially regulatory function, have been proposed [2].

B-cell differentiation has been become well characterized in recent years, primarily though studies in primary immune deficiencies in man. Tools of understanding B-cell differentiation were developed in mice, through studies of transgenic or knock out models, as B-cell function in man is very similar to mice. Therefore we will discuss findings and mechanisms primarily described in mice.

B-cells production in adults is a lifelong process, initiated in the bone marrow (BM), the primary lymphoid organ of B-cells. These cells originate from pluripotent haematopoietic stem cells (HSC), further subdivided into three subgroups: (1) long-term HSC (LT-HSC) with life-long self-renewal capacity, (2) short-term HSC (ST-HSC) with limited capacity, and (3) multipotent progenitors (MMP) capable of giving rise to all blood cell-lineages, which are not self-renewed. These different subgroups of stem cells can be characterized with flow cytometric analysis by determining the expression or absence of markers as (Lin-), Thy1.1, Sca-1, c-kit, CD34 and FLT3 [3]. MMP give rise to lymphoid-primed multipotent progenitors (LMPPs) followed by common lymphoid progenitors (CLPs) that can generate both B and T-cells.

Subsequently the lineage specific marker CD45R/B220 is expressed giving rise to B-cell precursors, although the exact intermediate cell population is still debated. In the BM, reticular cells (the most abundant stromal cell type) and osteoblasts generate specific microenvironmental niches for B-cells development. A sophisticated network delivers the necessary factors for the B-cell development. These factors include CXC-chemokine ligand 12 (CXCL12), FLT3 ligand (FLT3L), IL-7, stem-cell factor (SCF) and receptor activator of nuclear factor-kB ligand (RANKL). IL-7 plays a central role, and was first identified as a growth factor for B-cell progenitors. This interleukin acts though IL-7R and its biological actions include commitment, survival, proliferation and maturation, plus initial immunoglobulin (Ig) gene rearrangement [4].

Furthermore, development of B-cell precursors requires the expression of several transcription factors, as assessed in genetically modified mice. So far, PU.1, Ikaros, E2A, Bcl11a, early B-cell factor (EBF) and paired box protein 5 (Pax-5) have been showed to be involved in commitment and/or specification of B-lineages. They lead to several cellular processes, including activation of the locus for the recombination activating genes (RAG) 1 and 2, leading to expression their Rag1-2 recombinase indispensable for V (D) J recombination.

B-cell precursors are characterized by the expression of various surface markers (B220, CD19, CD24, CD43, and IL-7Rα/CD127) and the stepwise and ordered rearrangement of Ig gene segments. The earliest committed B-cell precursors are pre-pro-B-cells. These cells have their immunoglobulin loci in germline configuration, but despite this they do not express components of the B-cell receptor (BCR). The next level is pro-B-cells (early and late), where V (D) J recombination is initiated. Late pro-B-cell synthesize membrane-anchored heavy chain of μ (HCμ) and develop into pre-B-cells, which further divide into large and small subpopulations of cells. Large pre-B-cells undergo a limited clonal expansion resulting in assembly of pre-B-cell receptor (pre-BCR). This is the first differentiation checkpoint, as cells that fail to assembly pre-BCR are deleted. Pre-BCR is composed by two HCμ associates with the surrogate light chain (SLC) consisting of VpreB and λ5 chains; and the Igα/Igβ transducting complex. When proliferation stops, the cells are transformed to small pre-B-cells. An induction of Ig light chain (IgL) gene rearrangement follows, which allows the cells to form a complete BCR, composed by Igμ and IgL chains, together with Igα/Igβ, which constitutes the receptor in an IgM-positive immature B-cell [5–7]. This is the final checkpoint before the

cell is leaving the BM. Immature B-cells with potential reactivity to self-antigens are inactivated though deletion (apoptosis), anergy or receptor editing, a procedure known as negative selection. Indeed, the majority of new B-cells formed in the BM, fail to survive and exhibit a short life-span of 1–4 days [8]. The B-cells that do not react to self-antigen, are allowed to leave the BM, after increasing their expression of IgM, and these cells are called immature (transitional) B-cells.

However, even when immature B-cells leave the BM, they still face the possibility of deletion by possible migration to lymph nodes or sites of inflammation, encouraging peripheral self-antigen. By contrast, immature (transitional) B-cells that traffic directly to the spleen will undergo the next maturation steps. In order to achieve that, immature B-cells has developed several specific mechanisms to home to the spleen. For example immature B-cells express the chemokine receptor CCR2 that prevent them from homing to lymph nodes, allowing these cell to traffic to the spleen [9].

In spleen transitional B-cells start to express surface IgD, the complement receptor CD21, and CD23 (FcεRII). These cells can been divided into two subgroups; T1 (IgM^{high} IgD^{low} CD23^{low} CD21/35$^-$) and T2 (IgM^{high} IgD^{high} CD23$^+$ CD21/35^{high}), although overlapping groups have been proposed [10]. T1 cells remain at the PALS (periarteriolar lymphoid sheaths) where they are still under negative selection by self-antigens trapped by the spleen. The survivals T1 develop into T2 found in the primary follicles of the spleen.

The successful transit of immature B-cells to mature ones is thus under tight control. A sufficient BCR signal is essential for development of T1 into T2 and then into mature B-cells. Both the tyrosine phosphatase CD45 and co-receptor CD22 modulate further the BCR initiated signals. The microenvironment in the spleen also plays an important role. For example; the recently discovered B-cell-activating factor (BAFF) belongs to the TNF family and enhance B-cell survival as well as speeding up maturation. This factor is expressed by several cells in the spleen, including monocytes, macrophages and dendritic cells. The three receptors for BAFF (BCMA, TACI and BR3) are expressed by B-cells [11, 12].

Mature B-cells can be divided in three broad populations. The majority (80–90% of adult mouse spleen B-cells) will end up as follicular (FO) (IgM^{low} IgD^{high} CD23$^+$ CD21/35^{int}) followed by marginal zone (MZ) (IgM^{low} IgD^{high} CD23$^-$ CD21/35^{high}) B-cells (5–10%). FO B-cells represents the mature circulating B-cells. These cells migrate to and within secondary lymphoid organs such as lymph nodes under the influence of specific signals, identified as the Switch Associated Protein 70 (SWAP-70) [13]. In the lymph node, the B-cell can encounter antigen, and with T-cell help, they establish a germinal center in the lymph node follicles. There they proliferate and undergo affinity maturation and Ig class-switch recombination. Essential are the interactions with T-helper cells (CD40L-CD40 & ICOS-ICOSL), accompanied by secreted cytokines. Follicular dendritic cells participate by antigen impound and expression of complement receptors (CD21, CD35). Plasma cell formation is also under the control of various transcription factors as the B-lymphocyte-induced maturation protein 1 (BLIMP1). Eventually plasma cells and memory B-cells exit the germinal center, and re-enter the circulation entering the long-live B-cell pool.

Furthermore FO B-cells have also the capacity for an early-response after encounter antigen and receive T-cell helping periphery by forming extrafollicular foci of plasmablasts and plasma cells. However, these are short-lived cells that soon undergo apoptosis *in-situ* [14].

The marginal zone B-cells (MZ) do not circulate and they are located in marginal sinus. Their close contacts with MOMA-1^{pos} macrophages, that filter the blood, make them ideal to detect foreign antigens. Upon recognition of T-Cell-Independent antigens they start rapidly to proliferate and differentiate into plasma cells, producing low-affinity abs, probably an important first extensive line of defence against pathogens.

A third type, the B1 B-cells, is mainly present in the pleural, peritoneal cavities and spleen. Their progenitors are profuse in fetal liver, yet absent in adult BM. Importantly; B1 cells have a unique self-renewing capacity. They give the earliest antibody response; provided by natural preexisting antibodies. An interesting new function of these cells has been proposed. B-1a (CD19$^+$/CD5$^+$) cell deficient mice on a cockroach allergen-induced model revealed a potent regulatory role in airway inflammation, by suppression of allergen-sensitized T-cells [2]. Additionally, it was shown that peritoneal B-1a cells can produce IL-10 after antigenic stimulation.

In conclusion, many recent studies have described novel pathways and mechanisms of B-cells differentiation. Understanding the details of how B-cells start producing specific antibodies including allergen specific IgE can potentially give us tools for possible intervention and perhaps prevention of allergic disease.

References

1. Durandy A, Revy P, Imai KAF: Hyper-immunoglobulin M syndromes caused by intrinsic B-lymphocyte defects. Immunol Rev 2005; 203:67–79.
2. Lundy SK, Berlin AA, Martens TF, NW L: Deficiency of regulatory B-cells increases allergic airway inflammation. Inflamm Res 2005; 54:514–521.
3. Nagasawa T: Microenvironmental niches in the bone marrow required for B-cell development. Nat Rev Immunol 2006; 6:107–116.
4. Milne CD, Paige CJ: IL-7: A key regulator of B lymphopoiesis. Seminars in Immunology 2006; 18(1):20–30.
5. Hardy RR, Hayakawa K: B-cell development pathways. Ann Rev Immunol 2001; 19:595–621.
6. Meffre E, Casellas RCN: Antibody regulation of B-cell development. Nat Immunol 2000; 1:379–385.
7. Vettermann C, Herrmann K, Jack H-M: Powered by pairing: the surrogate light chain amplifies immunoglobulin heavy chain signaling and pre-selects the antibody repertoire. Seminars in Immunology 2006; 18:44–55.
8. Hao Z, Rajewsky K: Homeostasis of peripheral B-cells in the absence of B-cell influx from the bone marrow. J Exp Med 2001; 194:1151–1164.
9. Flaishon L, Becker-Herman S, Hart G, Levo Y, Kuziel WA, Shachar I: Expression of the chemo-

kine receptor CCR2 on immature B-cells negatively regulates their cytoskeletal rearrangement and migration. Blood 2004; 104:933–941.

10. Loder F, Mutschler B, Ray RJ, Paige CJ, Sideras P, Torres R, Lamers MC, Carsetti R: B-cell development in the spleen takes place in discrete steps and is determined by the quality of B-cell receptor-derived signals. J Exp Med 1999; 190:75–90.

11. Carsetti R, Rosado MM, Wardmann H: Peripheral development of B-cells in mouse and man. Immunol Rev 2004; 197:179–191.

12. Matthew TD, Srivastava B, Allman D: Regulation of peripheral B-cell maturation. Cellular Immunology 2006; 239:92–102.

13. Pearce G, Angeli V, Randolph GJ, Junt T, von Andrian U, Schnittler H-J, Jessberger R: Signaling protein SWAP-70 is required for efficient B-cell homing to lymphoid organs. Nat Immunol 2006; 7:827–834.

14. Shapiro-Shelef M, Calame K: Regulation of plasma-cell development. Nature Reviews Immunology 2005; 5:230–242.

Apostolos Bossios

Lung Pharmacology Group, Guldhedsgatan 10A, SE-41346, Gothenburg, Sweden, Tel. +46 31 3423136, Fax +46 31 413290, E-mail apostolos.bossios@gu.se

Parasites and Allergy: From Mice to Man

A.M. Dittrich[1,2] and E. Hamelmann[1]

[1]Department of Pediatric Pneumology and Immunology, Charité University-Medicine, Berlin, Germany, [2]Currently: Department for Immunobiology, Yale University School of Medicine, New Haven, CT, USA

Summary: Even though the inverse relationship between parasitic infections and allergic diseases has been recognized for quite some time, many of the underlying aspects remain unresolved. This review summarizes, on the basis of the epidemiological studies, the published findings from animal studies investigating the effects of parasitic infections on allergic immune responses. The emphasis lies on the dissection of the immunological mechanisms of parasite immune modulation that has been provided so far. Both the epidemiological and the animal studies provide a strong basis to rely on when designing new human interventional trials which will constitute the ultimate proof of concept for the immune modulating properties of parasites and will form the basis for novel therapeutic concepts for treatment of allergies.

Keywords: allergy, parasite, helminth, rodent, immunomodulation

The fact that allergic diseases, among them bronchial asthma, have increased considerably in industrialized countries in the past decades, is a well-acknowledged entity. However, the epidemiological and immunological basis for this phenomenon remains only partly understood. Still the most intriguing theories for this is given by the so-called hygiene hypothesis [1], based on the observation of a negative correlation between allergic diseases and childhood infections. In developing countries, there is a considerably lower prevalence of allergic diseases, and there is even a decline in allergy rates between rural and urban areas within one country regardless of its developmental status [2].

Initially, the increase in allergic diseases was attributed to an insufficient balance between Th1 and Th2 immunity due to a lack of Th1-promoting infections in industrialized countries. However, recent observations have challenged this explanation. Firstly, Th1 diseases such as type 1 diabetes have also been progressively increasing in the past few decades, suggesting a common denominator underlying the increase of both Th1 and Th2 diseases instead of an imbalance between Th1 and Th2 immune responses [3]. Secondly, the occurrence of helminth infections and allergic diseases, both conditions being accompanied by strong Th2 immune responses, are nearly exclusive or at least negatively associated [reviewed in 4], an observation that has been confirmed in developed countries [5]. The hygiene hypothesis therefore has to be modified in order to state that a robust regulatory network induced by a high overall infection rate, regardless of the nature of its immunological skewing, is central to the balance and the prevention of either Th1 and/or Th2 diseases [6].

The epidemiological studies on helminth infections support this explanation, at their best intertwining epidemiological observations and immunological analyses [6]. Epidemiological studies have their shortcomings, though when it comes to dissecting the mechanism(s) of the relationships they observe. At this point, animal studies constitute an invaluable tool to complement epidemiology and generate the "proof-of-concept." Recent studies in mouse models have

Table 1. Animal studies on the relationship between parasitic infections and allergic diseases.

Reference	Parasite	Disease model [species/ antigen/phenotypee]	Main effects	Regulatory mechanism
Price et al. Parasite Immunol. 1984	*Nematospiroides dubius/Nippostrongylus brasiliensis*	Mouse/OVA/allergic sensitization	Allergen-specific IgG↓	–
Price et al. Exp Parasitol 1987	*N. dubius/Nippostrongylus brasiliensis*	Mouse/OVA/DTH	DTH↓ Allergen-specific IgG/IgM$_{serum}$→	–
Wang et al. Clin. Exp. Allergy 2001	*Strongyloides stercoralis*	Mouse/OVA/allergic airway inflammation	Eotaxin$_{Lung}$↓ OVA-spec. IgE$_{BAL}$↓	–
Lima et. al. Clin. Exp. Allergy 2002	*Ascaris suum*	Mouse/Egg White-OVA/allergic airway inflammation	Allergen-specific IgE$_{serum\ and\ BAL}$↓ Airway Reactivity↓ Airway inflammation↓ IL-4, -5, Eotaxin$_{BAL}$↓	–
Bashir et al. J Immunol. 2002	*Heligmosomoides polygyrus*	Mouse/peanut extract/food allergy-anaphylaxis	Allergen-specific IgE$_{serum}$↓ Plasma histamine↓ Anaphylaxis Score↓ Allergen-specific IL-13↓	IL-10
Negrão-Corrêa et. al. Inf.Imm. 2003	*Strongyloides venezuelensis*	Rat/OVA/allergic airway inflammation	Effect on AHR depends on kinetics [→ and ↓]	–
Mangan et. al. JI 2004	*Schistosoma mansonii*	Mouse/Pen-V-OVA-BSA/anaphylaxis	Anaphylaxis Score↓ Plasma histamine↓	Regulatory B-cells via secretion of IL-10
Pinto et. al. Parasite Imm. 2004	*Angiostrongylus costaricensis*	Mouse/OVA/allergic airway inflammation	Eosinophils$_{BAL}$↓ Total BAL cell counts→	
Wohlleben Int. Imm. 2004	*Nippostrongylus brasiliensis*	Mouse/OVA/allergic airway inflammation	Airway Hyperreactivity↓ Eotaxin$_{Lung}$↓ Allergen-specific IgE and IgG1$_{serum}$→ Allergen-specific IgE and IgG1$_{BAL}$	IL-10
Wilson et. al. J Exp. Med. 2005	*Heligmosomoides polygyrus*	Mouse/OVA&Der p 1/allergic airway inflammation	Airway inflammation↓ Allergen-specific IgE$_{serum}$→ IL-5, Eotaxin$_{BAL}$↓ CD4$^+$/CD25$^+$/Foxp3$^+$ cells↑	CD4$^+$/CD25$^+$/Foxp3$^+$ T reg cells IL-10 not involved
Oshiro et. al. Imm. Cell Biol. 2006	*Ascaris suum* [PAS-1 = A. suum component]	Mouse/OVA/DTH	DTH↓ Allergen-specific IgE and IgG1$_{serum}$	

OVA: ovalbumin
BSA: bovine serum albumin
DTH: delayed type of hypersensitivity

shed light on possible mechanisms by which parasites suppress allergic reactivity; however they also suggest that the picture is complex and is far from being completely understood [7–17]. Table 1 provides a summary on animal studies performed so far regarding parasites and allergy. Some results of these studies seem controversial as clear differences and contradictions can be noted, however common denominators can also be observed and shall be discussed in the following.

The oldest published animal studies analyzing the effect of a parasitic infection on a subsequent or concomitant allergic sensitization show a reduction of allergen-specific immunoglobulin secretion [8]. Most studies so far have confirmed this findings and added analyses of other aspects that constitute the allergic phenotype. They assert that parasites can suppress all main allergic disease entities that can be satisfactorily modeled in animals, e.g., delayed type hypersensitivity reactions [7, 17] food allergy [11], anaphylaxis [11, 13] and bronchial asthma [9, 10, 12, 14–16]. Some authors have advanced to study the mechanisms underlying this suppression pointing toward downregulation of Th2 effector cytokine responses to allergen. Studies investigating mediators – soluble and cellular – responsible for this suppression of Th2 responses to allergen are limited, though. Some studies showed that IL-10 mediates the suppressive effects in their systems [11, 13, 14], while others cannot find a role for IL-10 in their system [16]. Similarly, only Mangan et al. and Wilson et.al addressed the possible cell types involved in the suppression and also came to different conclusions. This might be due to differences in the models employed, both on the host side (anaphylaxis vs. airway inflammation) and/ or the parasite side (Schistosoma mansonii vs. Heligsomoides polygyrus). Our own studies with yet another parasite (Litomosoides sigmodontis) in a mouse model of allergic airway disease seem to confirm Wilson's data as they also show an increase in numbers and function of regulatory T-cells (Treg). Interestingly and yet unreported, we observed great increases in allergen-specific TGF-β secretion suggesting yet another mediator responsible for the suppressive effect of this particular infection.

More work in animals models is required to really understand the complex mechanisms of immune evasion that parasites have developed during the centuries of co-evolution with their host. Only a more complete understanding of the mechanisms involved will eventually enable us to exploit the benefits of parasite infections without having to accommodate their detrimental consequences. To this end, the identification of parasitic components with immunomodulatory functions, as attempted by Oshiro et al. [17] should allow easier control of dosage and effect and should therefore constitute an important venue of future research.

Interestingly, animal studies have also shown that the immunomodulatory properties of parasites are not limited to allergic diseases, as parasite infections have also been shown to suppress inflammatory bowel diseases, neurological autoimmune diseases, type I diabetes, rheumatoid arthritis and transplant rejection [18–22]. Translating these animal findings to clinical studies is far more advanced in fields other than allergic diseases. Human interventional studies with eggs from Trichuris suis, a pig-parasite, have shown favorable effects on Crohn's disease and ulcerative colitis [23]. This has led researchers to attempt similar studies aimed at reducing airway hyperresponsiveness [24]. Carefully designed human and animal studies on the relationship of allergic diseases and parasitic infections are urgently needed: To shed light on the the mechanisms employed by parasites for immune modulation; and to correctly assess their potential for novel modes of anti-allergic therapies.

References

1. Strachan DP: Hay fever, hygiene, and household size. BMJ 1989; 299:1259–1260.
2. The International Study of Asthma and Allergies in Childhood [ISAAC] Steering Committee. Worldwide variation in prevalence of symptoms of asthma, allergic rhinoconjunctivitis, and atopic eczema: ISAAC. Lancet 1998; 351:1225–1232.
3. Stene LC, Nafstad P: Relation between occurrence of type 1 diabetes and asthma. Lancet 2001; 357:607–608.

4. Yazdanbakhsh M, van den Biggelaar A, Maizels RM: Th2 responses without atopy: immunoregulation in chronic helminth infections and reduced allergic disease. Trends Immunol 2001; 22:372–377.

5. Schafer T, Meyer T, Ring J, Wichmann HE, Heinrich J: Worm infestation and the negative association with eczema [atopic/nonatopic] and allergic sensitization. Allergy 2005; 60:1014–1020.

6. Yazdanbakhsh M, Kremsner P, van Ree R: Allergy, parasites, and the hygiene hypothesis. Science 2002; 296:490–494.

7. Price P, Turner KJ: Immunological consequences of intestinal helminth infections. Humoral responses to ovalbumin. Parasite Immunol 1984; 6:499–508.

8. Price P, Turner KJ: Nematospiroides dubius and Nippostrongylus brasiliensis: delayed type hypersensitivity responses to ovalbumin in the infected mouse. Exp Parasitol 1987; 63:21–31.

9. Wang CC, Nolan TJ, Schad GA, Abraham D: Infection of mice with the helminth Strongyloides stercoralis suppresses pulmonary allergic responses to ovalbumin. Clin Exp Allergy 2001; 31:495–503.

10. Lima C, Perini A, Garcia ML, Martins MA, Teixeira MM, Macedo MS: Eosinophilic inflammation and airway hyper-responsiveness are profoundly inhibited by a helminth [Ascaris suum] extract in a murine model of asthma. Clin Exp Allergy 2002; 32:1659–1666.

11. Bashir ME, Andersen P, Fuss IJ, Shi HN, Nagler-Anderson C: An enteric helminth infection protects against an allergic response to dietary antigen. J Immunol 2002; 169:3284–3292.

12. Negrão-Corrêa D, Silveira MR, Borges CM, Souza DG, Teixeira MM: Changes in pulmonary function and parasite burden in rats infected with Strongyloides venezuelensis concomitant with induction of allergic airway inflammation. Inf Imm 2003; 71:2607–2614.

13. Mangan NE, Fallon RE, Smith P, van Rooijen N, McKenzie AN, Fallon PG: Helminth infection protects mice from anaphylaxis via IL-10-producing B-cells. J Immunol 2004; 173:6346–6356.

14. Wohlleben G, Trujillo C, Muller J, Ritze Y, Grunewald S, Tatsch U, Erb KJ: Helminth infection modulates the development of allergen-induced airway inflammation. Int Immunol 2004; 16:585–596.

15. Pinto LA, Pitrez PM, Fontoura GR, Machado DC, Jones MH, Graeff-Teixeira C, Stein RT: Infection of BALB/c mice with Angiostrongylus costaricensis decreases pulmonary inflammatory response to ovalbumin. Parasite Immunol 2004; 26:151–155.

16. Wilson MS, Taylor MD, Balic A, Finney CA, Lamb JR, Maizels RM: Suppression of allergic airway inflammation by helminth-induced regulatory T-cells. J Exp Med 2005; 202:1199–1212.

17. Oshiro TM, Enobe CS, Araujo CA, Macedo MS, Macedo-Soares MF: PAS-1, a protein affinity purified from Ascaris suum worms, maintains the ability to modulate the immune response to a bystander antigen. Immunol Cell Biol 2006; 84:138–144.

18. Moreels TG, Nieuwendijk RJ, De Man JG, De Winter BY, Herman AG, Van Marck EA, Pelckmans PA: Concurrent infection with Schistosoma mansoni attenuates inflammation induced changes in colonic morphology, cytokine levels, and smooth muscle contractility of trinitrobenzene sulphonic acid induced colitis in rats. Gut 2004; 53:99–107.

19. La Flamme AC, Ruddenklau K, Backstrom BT: Schistosomiasis decreases central nervous system inflammation and alters the progression of experimental autoimmune encephalomyelitis. Infect Immun 2003; 71:4996–5004.

20. Zaccone P, Fehervari Z, Jones FM, Sidobre S, Kronenberg M, Dunne DW, Cooke A: Schistosoma mansoni antigens modulate the activity of the innate immune response and prevent onset of type 1 diabetes. Eur J Immunol 2003; 33:1439–1449.

21. McInnes IB, Leung BP, Harnett M, Gracie JA, Liew FY, Harnett W: A novel therapeutic approach targeting articular inflammation using the filarial nematode-derived phosphorylcholine-containing glycoprotein ES-62. J Immunol 2003; 171:2127–2133.

22. Ledingham DL, McAlister VC, Ehigiator HN, Giacomantonio C, Theal M, Lee TD: Prolongation of rat kidney allograft survival by nematodes. Transplantation 1996; 61:184–188.

23. Elliott DE, Summers RW, Weinstock JV: Helminths and the modulation of mucosal inflammation. Curr Opin Gastroenterol 2005; 21:51–58.

24. Falcone FH, Pritchard DI: Parasite role reversal: worms on trial. Trends Parasitol 2005; 21:157–160.

Eckard Hamelmann

Department of Pediatric Pneumology and Immunology, Charité-Campus Virchow Klinikum, Charité Universitätsmedizin Berlin, Augustenburger Platz 1, D-13353 Berlin, Germany, Tel. +49 30 450-559-498, Fax +49 30 450-559-951, E-mail eckard.hamelmann@charite.de

C3a and C4a: Complement Split Products Identify Patients with Hyperacute Lyme Disease

R. Shoemaker[1], P. Giclas[2], C. Crowder[3], D. House[1], and M.M. Glovsky[4]

[1]Center for Research on Biotoxin Associated Illnesses, Pocomoke, MD, [2]National Jewish Medical and Research Center, Denver, CO, [3]UC Irvine, Irvine, CA, [4]Quest Diagnostics Nichols Institute, Department of Immunology, San Juan Capistrano, CA, all USA

Summary: Lyme disease, discovered more than 30 years ago, is the most prevalent arthropod-borne illness in the United States and Europe. Lyme disease is caused by a spirochete, *Borrelia burgdorferi*, and spread by the bite of ticks of the *Ixodes ricinus* complex [1]. Laboratory diagnosis of Lyme disease within the first few weeks of infection is inadequate because it requires the presence of antibody to *B burgdorferi*, confirmed by Western blot showing antibody reactivity to several proteins of the organism [2]. After infection, 2 to 3 weeks are required for antibody production and Western blot reactivity. Not all patients are positive by antibody measurement. Lyme disease generally manifests with flu-like symptoms of fever, malaise, headaches, arthralgia, and myalgia. A typical skin rash, erythema migrans chronicum (EMC), appears in < 50% of Lyme disease patients [3]. Both the innate and the adaptive immune responses are needed to control *B burgdorferi* infection [1]. To explore early innate immune responses in acute Lyme disease, we studied complement components and activation products in patients seen soon after tick bites. Patients presenting with typical Lyme symptoms 2 to 4 days after tick bite, with or without EM, were included. Control subjects were healthy individuals and patients with tick bites but no illness. Complement components and complexes, including C2, C3, C4, Factor B, C4d, and immune complexes (C1q binding and C3d containing), were similar in Lyme disease patients and control subjects. However, Lyme disease patients had significantly higher levels of C4a and C3a (split products of C4 and C3) than did control subjects ($p < .05$). All Lyme disease patients but only 3 control subjects had elevated levels of C3a, C4a, or both. Thus, testing for C3a and C4a may provide useful markers to detect Lyme disease in the early stages.

Keywords: Lyme disease, complement diagnostic markers, C4a, C3a

Introduction

Lyme disease, an increasingly common infectious disease, is caused by infection with the tick-borne spirochete *Borrelia burgdorferi*. Currently, no test is available to diagnose acute Lyme disease. Innate and acquired immune-mediated responses are important for eradicating the spirochete (Figure 1). Innate immune responses, especially complement, could serve as a marker of illness in patients seen shortly after a tick bite.

Rationale for Use of Complement Split Product Assays to Aid in Diagnosis of Lyme Disease

- Plasma C3a and C4a rise rapidly after activation

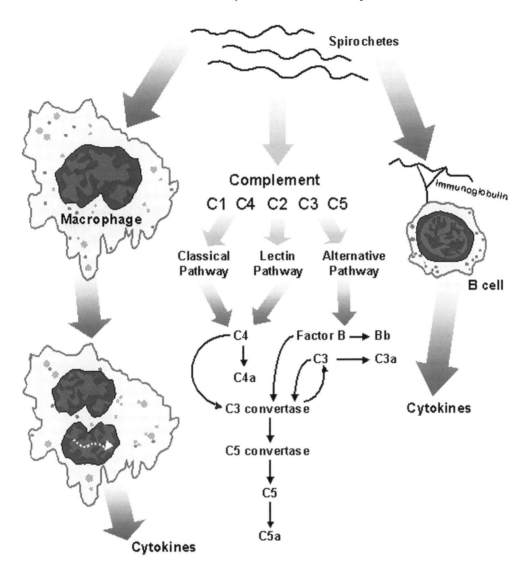

Figure 1. Innate immune response to *Borrelia burgdorferi*. *B burgdorferi* spirochetes activate complement in the plasma and generate C4a by the classical and lectin pathways. The alternative pathway is activated, possibly by spirochete membrane lipopolysaccharides, and generates the split products Bb and C3a from factor B and C3. C5a is also produced by cleavage of C5. Macrophages and B- and T-lymphocytes are activated and release proinflammatory cytokines.

- Elevated levels of C4a:
  - fall with successful treatment
  - are maintained absent treatment
  - are short-lived; ongoing high levels may reflect ongoing stimulus for production

Relevance of C3a

- Chemotactic for eosinophils
- Smooth muscle constriction

- Releases proinflammatory compounds from WBCs: oxidants, leukotrienes, enzymes
- Specific receptor (C3aR) on many cell types, including smooth muscle, adipocytes, endothelial cells in lung, brain, liver, kidney, some T-cells
- Amplification loop from alternative pathway generates large amounts C3a

Relevance of C4a

- Generated by cleavage of C4
- Formed by activation of classical pathway or lectin pathway, but NOT alternative pathway

Purpose

In this case-control study we investigated the utility of C3a and C4a measurement for detection of acute Lyme disease.

Method

Patients

Thirty-one consecutive patients with acute Lyme disease, 14 with and 17 without an erythema chronicum migrans (ECM) skin rash seen by a physician within 96 h of a tick bite, were matched with 20 consecutive tick-bite patients (2–4 days after bite) without Lyme disease symptoms or ECM and 37 apparently healthy patients undergoing routine physical examinations. Individuals with any of the following were excluded from the study: antibiotic usage at time of bite; previous tick bite or Lyme disease in the past 30 days; presence of other inflammatory conditions; previously elevated C3a or C4a; or diagnosed lupus or pancreatitis. This study was approved by an institutional review board and all participants provided informed written consent.

Laboratory Methods

Factor B, C4, and C3 complement proteins were determined by nephelometry using specific anti-sera. Immune complexes binding C1q (Binding site, San Diego, CA) and containing C3d (IBL-Diagnostics, Hamburg, Germany) were tested with ELISA kits. C2 protein was determined by diffusion in antibody-impregnated agar gels. Levels of C3a des Arg (Quidel Labs, San Diego, CA) and C4a des Arg (Pharmingen BD, San Jose, CA) were determined with kits.

In Vitro Testing

Pure cultures of *B burgdorferi* and *B hermsii* were added to normal human serum. C3a, C4a, and split products of factor B and C5 were measured at 60 minutes.

Results

Levels of C2, C3, C4, and factor B did not differ significantly between patients with Lyme disease (with or without ECM) and control subjects (with or without tick bite); none of the subjects had decreased levels of these markers.

Patients with acute Lyme disease had significantly higher levels of C3a and C4a than did tick-bite and healthy control subjects (data not shown). All patients with acute Lyme disease had elevated levels of C3a (>368 ng/mL), C4a (>745 ng/mL), or both. Among ECM-positive patients with acute disease, 10 of 10 had increased C4a and 12 of 12 had increased C3a levels. Among ECM-negative patients with acute disease, 10 of 17 (59%) had elevated C3a and 13 of 15 (87%) had elevated C4a. None of the healthy controls and few of the tick-bite controls had elevated levels of C3a or C4a.

Addition of *B burgdorferi* or *B hermsii* to normal human serum led to *in vitro* activation of complement by both the classical and alternative pathways (data not shown).

Conclusions

- C3a and C4a levels were significantly higher in patients with acute Lyme disease than in tick-bite and healthy control subjects.
- Elevated C3a or C4a levels were present in all patients with acute Lyme disease and absent in almost all control subjects.
  - C3 and C4 are generally decreased in SLE and other immune complex diseases but were normal in all patients with Lyme disease.
- C3a and C4a measurements are relevant tests currently available for differentiating patients with acute Lyme disease from individuals with tick-bite without Lyme disease.

- *B burgdorferi* and *B hermsii* activate both the classical and alternative complement pathways in normal human serum, consistent with our findings of complement activation in patients with Lyme disease.

References

1. Steer AC, Coburn J, Glickstein L: The emergence of Lyme disease. J Clin Invest 2004; 113:1093–1109.

2. Engstrom EM, Shoop E, Johnson RC: Immunoblot interpretation criteria for serodiagnosis of early Lyme disease. J Clin Micro 1995; 33:419–427.

3. Steer AC: Lyme disease. N Engl J Med 2001; 345:115–125.

M. Michael Glovsky

960 E. Green St. Pasadena, CA 91106, USA, E-mail yksvolg@caltech.edu

Plasma Cell Differentiation and Immunoglobulin Secretion

Are Induced by Interleukin-4 and Anti-CD40 and Differ in Cord Blood and Adult Naïve B-Cells

L. Hummelshoj[1], L.P. Ryder[2], and L.K. Poulsen[1]

[1]*Laboratory of Medical Allergology, Allergy Clinic and* [2]*Tissue Typing Laboratory, Department of Clinical Immunology, both National University Hospital, Copenhagen, Denmark*

Summary: *Background:* Cord blood (CB) B-cells produce low amounts of antibodies indicating immaturity of the cells or the environment they reside in. Our aim was to investigate class switch recombination and plasma cell differentiation to IgE and IgG_4 in IgD^+ B-cells from CB in comparison to adult peripheral blood (PB). *Methods:* IgD^+ B-cells from CB and PB were stimulated with IL-4 and anti-CD40. After 4 or 12 days of stimulation, germline transcripts (GLTs), AID, XBP-1, CD38, CD138, intracellular IgE and XBP-1 and secreted immunoglobulins were measured. *Results:* After 4 days of stimulation, ε and $\gamma4$ GLTs were induced in both CB and PB B-cells. No significant differences were observed in the levels of AID between the two groups. After 12 days of stimulation, secretion of IgE and IgG_4 were induced to a similar level in both groups whereas IgG were only significantly upregulated in CB-cells. Both groups displayed a low but detectable IgA. The plasma cell markers CD38 and CD138 were highly upregulated in stimulated CB-cells compared to stimulated PB-cells whereas XBP-1 was expressed at a similar level in the two groups. *Conclusion:* IL-4 and CD40-ligation increased the secretion of IgE and IgG_4 in both CB and PB B-cells. Thus naïve CB B-cells can easily be affected to switch to IgE and IgG_4, but are more easily further differentiated to become IgE but not IgG_4 producing plasma cells compared to PB-cells.

Keywords: plasma cell, human, IL-4, AID, XBP-1, IgE, class switch recombination

Introduction

B-cells undergo immunoglobulin (Ig) somatic hypermutation to increase the antibody (Ab) affinity and Ig class switch recombination (CSR) to change effector functions [1, 2]. Antigen binding to the membrane bound Ab together with cytokine and T-cell stimulation promote switching to another Ab class by somatic DNA recombination that link the rearranged VDJ region with one of the downstream H chain constant (CH) region genes

($C\gamma3$, $C\gamma1$, $C\alpha1$, $C\gamma2$, $C\gamma4$, $C\varepsilon$, $C\alpha2$) [3]. The process of Ig differentiation proceeds in three steps: 1) transcription of the germline transcript (GLT), 2) DNA class switch recombination (CSR), and 3) the B-cell differentiation into an Ig secreting plasma cell that is accompanied by major changes in the cell surface phenotype including the modulation of surface Igs, CD38, CD138 and the transcription factor X-box binding protein I (XBP-1), the latter which is essential for the differentiation into plasma cells [4, 5].

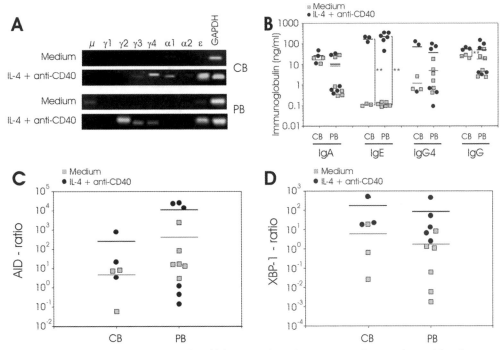

Figure 1. PCR analysis of germline transcripts (GLTs) (A), ELISA analysis of IgA, IgE, IgG and IgG₄ production (B), real-time PCR analysis of AID (C) and real-time PCR analysis of XBP-1 (D). Naïve IgD⁺ B-cells were stimulated for 4 days (A and C) or 12 days (B and D) with anti-CD40 Ab in the presence of IL-4. Secreted Ig was quantified in day 12 supernatants. Results are shown for three or six independent experiments with the horizontal lines representing the means. Observations below the detection limit were given the value of the detection limit. **: $p < .01$ (B). cDNA was conducted and GLTs, AID and XBP-1 were measured. Each GLT PCR was performed on cDNA pooled from three or six patients followed by electrophoresis on a 2% agarose gel (A). For AID and XBP-1, the results are standardized to the housekeeping gene b-actin and expressed as the ratio to the unstimulated cultures (C and D).

Cord blood (CB) B-cells produce almost no antibodies except the immunoglobulin (Ig)M isotype, indicating immaturity of the cells or the environment they reside in. Our aim was to investigate immunoglobulin class switch recombination to IgE and IgG₄ in naïve IgD⁺ B-cells in CB in comparison to adult peripheral blood (PB). We isolate naïve B-cells from buffycoats by positive selection for IgD. Such cells have not yet undergone class switching and are therefore suitable for examining the effects of cytokines and anti-CD40 on the class switch recombination and further differentiation into plasma cells.

Material and Methods

IgD⁺ B-cells from CB and PB were purified by positive selection using specific anti-IgD

mAb-coated magnetic beads as previously described [6]. Purity was routinely >90%. Cells (5×10^5 cells/ml) were stimulated with 10 ng/ml IL-4 (R&D Systems, Abingdon, U.K.) and 0.5 µg/ml anti-CD40 (Immunotech, Marseille, France) in the presence of irradiated CD32 transfected fibroblast. After 4 days of stimulation, the lymphocytes were analyzed for germline transcripts (GLTs) and Activation-Induced Deaminase (AID) by traditional and real-time PCR, respectively. After 12 days of stimulation, surface CD38 and CD138 and intracellular IgE and XBP-1 were measured by flow cytometry. Furthermore, XBP-1 mRNA were analyzed by real-time PCR and secreted IgA, IgE, IgG₄ and total IgG were measured by ELISA.

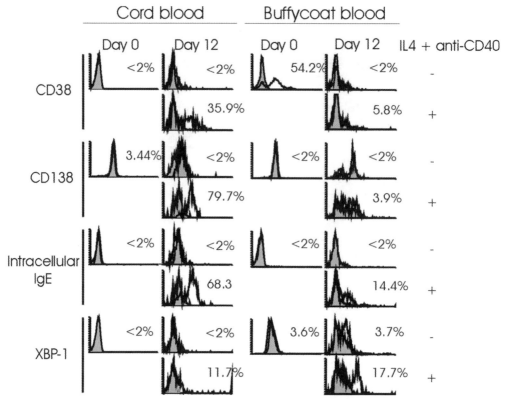

Figure 2. Flow cytometric analysis of the expression of CD38, CD138, intracellular IgE and intracellular XBP-1. Naïve IgD⁺ B-cells were stimulated and cultured for 12 days with anti-CD40 Ab in the presence of IL-4. Results are depicted as white histograms overlaying the isotype control (gray area) and are expressed in percent positive cells. One representative experiment out of three or six is shown. Isotype controls were gated at 2% and viable B-cells were gated according to low side-scatter and propidium iodide staining. Each histogram represents 5000 analyzed cells.

Results

After 4 days of stimulation with IL-4 and anti-CD40, CB and PB B-cells both up-regulated ε and γ4 GLTs compared to unstimulated samples (Figure 1A). PB B-cells furthermore up-regulated γ2 and γ3 GLTs that was not found in the CB B-cells. Low amount of GLTs were observed in the un-stimulated cells.

Using real-time PCR we measured the expression of AID, which has been found to be necessary for class switch recombination. After 4 days of culture with IL-4 and anti-CD40, CB and PB B-cells both up-regulated AID compared to unstimulated samples, however not significantly (Figure 1B).

After 12 days of stimulation with IL-4 and anti-CD40, IgA, IgE, IgG₄ and total IgG were measured by ELISA. Naïve CB B-cells did not

by themselves produce IgE or IgG₄ whereas it was possible to detect both IgA (15.2 ± 4.9 ng/ml) and IgG (21.65 ± 3.5 ng/ml) (Figure 1C). Addition of IL-4 and anti-CD40 significantly enhanced both IgE (152.7 ± 41.7 ng/ml) and IgG₄ (64.1 ± 24.2 ng/ml) production whereas only a minor increase was observed for IgA (24.9 ± 16.4 ng/ml) and IgG (50.8 ± 8.7 ng/ml). The level of Igs produced was found to be comparable to the adult B-cells.

After 12 days of stimulation with IL-4 and anti-CD40, CD38, CD138, intracellular IgE and XBP-1 were measured by flow cytometry (Figure 2). The plasma cell markers in CB B-cells were significantly differently up-regulated compared to PB B-cells. Both CD38 (35.9%), CD138 (79.7%) and intracellular IgE (68.3%) were found to be highly up-regulated. XBP1 (11.7%) however, were found in a lower level compared to the adult B-cell stimulations.

Using real-time PCR we measured the expression of XBP-1, which has been found to be necessary for plasma cell differentiation. After 12 days of culture with IL-4 and anti-CD40 CB and PB-cells both up-regulated XBP-1 compared to unstimulated samples, however not significantly (Figure 1D). The levels found in PB were comparable with the levels found in CB.

Discussion

Contrary to the adult B-cells we did not detect any CD38 positive cells in freshly isolated B-cells from cord blood. This observation might reflect the difference in differentiation stage between the cord blood B-cells and more developed adult B-cells. We also found naïve B-cells from cord blood being able to differentiate into CD38$^+$ CD138$^+$ IgE$^+$ plasma cells to a much higher level compared to the buffycoat B-cells. However, the amount of secreted IgE was the same in the two groups. Taken together, these findings indicate that B-cells from cord blood are initially "more naïve" but on the other hand more easily stimulated into plasma cells although their ability to produce Igs might be less effective compared to the adult B-cells.

References

1. Heyzer-Williams LJ, Heyzer-Williams MG: Antigen-specific memory B-cell development. Annu Rev Immunol 2005; 23:487–513.
2. Duchosal MA: B-cell development and differentiation. Semin Hematol 1997; 34:2–12.
3. Stavnezer J: Molecular processes that regulate class switching. Curr Top Microbiol Immunol 2000; 245:127–168.
4. Reimold AM et al.: Plasma cell differentiation requires the transcription factor XBP-1. Nature 2001; 412:300–307.
5. Shapiro-Shelef M, Calame K: Regulation of plasma-cell development. Nat Rev Immunol 2005; 5:230–242.
6. Hummelshoj L, Ryder LP, Poulsen LK: The role of the interleukin-10 subfamily members in immunoglobulin production by human B-cells. Scand J Immunol 2006; 64:40–47.

Lone Hummelshoj Jensen

National University Hospital, Laboratory of Medical Allergology, Allergy Clinic 7551, Blegdamsvej 9, DK-2100 Copenhagen O, Denmark, Tel. +45 35 457593, Fax +45 35 457581, E-mail l.hummelshoj@rh.dk

Single Nucleotide Polymorphisms of CD14

Are Associated with the Development of Respiratory Syncytial Virus Bronchiolitis in Japanese Children

Y. Inoue[1], N. Shimojo[1], E.J. Campos [1], A. Yamaide[2], S. Suzuki[3], T. Arima[1], T. Matsuura, M. Tomiita[1], M. Aoyagi[3], A. Hoshioka[2], A. Honda[4], and Y. Kohno[1]

1Department of Pediatrics, Graduate School of Medicine, Chiba University, Chiba, 2Chiba Children's Hospital, 3Shimosizu Hospital, 4Asahi Central Hospital, all Japan

Summary: *Background:* Respiratory syncytial virus (RSV) is the most important cause of lower respiratory tract disease in infant, and is also well known as the risk factor for the development of recurrent wheezing and bronchial asthma. In recent times, it was reported that the fusion protein of RSV binds to Toll like receptor 4 (TLR4) and CD14 and initiates Th1 response. In this study, we investigated whether genetic variations of these molecules are associated with the development of RSV bronchiolitis and recurrent wheezing after RSV bronchiolitis in Japanese population. *Methods:* We genotyped several SNPs of TLR4 and CD14 gene by PCR restriction fragment length polymorphism genotyping method, and investigated a relation between these SNPs and the development of RSV bronchiolitis or recurrent wheezing after RSV bronchiolitis in Japanese children. *Results:* We did not find the Asp299Gly and Thr399Ile of the TLR4 gene in the Japanese population. We found that the distribution of genotype of CD14 159 C/T in children with RSV bronchiolitis is same with that in controls. In contrast, the distribution of genotype of CD14 550 C/T in children with RSV bronchiolitis were significantly different from those in controls. Between infants with recurrent wheezing after RSV bronchiolitis and those without recurrent wheezing, there was no difference in the distribution of CD14 SNPs. *Conclusion:* Genetic traits relating CD14 550 C/T but not TLR4 might be important for the development of RSV bronchiolitis in the Japanese population.

Keywords: gene polymorphism, respiratory syncytial virus, bronchiolitis, asthma, innate immunity, toll like receptor, CD14

Introduction

Respiratory syncytial virus (RSV) is the most important cause of lower respiratory tract disease in infants, and is also well known as the risk factor for the development of recurrent wheezing and bronchial asthma [1]. Although the precise mechanisms for the development of asthma and allergy by RSV infection are not clear, suppressed IFN-γ production and increased IL 10 production during RSV infection may cause relative dominance of Th2 cytokine. Therefore, some differences of immune responses to RSV in infancy may be associated with the development of severe RSV infection and following asthma and allergy. In recent times, it was reported that the fusion protein of RSV binds to Toll like receptor 4 (TLR4) and CD14 [2], and the genetic variations of these molecules were associated with the development and the severity of RSV bronchiolitis [3]. In this study, we investigated whether genetic variations of these molecules are associated with the development of RSV bronchiolitis and recurrent wheezing after RSV bronchiolitis in Japanese population.

Subjects and Methods

The study population was recruited at Chiba University Hospital, Chiba Children's Hospital, Shimosizu Hospital and Asahi Central Hospital. We recruited 48 RSV bronchiolitis patients who were hospitalized because of severe RSV bronchiolitis and 80 healthy controls. RSV bronchiolitis was diagnosed by wheezing and presence of RSV antigen in nasopharyngeal secretion. Exclusion criteria included cardiac diseases, chronic respiratory diseases, previous wheezing episode, age > 24 months, prematurity. DNA was extracted from peripheral blood collected with EDTA by use of QIAamp DNA Blood Kit (Qiagen) or buccal cells by use of BuccalAmp DNA Extraction Kit (EPICENTRE), according the manufacture's instructions respectively. Genotyping of the TLR4 Asp299Gly and Thr399Ile was performed according to a protocol described elsewhere [3]. Genotyping of the CD14 159 C/T and 550 C/T were performed according to a protocol described elsewhere [3, 4]. We investigated a relation between these SNPs and the development of RSV bronchiolitis or recurrent wheezing after RSV bronchiolitis in Japanese children. All statistical analyses were performed using the program package SNPAlze ver. 4.1 (Dynacom Co. USA). The chi-square (χ^2) test and Fisher's exact test were used to compare differences in genotype or allele frequency among groups. Odds ratio, confidence intervals and p values were calculated, and p values < .05 were considered to be significant.

Results

We did not find the Asp299Gly and Thr399Ile of the TLR4 gene in the Japanese population. We found that the distribution of genotype of CD14 159 C/T in children with RSV bronchio-

Table 1. Number of subjects.

	CC	CT + TT
Healthy controls	54	65
RSV bronchiolitis patients	38	15

litis is same with that in controls. On the other hand, the distribution of genotype of CD14 550 C/T in children with RSV bronchiolitis was significantly different from those in controls (p = .007). Compared with controls, the frequency of CC genotype (p = .003, odds ratio 2.92, Table 1) and C allele (p = .027, odds ratio 2.02) were significantly higher in children with RSV bronchiolitis. Between infants with recurrent wheezing after RSV bronchiolitis and those without recurrent wheezing, there was no difference in the distribution of CD14 SNPs.

Discussion

Our present data showed for the first time the relationship between CD14 C 550 C/T and development of RSV bronchiolitis in Japanese population. The finding is in contrast to previous reports in western country [3]. This might be due to absence of TLR4 polymorphisms in Japanese population and/or different environmental factors that are associated with innate immune response via TLR4/CD14 recognition. Thus contribution of genetic polymorphisms in innate immune response to microbes including RSV varies among ethnics and environment.

References

1. Sigurs N, Gustafsson PM, Bjarnason R, Lundberg F, Schmidt S, Sigurbergsson F, Kjellman B: Severe respiratory syncytial virus bronchiolitis in infancy and asthma and allergy at age 13. Am J Respir Crit Care Med 2005; 171:137–141.
2. Kurt Jones EA, Popova L, Kwinn L, Haynes LM, Jones LP, Tripp RA, Walsh EE, Freeman MW, Golenbock DT, Anderson LJ, Finberg RW: Pattern recognition receptors TLR4 and CD14 mediate response to respiratory syncytial virus. Nat Immunol 2000; 1:398–401.

3. Tal G, Mandelberg A, Dalal I, Cesar K, Somekh E, Tal A, Oron A, Itskovich S, Ballin A, Houri S, Beigelman A, Lider O, Rechavi G, Amariglio N: Association between common Toll like receptor 4 mutations and severe respiratory syncytial virus disease. J Infect Dis 2004; 189:2057–2063.

4. Guerra S, Carla Lohman I, LeVan TD, Wright AL, Martinez FD, Halonen M: The differential effect of genetic variation on soluble CD14 levels in human plasma and milk. Am J Reprod Immunol 2004; 52(3):204–211.

Yuzaburo Inoue

Department of Pediatrics, Graduate School of Medicine, Chiba University, 1–8–1 Inohana Chuou-ku, Chiba City, Chiba, Japan 260-8670, Tel. +81 43 226-2144, Fax +81 43 226-2145, E-mail yuzaburo@cf6.so-net.ne.jp

CD8 T-Cell – Dendritic Cell Cross-Talk

K.L. Wong and D.M. Kemeny

Immunology Program and Department of Microbiology, National University of Singapore, Singapore

Summary: *Background:* We previously established that CD8 T-cells suppress in vivo IgE responses by inducing dendritic cells (DC) to produce interleukin (IL)-12. *Methods:* To investigate how CD8 T-cells could induce DCs to produce IL-12, we established an *in vitro* cell culture system in which CD8 T-cells from OT-I transgenic mice were cocultured with splenic dendritic cells that were pulsed with $^{257-264}$OVA peptide. *Results:* We find that both naive and activated CD8 T-cells could induce the upregulation of surface costimulatory markers CD40 and CD86 on DCs. However, only activated, but not naïve, CD8 T-cells induced DCs to produce IL-12p70. *Conclusion:* This study describes a novel positive feedback loop which can occur during cell mediated immunity whereby previously activated CD8 T-cells stimulate DCs to produce IL-12p70.

Keywords: CD8 T-cells, dendritic cells, interleukin-12

Introduction

CD8 T-cells have been shown to inhibit IgE responses [1, 2]. Using the prototype allergen ovalbumin (OVA), it was established that the IgE suppressive CD8 T-cells were OVA-specific, expressed the $\alpha\beta$ T-cell receptor (TCR) and were MHC-I restricted [3]. CD8 T-cell mediated suppression of IgE responses was also found to be dependent on dendritic cell derived IL-12 [4]. The ability of CD8 T-cells to downregulate Th2 and IgE responses could be attributed to their ability to "license" DCs for the effective priming of Th1 responses [5]. Consistent with this, CD8 T-cells produce IFN-γ during early interactions with DCs, which cooperates with CD40L expressing CD4 T-cells to induce IL-12 for the development of Th1 responses [6]. To investigate the ability of CD8 T-cells to induce IL-12, we used an OVA transgenic system in which CD8 T-cells from OT-I mice recognize the OVA peptide$^{257-264}$ in the context of H-2K^b. This allowed us to investigate how CD8 T-cells influence DCs during a peptide specific interaction. Furthermore, we observed that only CD8 T-cells from OVA primed mice, but not CD8 T-cells from nonimmunized mice, could suppress IgE responses via induction of DC IL-12 [4]. Hence we speculate that CD8 T-cells may need to be activated prior to acquisition of the ability to induce IL-12 production by DCs. In this study, we developed an *in vitro* system whereby peptide pulsed splenic DCs were cocultured with OT-I derived CD8 T-cells, and show that whereas both naïve and activated CD8 T-cells could induce DCs to mature, only activated CD8 T-cells could induce DCs to produce IL-12p70.

Materials and Methods

CD8 T-cells were obtained from spleens of naïve OT-I mice. CD8 T-cells were purified by density centrifugation using Ficoll-Hypaque (Amershan Biosciences) at 600 × g at room temperature for 20 min without braking, followed by positive selection using anti-CD8α MACS beads (Miltenyi Biotech). Activated CD8 T-cells were obtained by stimulation *in vitro* with 10 ng/ml PMA and 400 ng/ml ionomycin (Sigma) for two days. Dendritic cells were obtained from naïve

A

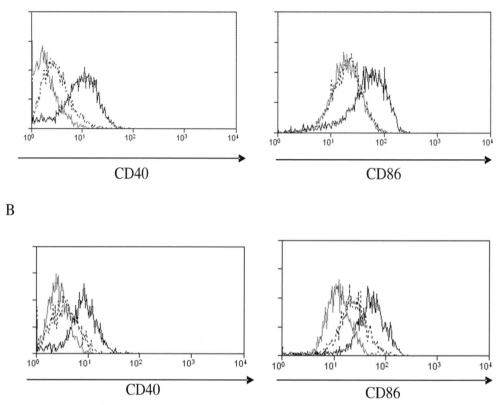

Figure 1. Upregulation of surface costimulatory molecules on DCs by CD8 T-cells (A) Upregulation of CD40 and CD86 by naïve CD8 T-cells (B) Upregulation of CD40 and CD86 by activated CD8 T-cells. Gray lines = DC + SIINFEKL peptide. Dotted lines = DC + CD8 T-cells. Black lines = DC + SIINFEKL peptide + CD8 T-cells.

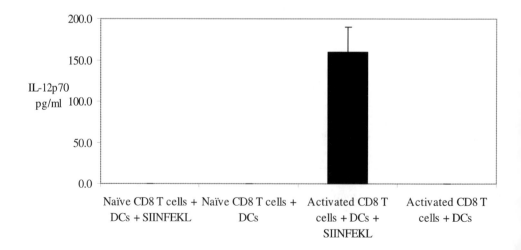

Figure 2. Activated but not naïve CD8 T-cells induced DCs to produce IL-12p70.

C57BL/6 spleens. DCs were purified by density centrifugation with 1.062 g/ml optiprep (Sigma) at 1700 × g for 10 min at 4 °C without braking, followed by positive selection using anti-CD11c MACS beads. For co-cultures, splenic DCs were pulsed with 1 μM of SIIN-FEKL peptide and subsequently washed prior to addition of OT-I CD8 T-cells in 96 well U-bottomed wells. Cells were incubated overnight and the expression of CD40 and CD86 on CD11c⁺ cells were analyzed by FACS, and the levels of IL-12p70 in supernatants were analyzed by ELISA after over-night co-culture. The medium used was RPMI 1640 supplemented with 1% nonessential amino acids, 5 μM β-mercaptoethanol, 1.0 mM sodium pyruvate, 2.0 mM L-glutamine, 100 μg/ml streptomycin and 100 IU/ml penicillin and 10% FCS (Hyclone).

Results

We first investigated whether CD8 T-cells cause DCs to upregulate surface costimulatory molecules during a peptide specific CD8-DC interaction. Control DCs, which were cultured without CD8 T-cells showed constitutive expression of CD86, consistent with the fact that splenic DCs spontaneously mature after isolation. When DCs where co-cultured with naïve CD8 T-cells without peptide, moderate upregulation of CD40 but not CD86 was observed (Figure 1A) and when previously activated CD8 T-cells were used expression of both CD40 and CD86 was increased. Significant upregulation of CD40 and CD86 on DCs was evident when peptide pulsed DCs where co-cultured with either naïve or activated CD8 T-cells. This demonstrated that both naïve and activated CD8 T-cells could upregulate surface costimulatory molecules on DCs during a peptide specific CD8 T-cell with DCs. We next compared the ability of naïve and activated CD8 T-cells to induce DCs to produce IL-12p70. Results showed that only activated but not naïve CD8 T-cells induced DCs to produce IL-12p70 during a peptide specific interaction. Control cultures of CD8 T-cells with DCs without peptide demonstrated that production

of IL-12p70 required a peptide specific interaction between activated CD8 T-cells and DCs (Figure 2). No IL-12p70 was detected with cultures containing only peptide pulsed DCs or CD8 T-cells with peptide (data not shown).

Discussion

The study shows that whereas both naïve and activated CD8 T-cells could upregulate costimulatory molecules on DCs during a peptide specific interaction, only activated CD8 T-cells could induce DCs to produce IL-12p70. We hence describe a novel positive feedback loop during cell mediated immunity whereby activated CD8 T-cells induce DCs to produce IL-12p70. The observation that activated, but not naïve CD8 T-cells could induce DCs to produce IL-12, is consistent with the notion that an effective immunological response would seek to augment itself via crosstalk and positive feedback among immune cells [5].

References

1. Renz H, Lack G, Saloga J, Schwinzer R, Bradley K, Loader J, Kupfer A, Larsen GL, Gelfand EW: Inhibition of IgE production and normalization of airways responsiveness by sensitized CD8 T-cells in a mouse model of allergen-induced sensitization. J Immunol 1994; 152:351–360.
2. Holmes BJ, MacAry PA, Noble A, Kemeny DM: Antigen-specific CD8⁺ T-cells inhibit IgE responses and interleukin-4 production by CD4⁺ T-cells. Eur J Immunol 1997; 27:2657–2665.
3. MacAry PA, Holmes BJ, Kemeny DM: Ovalbumin-specific, MHC class I-restricted, α β-positive, Tc1 and Tc0 CD8⁺ T-cell clones mediate the *in vivo* inhibition of rat IgE. J Immunol 1998; 160:580–587.
4. Thomas MJ, Noble A, Sawicka E, Askenase PW, Kemeny DM: CD8 T-cells inhibit IgE via dendritic cell IL-12 induction that promotes Th1 T-cell counter-regulation. J Immunol 2002; 168: 216–223.
5. Kalinski P, Moser M: Consensual immunity: success-driven development of T-helper-1 and T-helper-2 responses. Nat Rev Immunol 2005; 5: 251–260.

6. Mailliard RB, Egawa S, Cai Q, Kalinska A, Byk-
ovskaya SN, Lotze MT, Kapsenberg ML, Storkus
WJ, Kalinski P: Complementary dendritic cell-
activating function of CD8$^+$ and CD4$^+$ T-cells:
helper role of CD8$^+$ T-cells in the development of
T helper type 1 responses. J Exp Med 2002;
195:473–483.

David M. Kemeny

#03–05 Centre for Life Sciences (CeLS), 28 Medical Drive, Sin-
gapore 117456, Tel. +65 65165518, Fax +65 67782684, E-mail
mickdm@nus.edu.sg

Maternal Smoking in Pregnancy

Suppresses Neonatal TLR-Mediated Microbial Responses, and This Effect Is Increased by Maternal Allergy

S.L. Prescott and P.S. Noakes

School of Paediatrics and Child Health, Princess Margaret Hospital for Children, University of Western Australia, Perth, Australia

Summary: *Background:* Early life exposures have critical effects on the developing immune system and can increase allergic predisposition. In particular, there is mounting interest in factors that influence developing responses to microbial agents. This study addressed the interactive effects of two major maternal factors on early Toll-like receptor (TLR)-mediated microbial responses, namely maternal allergy and smoking in pregnancy. *Methods:* In a prospective birth cohort ($n = 122$), we compared cord-blood immune responses of neonates of smoking ($n = 60$) and nonsmoking ($n = 62$) mothers. These groups included equal numbers of allergic women (50% and 49% respectively). Neonatal cytokine responses were assessed to optimal doses of TLR2 ligand (Pansorbin 0.1%), TLR3 ligand (Poly [I:C] 30 µg/ml), TLR4 ligand (lipopolysaccharide [LPS] 10 ng/ml) and TLR9 ligands (CpG C 1.66 µg/ml). *Results:* Maternal allergy did not have consistent independent effects on TLR responses, although there was a trend for lower TLR2 (IL-6 and IL-10) and TLR4 responses (IL-10) responses in neonates of atopic mothers. Infants of smoker showed significantly attenuated TLR-mediated responses compared to infants of nonsmokers, including lower responses following TLR2 (TNFα $p = .004$; IL-6 $p = .045$; IL-10 $p = .014$), TLR3 (TNFα $p = .044$) TLR4 (TNFα $p = .034$) and TLR9 (IL-6 $p = .046$) activation. The inhibitory effects of smoking on TLR responses were significantly greater if mothers were atopic. This potentiating effect of maternal allergy was most apparent for TLR2 (IL-6), TLR3 (TNFα) and TLR4 (TNFα) responses. *Conclusions:* Maternal smoking in pregnancy also has significant effects on innate immune function that could contribute to increased risk of respiratory infections and asthma. These effects appear greater if mothers are allergic. This highlights that other early life interactions are highly relevant to the "hygiene hypothesis."

Keywords: smoking, pregnancy, cord blood, toll-like receptors, neonates, immune development

Introduction

Subtle disorders of immune function in early infancy have been implicated in the increasing susceptibility to allergic disease [1–4], presumably through early immaturity of regulatory immune function. There is accumulating evidence that activation of the immune system through innate Toll-like receptors (TLR) pathways is essential for normal immune maturation. The mounting burden of allergic T helper cell type 2 (Th2) mediated diseases and other forms of immune dysregulation, has lead to intense interest in factors that may either enhance or potentially inhibit early immune maturation through these pathways. While exposure to ambient microbial factors is known to enhance immune [5, 6], factors that could *inhibit* early immune maturation are less well documented. This study addressed the effects of two major maternal factors on early TLR-mediated microbial responses, namely *mater-*

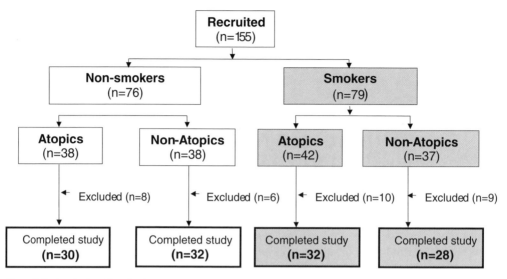

Figure 1. Study volunteer flow sheet.

nal allergy and *smoking in pregnancy*, and how these factors *interact* to influence neonatal innate immune function. While there is evidence that both of these factors can predispose to allergic airway disease, the mechanisms are not known. In addition to the well documented effects on *in utero* airway development [7–11], we and others have shown preliminary evidence that maternal smoking may also have effects on immune development [12, 13], including impaired Th1 function [13]. We speculate that the toxic effects of maternal smoking may affect development and function of innate TLR responses, and this may contribute to the well-documented susceptibility to both infection and asthma [14] in exposed infants. The main aim of this study was to examine this hypothesis, and to examine the interactive effects of these two common "exposures" in order to determine if infants at high risk of allergy (maternal allergy) are also more susceptible to any effects of maternal smoking on neonatal innate TLR-mediated immune responses.

Materials and Methods

Study Population

A prospective cohort of 122 women was pregnant women (*n* = 155), recruited from

both hospital obstetrician's rooms and antenatal clinics (including St John of God Hospital, King Edward Memorial Hospital and Osborne Park Hospital), between August 2002 and October 2004. The women were recruited into 4 approximately equal-sized groups according to both their allergy and smoking status (as shown on Figure 1). The 122 women who completed the study included approximately equal numbers of atopic smokers (*n* = 32), nonatopic smokers (*n* = 28), atopic nonsmokers (*n* = 30) and nonatopic nonsmokers (*n* = 32).

This allowed us to examine the relationship between maternal smoking, maternal allergic status and neonatal TLR responses. Maternal and family medical and allergy history and demographic information was collected using interview questionnaires administered at recruitment, usually during the last trimester. Subjects were excluded from analysis if they delivered preterm (< 36 weeks gestation), if there was any significant neonatal morbidity or disease or if cord blood was not collected at delivery

Cord blood was collected at delivery from the healthy full term neonates for the analysis of cytokine profiles. All women recruited into the study received verbal and written information about the study and signed written consent.

Maternal Atopic Status

Maternal allergy status was determined by detailed interview-questionnaire and allergen skin prick test (SPT) to common allergens including house dust mite, southern grass mix, mould mix, dog hair-dander and cockroach. A wheal size of ≥ 3 mm above the negative control was considered positive. Women were defined as allergic if they had a history of disease and one or more positive SPT.

Maternal Smoking Status

Maternal cigarette smoke exposure was determined by two methods: a) self-reporting as determined by the administration of a standardized health questionnaire and b) cotinine analysis from maternal blood measure by HPLC after solid phase extraction.

Cord Blood and TLR Functional Assays

Cord blood samples were collected from the placental vessels by venipuncture immediately after delivery. CBMC were cryopreserved after collection and subsequently batch analyzed. Upon thawing, CBMC were resuspended in AIM-V serum-free medium (Gibco Life Technologies, Grand Island, NY, USA) and cultured either alone or together with together with optimal stimulating doses of specific microbial ligands for TLR2 (Pansorbin 0.1% Calbiochem®), TLR3 (poly (I:C) 30 µg/ml, Sigma), TLR4/CD14 (lipopolysaccharide [LPS] 10 ng/ml), and TLR9 (cytosine-phosphate-guanine [CpG C] oligodeoxynucleotides, 1.66 µg/ml; Coley Pharmaceutical Group, Ottowa, Ontario, Canada). CBMC were resuspended at 2.5×10^5 cells in 250 µl (for 24 h at 37 °C in 5% CO_2) for all stimuli except for CpG (at 5×10^5 CBMC in 250 µl for 48 h). Supernatants were assayed for the presence of IL-6, IL-10 and TNFα employing commercial time resolved fluorometry (TRF) assays using matched antibody pairs from Pharmingen (Becton Dickinson, San Jose, CA, USA). The detection limits for the assays were 2.5 pg/ml for all cytokines.

Statistical Analysis

Where possible, cytokine data were log-natural transformed to obtain a log normal distribution and described by the geometric mean and 95% confidence intervals. Relationships between categorical variables were analyzed using Pearson's χ^2 test. Comparisons between continuous variables were determined by an independent Students t-test (parametric data) or Mann-Whitney U-test for nonparametric data. Nonparametric correlations were determined by Kendall's tau b to avoid "ties" in the data where a proportion of the variables of interest shared "zero" values. Multiple regression modelling was used to assess the effects of potential confounding factors. A p value < .05 was considered statistically significant for all analyses. All statistical analyses were performed using SPSS software (Version 11 for Macintosh). The interpretation of the interactive plots is outlined in the Results.

Results

Characteristics of the Study Population

Of the 155 women who registered interest, 122 completed the study. Figure 1 illustrates the flow of participants through the study. 29 women who registered interest were excluded because of missed cord blood collections. There were no significant differences in gestation, maternal age, delivery method, neonatal growth parameters, Apgar scores or infant gender between the study groups.

The Effects of Maternal Allergy Status in Neonatal TLR Function

When the population was divided by atopic status, there were no differences in the proportion of smokers in each group [atopic group; smokers $n = 32$ (51.6%)/nonatopic group; smokers $n = 28$ (46.7%)]. This allowed us to initially compare these groups to examine the effects of maternal allergy on immune function, including TLR-mediated responses (Ta-

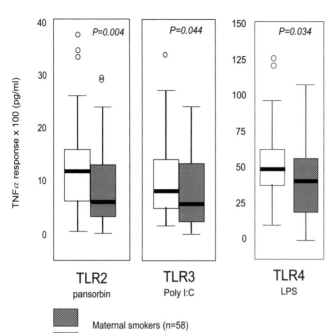

Figure 2. Effects of smoking on TNFα responses following TLR2, TLR3 and TLR4 ligation: Comparison of TNFα responses to TLR2, TLR3, and TLR4 stimulation in neonates born to smoking (shaded bars) and nonsmoking (clear bars) women. The cytokine levels shown are for the levels above unstimulated (control) cultures, and are expressed as median, IQR, 95% confidence intervals (pg/ml) as compared by the Mann Whitney U test. Significance levels are shown.

Table 1. Cord blood cytokine responses stimulated with TLR ligands (Pansorbin, poly (I:C), LPS and CpG OGN) from neonates born to atopic and nonatopic mothers[1].

Cytokine	Receptor (ligand)	Whole population				
		Atopics $n = 62$		Nonatopics $n = 60$		
		Median	IQR	Median	IQR	p^*
IL-6	TLR2 (Pansorbin)	13617	(7488, 21725)	15080	(9335, 24489)	.406
	TLR3 (poly I:C)	28993	(20032, 38420)	28417	(18084, 36387)	.466
	TLR4 (LPS)	29510	(18749, 38107)	31977	(23112, 36842)	.875
	TLR9 (CpG B#)	689	(543.78, 835.86)	621	(476.24, 765.83)	.505
	TLR9 (CpG C#)	587	(431.27, 743.25)	612	(464.05, 761.28)	.814
IL-10	TLR2 (Pansorbin)	175	(93, 411)	314	(121, 494)	.060
	TLR3 (poly I:C)	547	(360, 885)	644	(337, 1081)	.462
	TLR4 (LPS)	284	(186, 527)	337	(189, 535)	.417
	TLR9 (CpG B#)	216	(189.91, 242.97)	212	(184.98, 240.30)	.843
	TLR9 (CpG C#)	247	(213.05, 281.42)	277	(236.88, 317.74)	.257
TNFα	TLR2 (Pansorbin)	964	(410, 1467)	1048	(426, 1712)	.383
	TLR3 (poly I:C)	706	(338, 1364)	661	(429, 1400)	.703
	TLR4 (LPS)	4355	(2624, 6119)	4847	(2839, 6429)	.643
	TLR9 (CpG B)	2.5	(2.5, 3.64)	2.5	(2.5, 4.68)	.663
	TLR9 (CpG C)	2.5	(2.5, 4.95)	2.5	(2.5, 2.94)	.333

[1]Data represent levels of cytokine above background in cell culture supernatants and is expressed as median and interquartile range (IQR) pg/ml. Differences between the two groups were determined by Mann-Whitney U-test (nonparametric data) or Students t-test (parametric data). #IL-6 and IL-10 CpG B and C cytokine levels expressed as geometric mean and 95% CI. *$p < .05$ is considered to be a significant difference between the groups.

Table 2. Comparison of TLR responses according to maternal allergy and smoking status[1].

Cytokine	Receptor (ligand)	Atopics (n = 30)		Nonatopics (n = 32)		
		Median	IQR	Median	IQR	p*
IL-6	TLR2 (Pansorbin)	13851	10920, 23893	17228	11375, 24159	.808
	TLR3 (poly I:C)	28741	22733, 38684	26260	18354, 33229	.181
	TLR4 (LPS)	29509	19200, 40275	31977	24699, 38283	.786
	TLR9 (CpG C#)	679	429.43, 929.68	725	474.60, 977.14	.791
IL-10	TLR2 (Pansorbin)	232	160, 403	354	189, 553	.067
	TLR3 (poly I:C)	638	428, 869	608	382, 1181	.617
	TLR4 (LPS)	289	234, 566	333	251, 476	.674
	TLR9 (CpG C#)	232	185.72, 279.28	305	245.35, 365.35	.056
TNFα	TLR2 (Pansorbin)	1140	556, 1525	1136	639, 1927	.649
	TLR3 (poly I:C)	867	491, 1386	703	502, 1465	.739
	TLR4 (LPS)	4818	3704, 7176	4846	3060, 6159	.565
	TLR9 (CpG C)	2.5	2.5, 5.4	2.5	2.5, 5.5	.703

Smoking Group

Cytokine	Receptor (ligand)	Atopics (n = 32)		Nonatopics (n = 28)		
		Median	IQR	Median	IQR	p*
IL-6	TLR2 (Pansorbin)	11705	4568, 20162	13111	9081, 25332	.308
	TLR3 (poly I:C)	28992	13288, 35927	30198	17577, 36956	.803
	TLR4 (LPS)	29202	10439, 34755	32064	19098, 36752	.544
	TLR9 (CpG C#)	494	298.94, 690.98	482	342.24, 623.14	.919
IL-10	TLR2 (Pansorbin)	132	69, 425	249	87, 404	.312
	TLR3 (poly I:C)	538	183, 1003	667	212, 1056	.652
	TLR4 (LPS)	263	124, 457	342	151, 544	.534
	TLR9 (CpG C#)	261	209.86, 314.08	245	190.65, 299.56	.648
TNFα	TLR2 (Pansorbin)	555	199, 1230	590	343, 1580	.418
	TLR3 (poly I:C)	525	200, 1339	603	285, 1352	.437
	TLR4 (LPS)	3677	1301, 5541	4657	2537, 6668	.297
	TLR9 (CpG C)	2.5	2.5, 3.98	2.5	2.5, 2.5	.066

[1]Data represents levels of cytokine above background in cell culture supernatants and is expressed as median and interquartile range (IQR) pg/ml. Differences between the two groups were determined by Mann Whitney U-test (nonparametric data) or Students t-test (parametric data). #IL-6 and IL-10 CpG B and C cytokine levels expressed as geometric mean and 95% CI. *p < .05 is considered to be a significant difference between the groups.

ble 1). Maternal allergy was associated with reduced neonatal IL-10 responses to TLR2 (Pansorbin) stimulation, although this did not reach statistical significance (p = .060) (Table 1). This relationship was more evident when smokers were excluded from the analysis (Table 2). There were no other relationships between maternal allergy and TLR-mediated immune responses when comparing the whole population.

The Effects of Maternal Smoking on Neonatal TLR Function

We confirmed reported smoking status with cotinine levels, which were significantly higher in the smoking group (p < .001). When the population was divided by smoking status (each group having similar proportions of allergic women), we observed that infants of smoking mothers (n = 60) showed significant

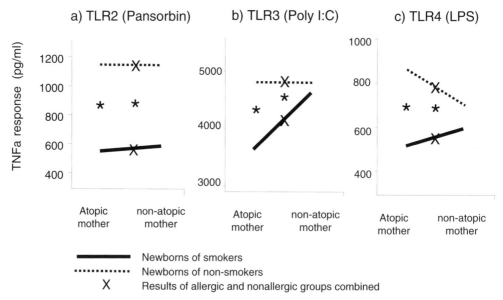

Figure 3. Interaction plots: the interactive effects of maternal smoking and maternal allergy on TNFα responses to a) TLR2, b) TLR3 and c) TLR4 stimulation. The lines show the median cytokine responses for nonsmokers (dashed lines) and smokers (continuous lines) while also comparing differences in effect in allergic women (left end of line) and nonallergic women (right end of line), or the effects in these groups combined ("X"). Groups were compared by the Mann Whitney U test and significant differences (*p < .05) are shown. A more detailed explanation of the interpretation of these interaction plots in the text.

attenuation of a number of aspects of innate TLR-mediated responses compared to infants of nonsmokers (*n* = 62), as described in more detail elsewhere [15]. This included significantly lower cytokine responses following TLR2 (TNFα *p* = .004; IL-6 *p* = .045; IL-10 *p* = .014), TLR3 (TNFα *p* = .044) TLR4 (TNFα *p* = .034) and TLR9 (IL-6 *p* = .046) activation. The differences in TNFα responses (to TLR2, 3 and 4) are shown on Figure 2.

Differential Effects of Maternal Smoking in Infants at High Risk of Allergy?

Next we determined if infants at high risk of allergy (maternal allergy) are also more susceptible to the effects of maternal smoking. We used interaction plots (Figure 3) to examine the effect of maternal allergy on the relationship between maternal smoking and immune responses. This allowed us to examine any change in these relationships according to maternal allergy (as indicated by the gradient of the "effect" lines). The degree of "separa-

tion" between each point of the "effect-line" indicates the effect of smoking on immune function (i.e., at the "allergic mother" or "non-allergic mother" ends of the line, or at the midpoint "x" which represents the effect when allergic and nonallergic groups are combined). Thus, the gradient of the lines indicates the effects of maternal allergy on immune function. Specifically, a "zero gradient" implies no effect of maternal allergy, whereas a steeper gradient indicates a change in the effect of smoking as a result of maternal allergic status. Parallel lines (regardless of gradient) indicate no interactive effects, whereas convergent/divergent lines indicate that the effects of maternal smoking vary with maternal allergy status.

Figure 3 illustrates these relationships for TNFα cytokine responses to TLR2 (Pansorbin), TLR3 (poly (I:C)) and TLR4 (LPS) ligands. While TNFα responses (to TLR2, 3 and 4 activation) were significantly attenuated in smokers, this was only seen in infants of atopic mothers or the combined group (for TLR2: *p* = .014, TLR3: *p* = .048, and TLR4: *p* = .014), with no significant effects of smoking in the

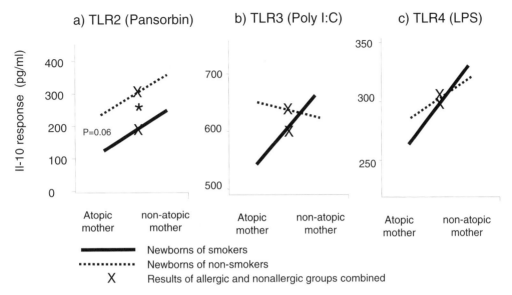

Figure 4. Interactive effects of maternal smoking and maternal allergy on IL-10 responses to a) TLR2, b) TLR3, and c) TLR4 stimulation. As for Figure 3, the lines show the median cytokine responses for nonsmokers (dashed lines) and smokers (continuous lines) while also comparing differences in effect in allergic women (left end of line) and nonallergic women (right end of line), or the effects in these groups combined ("X"). Groups were compared by the Mann Whitney U test and significant differences (*p < .05) are shown.

nonatopic group. These effects of maternal atopy were most apparent (divergent slopes) for TLR3 and TLR4 stimulation (Figure 3b and c respectively). Although there was a trend in the nonatopic group for smokers to have impaired TNFα responses to TLR2 this did not reach statistical significance (p = .094). These findings indicate that the effects of smoking on TNFα responses are significantly enhanced by maternal allergy. Thus, babies with atopic mothers who also smoked had the lowest TNFα responses to microbial agents and this was most evident compared with the subgroup of babies with nonatopic mothers who did not smoke (for TLR2: p = .011, TLR3: p = .081, and TLR4: p = .050).

As noted above, both maternal smoking (p = .014) and allergy (p = .06) were associated with attenuated IL-10 responses to TLR2 stimulation, however these effects were independent. This is illustrated on the interaction plot (Figure 4a) which shows sloping but parallel lines. Thus, IL-10 responses were lowest in babies who had allergic mothers who also smoked, most notably in comparison with babies with neither of these risk factors (non-

smoking nonatopic mothers) (p = .006). Although the effects of maternal smoking on neonatal TLR3 IL-10 responses appeared greater in the allergic group, this was not statistically significant (Figure 4b). There was a trend for lower TLR4 induced IL-10 with maternal allergy (Figure 4b) this was not statistically significant, and there was no difference in smokers and nonsmokers. For IL-6 responses (not shown) the attenuated responses to TLR2 stimulation (Pansorbin) in neonates of smoking mothers (p = .045) was also more evident if mothers were atopic (data not shown) although this was not significant (p = .069) probably because of the reduced numbers in the subgroup analysis.

Discussion

As two major risk factors for allergy and asthma, the purpose of this analysis was to determine the interactive effects of "maternal allergy" and "maternal smoking" on neonatal innate immune function. Our findings indicate that maternal smoking may have adverse effects on TLR mediated innate immune function, and that these effects may be more significant in neonates who also have allergic mothers.

The effects of smoking on neonatal TLR function in this population [15] is a novel finding, which has not been previously described to our knowledge. We speculate that these effects may not only contribute to the increased risk of infection [14], but also be implicated in the increased rates of other forms of chronic inflammatory respiratory disease seen in these children [16, 17]. Although the most recent systematic review by Strachan in 1998 [18] did not find any conclusive associations between "allergy" and parental smoking, this did not include the results of a more recent study by Kulig et al. which reported significantly higher risk of sensitization (odds ratio: 2.3, 95% C.I.: 1.1–4.6) in children exposure to maternal smoking compared with unexposed children [19]. Many previous studies have shown associations between parental smoking and allergic outcomes [19–27], although this has been variable. It is possible that more recently recognized genetic polymorphisms, which influence susceptibility to the effects of cigarette smoke [28], could account for some of the differences between studies.

Our current findings could provide an important pathway through which maternal smoking could potentiate the development of allergy. Innate immune pathways play an important role in mediating the protective environmental effects of microflora, as suggested by recent studies where microbial exposure in pregnancy was associated with increased gene TLR expression (of TLR2 and TLR4) and reduced risk of allergic sensitization (adjusted odds ratio 0.58; 95% CI 0.39–0.86) [5]. In the present study we have shown direct effects of smoking on neonatal APC function, detected as impaired innate responses to microbial stimulation. Other studies have also shown *in vitro* immunosuppressive effect of nicotine on APC (DC) function, including as antigen capturing, cytokine production (particularly IL-12 production), and eventually T-cell priming and polarization [29]. It could be argued that persistent immaturity of APC responses to

bacteria could interfere with microbial-driven Th1 maturation. This has implications for allergic risk, as impaired Th1 function in the perinatal period has been linked with allergic risk in many studies ([1–4] and others). At this stage it is not clear how long the effects of smoking on APC function might persist in the postnatal period, and further studies are needed to examine the longitudinal effects on the development of allergen-specific memory.

Our findings also suggest that children at "high risk" of allergy (with maternal allergy) may be more susceptible to these effects. Although the mechanisms are not clear, there is now preliminary evidence that high-risk neonates may have alterations in TLR expression [30] and function [31]. High risk neonates have also been noted to have altered generation of putative T regulatory cell populations after LPS stimulation, presumably through TLR4 pathways [32]. In our study we did not see any significant direct effects of maternal atopy on TLR2 responses, although there was a trend for lower IL-10 responses to Pansorbin ($p = .060$). While Smoking also had independent effects on TLR2 responses the effect of allergy was greatest if mothers also smoked (Figure 3). Although there was a nonsignificant trend for lower IL-10 responses following TLR4 activation (Figure 4), we did not see effects of maternal atopy on other TLR responses which is also consistent with the findings of Amoudruz et al. [31].

In summary, our findings lend support to the emerging hypothesis that both genetic and environmental exposures can influence early TLR mediated immune responses, and that this may have implications for subsequent allergy risk. We have shown that maternal smoking adversely effects neonatal TLR function, and that infants at high risk of allergy (maternal allergy) are also more susceptible to these effects. Follow-up studies are needed to determine if these factors make children more resistant to the protective effects of microbial stimuli. Our findings highlight the complexity of interactive effects in this period and demonstrated that other early factors are highly relevant to the "hygiene hypothesis."

Acknowledgments

We wish to acknowledge the staff and patients who assisted in this study. We are particularly grateful to the obstetricians and midwives at King Edward Memorial Hospital and St John of God Hospital, Subiaco, Western Australia. Finally, we wish to acknowledge Ms Elaine Pascoe for statistical advice. Prof. Prescott if funded by National Health and Medical Council (of Australia).

References

1. Kondo N, Kobayashi Y, Shinoda S et al.: Reduced interferon-γ production by antigen-stimulated cord blood mononuclear cells is a risk factor of allergic disorders – 6-year follow-up study. Clin Exp Allergy 1998; 28:1340–1344.
2. Tang MLK, Kemp AS, Thorburn J, Hill D: Reduced interferon-γ secretion in neonates and subsequent atopy. Lancet 1994; 344:983–985.
3. Rinas U, Horneff G, Wahn V: Interferon-γ production by cord blood mononuclear cells is reduced in newborns with a family history of atopic disease and is independent from cord blood IgE levels. Ped Allergy Immunol 1993; 4:60–64.
4. Prescott SL, Macaubas C, Smallacombe T, Holt BJ, Sly PD, Loh R, Holt PG: Reciprocal age-related patterns of allergen-specific T-cell immunity in normal vs. atopic infants. Clin Exp Allergy 1998; 28(Suppl. 5):39–44; discussion 50–51.
5. Ege MJ, Bieli C, Frei R et al.: Prenatal farm exposure is related to the expression of receptors of the innate immunity and to atopic sensitization in school-age children. J Allergy Clin Immunol 2006; 117:817–823.
6. Blumer N, Herz U, Wegmann M, Renz H: Prenatal lipopolysaccharide-exposure prevents allergic sensitization and airway inflammation, but not airway responsiveness in a murine model of experimental asthma. Clin Exp Allergy 2005; 35:397–402.
7. Brown RW, Hanrahan JP, Castille RG, Tager IB: Effect of maternal smoking during pregnancy on passive respiratory mechanics in early infancy. Pediatr Pulmonol 1995; 19:23–28.
8. Hanrahan JP, Tager IB, Segal MR, Tosteson TD, Vastile RG, Van Vunakis H, Weiss ST, Speizer FE: The effect of maternal smoking during pregnancy on early infant lung function. Am Rev Respir Dis 1992; 145:1129–1135.
9. Hoo A, Matthias H, Dezateux C, Costeloe K, Stocks J: Respiratory function among preterm infants whose mothers smoked during pregnancy. Am J Respir Crit Care Med 1998; 158:700–705.
10. Lodrup Carlsen KC, Jaakkola JJ, Nafstad P, Carlsen KH: In utero exposure to cigarette smoking influences lung function at birth. European Respiratory Journal 1997; 10:1774–1779.
11. Stick SM, Burton PR, Gurrin L, Sly PD, LeSouef PN: Effects of maternal smoking during pregnancy and a family history of asthma on respiratory function in newborn infants. Lancet 1996; 348:1060–1064.
12. Devereux G, Barker RN, Seaton A: Antenatal determinants of neonatal immune responses to allergens. Clin Exp Allergy 2002; 32:43–50.
13. Noakes PS, Holt PG, Prescott SL: Maternal smoking in pregnancy alters neonatal cytokine responses. Allergy 2003; 58:1053–1058.
14. Jedrychowski W, Flak E: Maternal smoking during pregnancy and postnatal exposure to environmental tobacco smoke as predisposition factors to acute respiratory infections. Environmental Health Perspectives 1997; 105:302–306.
15. Noakes P, Hale J, Thomas R, Lane C, Devadason SG, Prescott SL: Maternal smoking is associated with impaired neonatal Toll-like receptor (TLR) mediated immune responses. Submitted.
16. Chan-Yeung M, Dimich-Ward H: Respiratory health effects of exposure to environmental tobacco smoke. Respirology 2003; 8:131–139.
17. Monteil MA, Joseph G, Chang Kit C, Wheeler G, Antoine RM: Smoking at home is strongly associated with symptoms of asthma and rhinitis in children of primary school age in Trinidad and Tobago. Pan American Journal of Public Health 2004; 16:193–198.
18. Strachan DP, Cook DG: Health effects of passive smoking. 5. Parental smoking and allergic sensitization in children. Thorax 1998; 53:117–123.
19. Kulig M, Bergmann R, Klettke U, Wahn V, Tacke U, Wahn U: Natural course of sensitization to food and inhalant allergens during the first 6 years of life. J Allergy Clin Immunol 1999; 103:1173–1179.
20. Martinez FD, Antognoni G, Macri F, Bonci E, Midulla F, De Castro G, Ronchetti R: Parental smoking enhances bronchial responsiveness in nine-year-old children. Am Rev Respir Dis 1988; 138:518–523.
21. Weiss ST, Tager IB, Munoz A, Speizer FE: The relationship of respiratory infections in early childhood to the occurrence of increased levels of bronchial responsiveness and atopy. Am Rev Respir Dis 1985; 131:573–578.

22. el-Nawawy A, Soliman AT, el-Azzouni O, el-AmerS , Demian S, el-Sayed M: Effect of passive smoking on frequency of respiratory illnesses and serum immunoglobulin-E (IgE) and interleukin-4 (IL-4) concentrations in exposed children. J Trop Pediatr 1996; 42:166–169.

23. Wjst M, Heinrich J, Liu P, Dold S, Wassmer G, Merkel G, Huelsse C, Wichmann H: Indoor factors and IgE levels in children. Allergy 1994; 49:766–771.

24. Ronchetti R, Macri F, Ciofetta F, Indinnimeo L, Cutrera R, Bonci E, Antognoni G, Martinez FD: Increased serum IgE and increased prevalence of eosinophilia in 9-year-old children of smoking parents. J Allergy Clin Immunol 1990; 86(3 Pt 1):400–407.

25. Soyseth V, Kongerud J, Boe J: Postnatal maternal smoking increases the prevalence of asthma but not of bronchial hyperresponsiveness or atopy in their children. Chest 1995; 107:389–394.

26. Halonen M, Stern D, Lyle S, Wright A, Taussig LM, Martinez FD: Relationship of total serum IgE levels in cord and 9-month sera of infants. Clin Exp Allergy 1991; 21:235.

27. Lindfors A, van Hage-Hamsten M, Rietz H, Wickman M, Nordvall SL: Influence of interaction of environmental risk factors and sensitization in young asthmatic children. J Allergy Clin Immunol 1999; 104:755.

28. Kabesch M, Hoefler C, Carr D, Leupold W, Weiland SK, von Mutius E: Glutathione S transferase deficiency and passive smoking increase childhood asthma. Thorax 2004; 59:569–573.

29. Nouri-Shirazi M, Guinet E: Evidence for the immunosuppressive role of nicotine on human dendritic cell functions. Immunology 2003; 109:365–373.

30. Krauss-Etschmann S, Hartl D, Heinrich D et al.: Association between levels of Toll-like receptors 2 and 4 and CD14 mRNA and allergy in pregnant women and their offspring. Clin Immunol 2006; 118:292–299.

31. Amoudruz P, Holmlund U, Malmstrom V, Trollmo C, Bremme K, Scheynius A, Sverremark-Ekstrom E: Neonatal immune responses to microbial stimuli: is there an influence of maternal allergy? J Allergy Clin Immunol 2005; 115:1304–1310.

32. Haddeland U, Karstensen AB, Farkas AB et al.: Putative regulatory T-cells are impaired in cord blood from neonates with hereditary allergy risk. Pediatr Allergy Immunol 2005; 16:104–112.

S.L. Prescott

School of Paediatrics and Child Health, University of Western Australia, Princess Margaret Hospital for Children, GPO Box D184, Perth, Western Australia 6840

The Molecular Basis of IgE-Mediated Autoreactivity

R. Crameri, A. Limacher, A.G. Glaser, S. Zeller, C. Rhyner, and M. Weichel

Swiss Institute of Allergy and Asthma Research (SIAF), Davos, Switzerland

Summary: *Background:* IgE-mediated reactivity to self antigens is a phenomenon often observed in long lasting atopic diseases. Many of the structures involved in such reactions are phylogenetically conserved structures. *Methods:* The crystal structures of recombinantly produced allergens showing extended sequence homology to human proteins have been solved and compared to the crystal structures of the corresponding human proteins. *Results:* The crystal structures of MnSOD (Asp f 6) and cyclophilin (Asp f 11) of *Aspergillus fumigatus*, as well as the crystal structures of cyclophilin (Mala s 6) and thioredoxin (Mala s 13) of *Malassezia sympodialis* have now been solved. Extensive comparisons of these crystal structures with the crystal structures of the corresponding human enzymes revealed conserved folds and patches of conserved amino acids distributed all over the entire linear sequences of the molecules forming coherent, potentially conformational IgE-binding epitopes on the surface. In contrast to the extended sequence identity at the primary structure level, only 10–15% of the identical amino acids of the molecules are solvent exposed and thus able to contribute to antigen/antibody interactions. *Conclusions:* Reactivity to self antigens showing sequence homology with environmental recombinant allergens can clearly be traced back to conserved amino acid residues clustered on the surface of the IgE-binding molecules.

Keywords: allergy, allergens, cloning, crystal structures, autoreactivity, self antigens

Direct screening of a human lung cDNA library displayed on phage surface with solid-phase immobilized serum of patients suffering from long lasting allergic asthma and atopic eczema revealed more than 100 complete and partial sequences potentially encoding IgE-binding self-antigens [1]. Among these the phylogenetically highly conserved MnSOD, ribosomal P₂ protein, thioredoxin, heat shock protein, and cyclophilin, show relevant sequence identity to common environmental allergens [2–5]. The human self antigens MnSOD, cyclophilin A, B, and C, and thioredoxin produced as highly pure recombinant proteins show the expected enzymatic activity, and thus native like folding. They have been demonstrated to induce specific T-cell proliferation in PBMC's of individuals sensitized to homologous environmental allergens, to bind IgE in ELISA and Western blot analyses *in vitro*, and to induce immediate Type I hypersensitivity reactions in skin tests. These reactions,

so far only observed in chronic inflammatory forms of allergy like asthma [3], atopic eczema [6], and occupational exposure [7], are likely to contribute to the perpetuation of the allergy-related symptoms. The crystal structures of human MnSOD (PDB code 1ABM) cyclophilin (PDB code 2CPL) and thioredoxin (PDB code 1ERU) have been solved in contexts outside the field of allergy. In order to compare structural features on the surface of cross-reactive allergens, high-resolution crystal structures with all loops and surface residues well defined are a prerequisite. The solved structures of Asp f 6 (MnSOD), Mala s 6 (cyclophilin), and Mala s 13 (thioredoxin) with resolutions of 2 Å [2], 1.5 Å [8], and 1.41 Å [4], respectively, meet these requirements. While the only method allowing a complete definition of a B-cell epitope is co-crystallization of the allergen with a monoclonal antibody Fab fragment and solving the structure of the complex, a simple approach to identify potentially cross-reactive B-cell epitopes is the determination of shared features of cross-reactive allergens on sequence and structure level. Only conserved amino acids at primary structure level that are solvent exposed in cross-reactive structures are potentially involved in cross-reactivity. Asp f 6, Mala s 6, and Mala s 13 share 46%, 60%, and 45% sequence identity with human MnSOD, cyclophilin B, and thioredoxin at primary structure level, respectively. Combination of these data with data on the solvent exposure of these amino acid residues in the three-dimensional structures, and thus accessibility for antibody binding, allows identifying amino acids that are potentially involved in IgE-mediated cross-reactivity. Superposition of all three allergen structures with the structures of their human homologs reveals in all cases large structural similarities with minor deviations in a few loops. In spite of the high identity at primary sequence level, less than 30% of the identical amino acids are solvent-exposed to an extend allowing accessibility for antigen-antibody interactions. The identical solvent-exposed residues, dispersed over the whole length in the protein sequences, become clustered on a few continuous patches on the surface of the molecules. The solvent-accessible surface areas defined by these patches vary between $400–1000\,\text{Å}^2$ and are formed by 9–15 amino acid residues on different loops. These predicted B-cell epitopes are in agreement with the structure of known B-cell epitopes which occupy a buried surface in the range of $540–890\,\text{Å}^2$ and are formed by 10–20 amino acids [9]. We conclude that autoreactivity of the presented self antigens is due to 2–3 conformational B-cell epitopes formed by identical amino acids in the context of highly conserved backbone structures.

Acknowledgments

Work supported by the Swiss National Science Foundation grants no. 31–63382.00/2 and 310000–112540 and by the OPO-Foundation, Zürich.

References

1. Crameri R, Kodzius R, Konthur Z, Lehrach H, Blaser K, Walter G: Tapping allergen repertoires by advanced cloning technologies. Int Arch Allergy Immunol 2001; 124:43–47.
2. Flückiger S, Mittl PRE, Scapozza L, Fijten H, Folkers G, Grütter MG, Blaser K, Crameri R: Comparison of the crystal structures of the human manganese superoxide dismutase and the homologous Aspergillus fumigatus allergen at 2-Å resolution. J Immunol 2002; 168:1267–1272.
3. Mayer C, Appenzeller U, Seelbach H, Achatz G, Oberkofler H, Breitenbach M, Blaser K, Crameri R: Humoral and cell-mediated autoimmune reactions to human acidic ribosomal p_2 protein in individuals sensitized to Aspergillus fumigatus P_2 protein. J Exp Med 1999; 189:1507–1512.
4. Limacher A: Structural characterization of cross-reactive allergens. PhD Thesis No. 16075, Swiss Federal Institute of Technology (ETH) Zürich, 2005.
5. Limacher A, Kloer DP, Flückiger S, Folkers G, Crameri R, Scapozza L: The crystal structure of Aspergillus fumigatus reveals 3D domain swapping of a central element. Structure 2006, in press.
6. Schmid-Grendelmeier P, Flückiger S, Disch R, Trautmann A, Wüthrich B, Blaser K, Scheynius A, Crameri R: IgE-mediated and T-cell-mediated autoimmunity against manganese superoxide dismutase in atopic individuals. J Allergy Clin Immunol 2005; 115:1068–1075.
7. Weichel M, Glaser AG, Ballmer-Weber BK, Schmid-Grendelmeier P, Crameri R: Wheat and maize thioredoxins: a novel cross-reactive cereal allergen family related to baker's asthma. J Allergy Clin Immunol 2006; 117:676–681.
8. Glaser AG, Limacher A, Flückiger S, Scheynius A, Scapozza L, Crameri R: Cross-reactivity and crystal structure of the Malassezia sympodialis Mala s 6 allergen, a member of he cyclophilin pan-allergen family. Biochem J 2006; 396:41–59.
9. Padlan EA: X-ray crystallography of antibodies. Adv Protein Chem 1996; 49:57–133.

Reto Crameri

Head Molecular Allergology, Swiss Institute of Allergy and Asthma Research (SIAF), Obere Strasse 22, CH-7270 Davos, Switzerland, Tel. +41 81 410-08-48, Fax +41 81 410-08-40, E-mail crameri@siaf.uzh.ch

The Stromal Microenvironment Is a Potent Regulator of Dendritic Cell Function

A. Saalbach, C. Klein, U. Anderegg, C. Gebhardt, F. Kauer, M. Averbeck, and J.C. Simon

Dept. of Dermatology, Venerology and Allergology, Leipzig University Medical Center, Germany

Summary: *Background:* To trigger effective T-cell-mediated immune response dendritic cells (DC) have to migrate from peripheral tissues such as the epidermis via dermis into locally draining lymph nodes where they present antigen to naïve T-cells. During this migration DC undergo distinct phenotypic and functional changes termed collectively DC maturation. *Methods/Date Base:* Our recent findings that various components of the stromal microenvironment that DC encounter during their travel from peripheral epithelia to lymphoid tissues are reviewed in the light of its role in the regulation of immune function. *Results:* For the regulation of DC functions different components of the extracellular matrix are very important. Osteopontin (OPN) and Hyaluronan (HA) and small Hyaluronan fragments (sHA) interact with CD44 on DC. OPN induced chemotactic DC migration to lymph nodes and enhanced the DC capacity for Th1 polarization. Immunophenotypic maturation of human monocyte-derived DC and an increased allostimulatory capacity of DC were induced by sHA. Furthermore it could be shown that the local stromal microenvironment instruct DC to induce tissue-specific homing of T-cells. Beside the extracellular matrix stromal cells and their mediators are also potent regulators of DC functions. In interaction studies of DC with human dermal fibroblasts we could demonstrate that DC have the capacity to adhere specifically to the fibroblasts in vitro and in vivo via Thy-1 and ICAM-1 on fibroblasts and Mac-1 on DC. Moreover we found that the interaction of immature DC with fibroblasts induce the maturation of DC dependent on cell-cell contact as well as on soluble mediators. *Conclusion:* The stromal microenvironment actively participates in regulation of DC function resulting in the maturation, activation and/or differentiation of DC und thus, is involved in the control of immune responses.

Keywords: stromal microenvironment, dendritic cells

Functions of Dendritic Cells

Dendritic cells (DC) are the most potent antigen-presenting cells with key functions in induction of cell mediated immunity. They reside in and traffic through nonlymphoid peripheral tissues, continuously surveying the environment for invading microorganisms. Under steady-state conditions and in the absence of microbial stimulation or inflammation, apparently immature DC capture antigens (i.e., from apoptotic tissue cells), transport them to secondary lymphoid organs [1, 2] and are involved in the maintenance of tolerance. In contrast, the contact of DC with "danger signals" such as microbial agents or inflammatory mediators induces the maturation of DC resulting in an increase of their expression of major histocompatibility complex (MHC) molecules, co-stimulatory molecules, cytokines and an enhancement of their migratory capacity [3]. The mature DC migrate from the periphery to the T-cell zone of secondary lymphoid organs [4] where they induce T-cell dependent immune responses. As DC1 (high secretion of IL-12) or DC2 (low IL-12 secretion) they are able to polarize naïve T-helper (Th)-cells toward either a Th1 (IFN-γ secreting) or Th2 (IL-4 secreting) phenotype, respectively, thereby affecting the outcome of an immune response.

When traveling from peripheral to lymphoid tissues DC interact with the stromal microenvironment composed of different cells, the extracellular matrix and soluble mediators. There is accumulating evidence that components of the stromal microenvironment play an important role in the regulation of DC functions and in the priming of DC.

The Role of Osteopontin (OPN) in Dendritic Cell Migration and Activation

OPN, a molecule of the extracellular matrix is a highly acidic glycosylated phosphoprotein that contains an RGD integrin binding motif. It is secreted by a variety of nonimmune and immune cells. OPN is involved in bone formation, exerts chemotactic effects on T-cells and macrophages, and has been shown to have Th1 cytokine-like properties [5]. Weiss et al. [6] could show, that OPN is crucially involved in DC migration from the skin to regional lymph nodes during the sensitization phase of contact hypersensitivity (CHS). OPN interacts with both CD44 and αv on DC, thereby inducing chemotactic DC migration. Further, they show that OPN-deficient mice are compromised in their ability to attract DC to draining lymphatic organs and have an impaired CHS response to Trinitro-chloro-benzene (TNCB). Further it is known, that OPN functionally activates myeloid-type DC, augmenting their expression of HLA-DR, costimulatory molecules, and adhesion molecules, induces their Th1-promoting tumor necrosis factor α (TNF-α) and interleukin-12 (IL-12) secretion, and enhances their allostimulatory capacity [5].

The Role of Hyaluronan in Dendritic Cell Migration and Activation

Hyaluronan (HA) is a ubiquitous extracellular matrix component, present at high concentrations in the skin, where it is synthesized primarily by dermal fibroblasts and by epidermal keratinocytes. In normal skin, HA exists as a high molecular weight polymer but is cleaved into small fragments (sHA) at sites of inflammation [7, 8]. HA and sHA are able to interact with CD44 molecules on dendritic cells, but only sHA induced immunophenotypic maturation of human monocyte-derived DC (upregulation of HLA-DR, B7–1/2, CD83, downregulation of CD115) [7]. Likewise, only sHA increased DC production of the cytokines IL-1β, TNF-α, and IL-12 as well as their allostimulatory capacity [7, 8]. Furthermore we could show, that the activation of DC through sHA is mediated via the Toll-like receptor 4 (TLR-4) [9].

The Importance of Microenvironment and DC for T-Cell Homing

The transmigration of T-cells through the endothelial cell barrier into the tissue requires different adhesion molecules on the endothelial cells and the expression of corresponding receptors on T-cells (homing receptors). There are many evidences that DC apart from T-cell activation are also important for providing these T-cell-homing instructions recruiting T-cells to the inflamed tissue.

Among other things we could show, that the subcutaneous immunization of TNBS-derivatized DC into naïve syngeneic recipient mice resulted in a contact hypersensitivity responses (CHS), whereas intravenous injected TNBS-DC failed to induce CHS [10]. Further it showed up that intracutaneous, but not intravenous injection of bone marrow-derived dendritic cells induced skin-homing CD8+ T-cells with up-regulated E-selectin ligand expression. In contrast, intraperitoneal injection induced T-cells expressing the gut-homing integrin α4β7 [11]. Our results suggest a crucial role for the tissue microenvironment and dendritic cells in the instruction of T-cells for tissue-selective homing.

The Role of Stromal Cells and Their Soluble Mediators in Dendritic Cell Maturation and Differentiation

Stromal cells such as fibroblasts, endothelial cells or macrophages display different functional properties like migratory capacity, extracellular matrix production and degradation and contractility depending on anatomical site or disease status [12]. Thus, it seems plausible that DC may receive instructions from endothelial cells, stromal fibroblasts and their secreted products. Berthier et al. [13] showed, that soluble factors of fibroblasts inhibit the IL-12 production of spleenic DC and thus also the stimulation of type 1 immune responses. Furthermore recent evidences suggest that the stromal microenvironment directly affects the behavior and differentiation of DC. For example, endothelial cells are able to influence the differentiation and activation of DC [14, 15] and Zhang et al. [16] could show that the interaction of DC and endothelial-like spleenic stromal cells drives mature dendritic cells to differentiate into regulatory dendritic cells. This type of DC activates T-cells but inhibits the T-cell proliferation.

Also influences of the tumor microenvironment can affect DC. Thus Gabrilovich et al. [17] and Katsenelson et al. [18] show that the production of soluble factors by the tumor cells impairs the differentiation of DC from progenitor cells and thereby inhibits the antigen presentation.

These first data point out, that different tissue-microenvironments are involved crucially in maturation and differentiation of DC. Thus they are able to initiate, regulate or inhibit immune responses.

Fibroblasts are an extremely heterogeneous multifunctional cell population and their role in wound healing, developmental processes and tumor development is well established [19]. Nevertheless, immunologists have regarded fibroblast activation as relatively unimportant in regulating immune responses and have focused on cellular interactions between lymphocytes, macrophages and dendritic cells, which all generate antigen-specific responses [20]. However fibroblasts are capable of producing various paracrine immune modulators such as peptide growth factors, cytokines, chemokines and inflammatory mediators [21]. Additionally, they exhibit a pattern of adhesion receptors and costimulatory molecules such as CD40 [22]. Furthermore, there is abundant evidence that fibroblasts taken from diseased tissues display a fundamentally different phenotype compared with fibroblasts taken from normal tissues at the same anatomical site [23, 24]. In conclusion, fibroblasts represent not only purely structural elements but they are also active participants in the regulation of inflammation and immune responses.

We found that in vitro human DC have the capacity to adhere specifically to human dermal fibroblasts via the interaction of the β2-integrin on DC and Thy-1 (CD90) and ICAM-1 on fibroblasts. Moreover, in the dermis of an evolving cutaneous immune response such as allergic contact dermatitis, β2-integrin-positive DC are found in close apposition to Thy-1/ICAM-1-positive fibroblasts. Furthermore we could show that many maturation markers among them CD80, CD83, CD86, CD40 and HLA-DR were induced or up-regulated on DC upon co-culture with fibroblasts. Separation of DC and fibroblasts by transwell inserts revealed, that both direct cell-cell contact as well as soluble mediators are responsible for the fibroblast-induced maturation of DC. Based on preliminary results we suppose that adhesion mediated by β2-integrin on DC and Thy-1/ICAM-1 on fibroblasts results in a dramatic stimulation of autocrine TNF-α secretion by DC, which in turn induces full DC maturation.

Summary

The stromal microenvironment is a potent regulator of dendritic cell function. Besides the effects of extracellular matrix components like Hyaluronan, small Hyaluronan fragments and Osteopontin on dendritic cell migration and activation, the interaction of tissue microenvironment and dendritic cells plays a crucial role in the instruction of T-cell homing. Our recent data showed that stromal cells are involved in the regulation of maturation and differentiation of DC and thus in regulation of immune responses.

References

1. Balazs M, Martin F, Zhou T, Kearney JF: Blood dendritic cells interact with splenic marginal zone B-cells to initiate T-independent immune responses. Immunity 2002; 17:341–352.
2. Huang F-P, Platt N, Wykes M, Major JR, Powell TJ, Jenkins CD, MacPherson GG: A discrete subpopulation of dendritic cells transports apoptotic intestinal epithelial cells to T-cell areas of mesenteric lymph nodes. J Exp Med 2000; 191:435–444.
3. Tan JKH, O'Neill HC: Maturation requirements for dendritic cells in T-cell stimulation leading to tolerance versus immunity. J Leukoc Biol Aug 2005;78:319–324.
4. Sallusto F, Palermo B, Lenig D, Miettinen M, Matikainen S, Julkunen I, Forster R, Burgstahler R, Lipp M, Lanzavecchia A: Distinct patterns and kinetics of chemokine production regulate dendritic cell function. Eur J Immunol 1999; 29:1617–1625.
5. Renkl AC, Wussler J, Eggers T, Maier CS, Ahrens T, Martin S, Liaw L, Kon S, Uede T, Hirschfeld G, Simon JC, Weiss JM: Th1 cytokine-like properties of osteopontin on T-cells, macrophages, and dendritic cells in type 1 immune responses. Allergy Clin Immunol Int: J World Allergy Org 2002; Suppl. 2.
6. Weiss JM, Renkl AC, Maier CS, Kimmig M, Liaw L, Ahrens T, Kon S, Maeda M, Hotta H, Uede T, Simon JC: Osteopontin is involved in the initiation of cutaneous contact hypersensitivity by inducing Langerhans and dendritic cell migration to lymph nodes. J Exp Med 2001; 194:1219–1229.
7. Termeer C, Hennies J, Voith U, Ahrens T, Weiss JM, Prehm P, Simon JC: Oligosaccharides of hyaluronan are potent activators of dendritic cells. J Immunol 2000; 165(4):1863–1870.
8. Termeer C, Sleeman JP, Simon JC: Hyaluronan – magic glue for the regulation of the immune response? Trends Immunol 2003; 24(3):112–114.
9. Termeer C, Benedix F, Sleeman J, Fieber C, Voith U, Ahren T, Miyake K, Freudenberg M, Galanos C, Simon JC: Oligosaccharides of Hyaluronan activate dendritic cells via toll-like receptor 4. J Exp Med 2002; 195(1):99–111.
10. Lappin MB, Weiss JM, Delattre V, Mai B, Dittmar H, Maier C, Manke K, Grabbe S, Martin S, Simon JC: Analysis of mouse dendritic cell migration in vivo upon subcutaneous and intravenous injection. Immunology 1999; 98:181–188.
11. Dudda JC, Simon JC, Martin S: Dendritic cell immunization route determines CD8+ T-cell trafficking to inflamed skin: role for tissue microenvironment and dendritic cells in establishment of T-cell-homing subsets. J Immunol 2004; 172(2):857–863.
12. Parsonage G, Filer AD, Haworth O, Nash GB, Rainger GE, Salmon M, Buckley CD: A stromal address code defined by fibroblasts. Trends Immunol 2005; 26:150–156.
13. Berthier R, Rizzitelli A, Martinon-Ego C, Laharie AM, Collin V, Chesne S, Marche PN: Fibroblasts inhibit the production of interleukin-12p70 by murine dendritic cells. Immunology 2003; 108:391–400.
14. Randolph GJ, Beaulieu S, Lebecque S, Steinman RM, Muller WA: Differentiation of monocytes into dendritic cells in a model of transendothelial trafficking. Science 1998; 282:480–483.
15. Manna PP, Duffy B, Olack B, Lowell J, Mohanakumar T: Activation of human dendritic cells by porcine aortic endothelial cells: transactivation of naive T-cells through costimulation and cytokine generation. Transplantation 2001; 72:1563–1571.
16. Zhang M, Tang H, Guo Z, An H, Zhu X, Song W, Guo J, Huang X, Chen T, Wang J, Cao X: Splenic stroma drives mature dendritic cells to differentiate into regulatory dendritic cells. Nat Immunol 2004; 5:1124–1133, Epub 2004 Oct 10.
17. Gabrilovich DI, Chen HL, Girgis KR, Cunningham HT, Meny GM, Nadaf S, Kavanaugh D, Carbone DP: Production of vascular endothelial growth factor by human tumors inhibits the functional maturation of dendritic cells. Nat Med 1996; 2:1096–1103.
18. Katsenelson NS, Shurin GV, Bykovskaia SN, Shogan J, Shurin MR: Human small cell lung

carcinoma and carcinoid tumor regulate dendritic cell maturation and function. Mod Pathol 2001; 14(1):40–45.

19. Silzle T, Randolph GJ, Kreutz M, Kunz-Schughart LA: The fibroblast: sentinel cell and local immune modulator in tumor tissue. Int J Cancer 2004; 108:173–180.

20. Buckley CD, Pilling D, Lord JM, Akbar AN, Scheel-Toellner D, Salmon M: Fibroblasts regulate the switch from acute resolving to chronic persistent inflammation. Trends Immunol 2001; 22:199–204.

21. Smith RS, Smith TJ, Blieden TM, Phipps RP: Fibroblasts as sentinel cells. Synthesis of chemokines and regulation of inflammation. Am J Pathol 1997; 151:317–322.

22. Smith TJ: Insights into the role of fibroblasts in human autoimmune diseases. Clin Exp Immunol 2005; 141:388–397.

23. Hogaboam CM, Kunkel SL, Strieter RM, Taub DD, Lincoln P, Standiford TJ, Lukacs NW: Novel roles for chemokines and fibroblasts in interstitial fibrosis. Kidney Int 1998; 54:2152–2159.

24. Pap T et al.: Role of synovial fibroblasts in the pathogenesis of rheumatoid arthritis. Arthritis Res 2000; 2:361–367.

A. Saalbach

Department of Dermatology, Venerology and Allergology, Leipzig University Medical Center, Phillipp-Rosenthal-Str. 23–25, D-04103 Leipzig, Germany, E-mail derma@medizin.uni-leipzig.de

Induction and Efficacy of Cytolytic Regulatory T-Cells in Experimental Asthma

V. Carlier, L. Vanderelst, W. Janssens, M. Jacquemin, and J.-M. Saint-Remy

Center for Molecular and Vascular Biology, University of Leuven, Belgium

Summary: Allergen-specific regulatory T-cells were generated toward Der p 2. The phenotypic characterization of T clones identified cells belonging to the Th1 lineage but expressing markers of Tregs. Tregs were shown to be cytotoxic for antigen-presenting cells. Adoptive transfer of such clones before or after sensitization to Der p 2 in an experimental asthma model showed full prevention and highly significant suppression of both airway inflammation and nonspecific airway hyperreactivity.

Keywords: regulatory T-cells, asthma, cytotoxicity, Der p 2

Antigen-specific regulatory T-cells (Tregs) represent an attractive therapeutic strategy for allergic asthma, as such cells require cognate interaction with peptide for activation, and they are able to suppress T-cell response to other peptides of the same protein or even of other proteins.

In the course of studies on experimental asthma elicited with allergens of direct clinical relevance, we identified a proportion of T-cells recognizing an dominant epitope of Der p 2 (p21–35; [1]) that were difficult to maintain and expand in culture, unless IL-2 was added. The properties of the first clone obtained have been described [2]. The conditions under which T-cell clones sharing regulatory properties could be generated have been sought out in the mouse.

In Vitro Characterization of Treg Clones

Treg clones presenting the same phenotypic properties can now be consistently obtained. Such properties include high expression of CD25, CTLA-4, ICOS and GITR. Clones also express high levels of CD62L and CD103, which endow cells with the capacity to migrate to inflammatory sites and/or peripheral lymphoid organs. Resting cells show high levels of transcripts for Tbet and granzymes A and B, but not for Foxp3. The production of cytokines was evaluated by ELISA in supernatants from 3-day culture. High concentrations of IFN-γ were consistently found. IL-10 was undetectable or at very low concentrations. No IL-4, IL-5, TNF-α or TGF-β was found. Taken together, these regulatory T-cells present characteristic markers of Th1 cells (Tbet, granzyme B and IFN-γ production), but also markers typically used to identifying regulatory T-cells (CD25 hi, GITR and CTLA-4). Functional characteristics were evaluated in vitro. Upon cognate interactions with peptide presented into MHC-class II determinants, Tregs show rapid cytotoxicity on antigen-presenting cells, including B-cells and dendritic cells. Depending on the target cell, lysis is primarily dependent on Fas-FasL interaction or on secretion of granzymes. Blocking antibodies confirmed these findings. No inhibition of cytotoxicity was obtained with antibodies toward TGF-β.

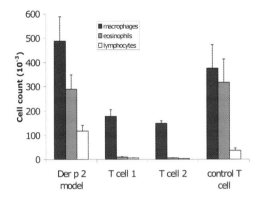

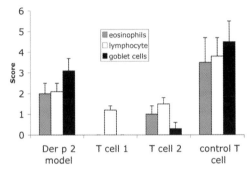

Figure 1. BALF cell composition and lung infiltrates in BALB/c mice sensitized to rDer p 2 and treated by rDer p 2 instillation. Treg clones were administered IV (2 × 10⁵ cells per mouse) prior to IP sensitization. The top panel shows the differential cell counts in BALF, including that of a control group injected with an unrelated T-cell clone. The bottom panel shows histology scores in the same groups of mice. Each group includes 6 to 8 mice.

Adoptive Transfer of Tregs in Experimental Asthma

A model of asthma was established in BALB/c mice using recombinant Der p 2 (rDer p 2) produced in Pichia pastoris. The protocol for inducing asthma included 3 IP sensitization with Der p 2 in alum followed by 2 series of 3 nasal instillations with Der p 2 carried out on 3 consecutive days one week apart. Broncho-alveolar lavage fluid (BALF) was evaluated for total cell content and cell differential. Lung tissues were stained with hematoxylin or PAS. Airway reactivity to increasing concentrations of methacholine administered by aerosol was assessed by whole body plethysmography and expressed as Penh values. Tregs were adoptively transferred to BALB/c mice either before (prevention) or after IP sensitization (suppression). 2×10^5 cells were injected once as a bolus in the tail vein. A control CD4$^+$ T-cell clone of unrelated specificity was also used. In the prevention setting, the 2 different Tregs completely prevented the increase in total cell numbers in BALF, while the control T-cell clone showed no modification as compared to mice receiving no T-cells. Only macrophages were identified in mice receiving Tregs. Lung examination showed little perivascular edema with minimum lymphocytes in the peribronchial spaces and virtually no eosinophils. No goblet cells were identified. Again the control cell line showed results identical to untreated mice. The results observed in the suppression experiments showed no increase in total cell numbers with the first Treg and a ± 30% increase of cell numbers with the second Treg clone, containing some eosinophils and lymphocytes. Histology examination showed some degree of perivascular and peribronchial edema with some infiltration made of eosinophils and lymphocytes, though the severity of infiltration was significantly reduced as compared to control mice. Some treated mice showed goblet cells. Airway reactivity to methacholine showed essentially no increase over that of the control mice in the prevention setting and very much reduced hyperreactivity in the suppression experiments. Results were consistent for the 2 Tregs.

Conclusion and Perspectives

T-cell clones raised to a common allergen show the capacity to prevent and suppress experimental asthma. They affect both lung inflammation and nonspecific hyperreactivity, which are considered as hallmarks of asthma. Interestingly, the phenotypic characterization of such clones identifies markers of Th1 and of regulatory T-cells, and as such they could represent a distinct subset of Tregs. Notably, their capacity to lyse antigen-presenting cells after cognate interaction and the absence of significant production of IL-10 and TGF-β distinguish them from other subsets of Tregs, such as Tr1 or Th3. The lack of Foxp3 transcription also identifies them as a separate subset from natural regulatory T-cells. Conditions under which CD4+ CD25+ cytotoxic Tregs can be elicited are being identified for further evaluation as a possible therapeutic approach for allergic asthma.

References

1. Wu B, VanderElst L, Carlier V, Jacquemin MG, Saint-Remy JMR: The Der p 2 allergen contains a universally immunogenic T-cell epitope. J Immunol 2002; 169:2430–2435.
2. Janssens W, Carlier V, Wu B, Vanderelst L, Jacquemin MG, Saint-Remy JMR: CD4+ CD25+ effector T-cells lyse antigen-presenting cells by Fas-FasL interaction in an epitope-specific manner. J Immunol 2003; 171:4604–4612.

Jean-Marie Saint-Remy

Center for Molecular & Vascular Biology, University of Leuven, Campus Gasthuisberg, Herestraat 49, B-3000 Leuven, Belgium, Tel. +32 16 345-791, Fax +32 16 345-990, E-mail jean-marie.saint-remy@med.kuleuven.ac.be

Antigen-Specific Expression of Lymphocyte Activation Markers CD69, CD25, and HLA-DR in Patients with Immediate Reactions to Amoxicillin

M.L. Sanz[1], P.M. Gamboa[2], R. Esparza[1], M.C. García-Aviles[1], M.R. Escudero[1], and A.L. De Weck[1]

[1]*Department of Allergology and Clinical Immunology, Clínica Universitaria, Universidad de Navarra, Pamplona, Spain,* [2]*Allergology Service, Hospital de Basurto, Bilbao, Spain*

Summary: We assessed the kinetic of the antigen-specific activation of T-cells in 36 patients with immediate reactions to amoxicillin and 16 controls, by the determination of the early activation marker CD69 and the late markers CD25 (IL2r) and HLA-DR. After *in vitro* incubation of the mononuclear cells isolated from peripheral blood with amoxicillin at 0, 4, 24, and 48 h, the cells were labeled with mononuclear antibodies: CD3 FITC, CD4 Percp Cy5.5, CD69 PE, CD25 PE, HLA-DR PE to be assessed subsequently by flowcytometry. Patients with immediate reactions to amoxicillin have an early activation of T CD4$^+$ cells that significantly increase the expression of CD69 and HLA-DR. Also we found a late activation with the increase of expression HLA-DR at 24 h.

Keywords: amoxicillin, lymphocyte activation markers, CD69, CD25, HLA-DR

Introduction

β-lactam drugs may induce both cellular and humoral allergic reactions, and there is evidence that T-cells play an important role in the pathogenesis of these reactions. In vitro T-cell response had been demonstrated in immediate and nonimmediate drug allergic reactions [1–4].

Amoxicillin is responsible for a major part of hypersensitivity reactions in drug allergy. While the exact mechanism is still a matter of debate, noncovalent drug presentation clearly leads to the activation of drug-specific T-cells [5–7].

The aim of this work was to assess the kinetic of the expression of early and delayed activation markers (CD69, CD25 and HLA-DR) in patients with immediate reactions to amoxicillin.

Material and Methods

Patients

Thirty-six patients with a well-documented history of amoxicillin allergy confirmed by a positive skin test, RAST, or controlled administration of the drug were included in the study. Eighteen atopic and nonatopic subjects with no history of adverse drug reactions and good tolerance to Amoxicillin established by negativity of skin test, RAST and controlled administration of oral Amoxicillin with the same methodology as for patients were selected as control group.

The study was approved by the institutional review board and informed consent was obtained from all subjects before carrying out the study.

Skin Test

Skin tests were performed using the usual techniques [8].

Cell Culture

Five milliliters of heparinized blood were obtained in BDvacuntainer® (Becton-Dickinson). Peripheral blood monuclear cells (PBLs) were isolated from heparinized blood by Ficoll-paque™ plus (Amersham Biosciences) by centrifugation at $1000 \times g$, for 20 min. 3×10^6 lymphocytes/ml were incubated with or without Amoxicillin (GlaxoSmithKline) at a final concentration of 0.625 mg/ml in a microwell plate in RPMI-1640 medium (GIBCO) supplemented with fetal calf serum (FCS), HEPES 25 mM and L-glutamine, in a kinetic study at 4, 24, and 48 h. As positive control we used 5 µg/ml phitohemglutinin A (PHA). As negative control we added RPMI supplemented culture media. As costimulators molecules we added 5 µg/ml CD28/CD49d (BD biosciences) at all the wells. Cells were incubated at 37 °C and 5% CO_2.

Phenotypic Immunofluorescence Analysis by Flow Cytometry

The lymphocytes were labeled with anti-CD3 FITC, CD4 PercPCy5.5, CD69-PE as early activation marker and with antibodies anti-CD3

Table 1. Lymphocyte activation markers in patients with immediate reactions to Amoxicillin (n = 36) and controls (n = 16).

		Time 0 h	Time 4 h		Time 24 h			Time 48 h		
		SI (mean ± SD)	SI (mean ± SD)	p^*	SI (mean ± SD)	p^*	p^{**}	SI (mean ± SD)	p^*	p^{**}	p^{***}
Patients	CD69	0.14 + 0.36	13.08 + 30.44	.001							
	CD25	2.13 + 2.41	1.12 + 0.62	ns	8.04 + 27.90	ns	.018	1.70 + 1.58	ns	.007	ns
	HLA-DR	1.61 + 1.8	1.11 + 0.9	.001	5.08 + 14.74	<.001	<.001	2.12 + 3.72	ns	<.001	ns
Controls	CD69	0.19 + 0.32	0.55 + 0.55	ns							
	CD25	0.69 + 0.51	1.40 + 1.72	ns	1.96 + 1.40	<.05	ns	2.65 + 3.80	ns	ns	ns
	HLA-DR	2.84 + 1.32	0.88 + 1.29	ns	1.75 + 3.91	ns	ns	4.65 + 12.82	ns	ns	ns

SI: Stimulation Index. p^* with respect to time 0 h, p^{**} with respect to time 4 h, p^{***} with respect to time 24 h.

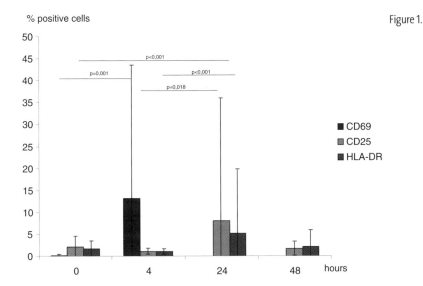

Figure 1.

FITC, CD4 PercPCy5.5 CD25-PE (IL-2r) and HLA-DR-PE as late activation markers.

The acquisition of the data was made in a FACScan (Becton Dickinson) with cell quest software, and the analysis was made with Paint-a-Gate software (BD).

Negative isotype controls were used to verify the staining specificity of the antibodies used.

Statistical Analysis

Comparisons between the groups were made using nonparametric statistical analysis (Kruskal-Wallis and Mann-Whitney tests).

Results

In the group of patients the CD69 expression increased significantly at 4 h of culture with amoxicillin. At 24 h of culture we found a significant increase of CD25 (IL2r) and HLA-DR (Table 1). In the control group only a slight increase of CD25 expression was observed at 24 h (Figure 1).

Discussion

β-lactam drugs may induce both cellular and humoral allergic reactions, and there is evi-

dence that T-cells play an important role in the pathogenesis of these reactions [9].

A T-cell activation has been described in 64.5% of the patients with immediate allergic reactions to β-lactams studied by lymphocyte transformation test (LTT). The high expression of CD69 on NK cells in Dermatophagoides pteronyssinus-stimulated cultures in allergic patients, described by Werfel et al [10] suggests that these cells are easily activated by cytokines from antigen-stimulated T-cells.

In our culture medium we included the costimulator molecules CD28 and CD49d to potentiate the T-cell activation, according to results obtained previously [11].

The CD4$^+$ CD25$^+$ cells increase at 24 h of culture, maybe related with the presence of regulator T-cells.

These results, together with the results obtained in this kind of patients regarding the CD63 expression in basophils after antigen-specific stimulation with β-lactams [12] contribute to a better understanding of the immunological mechanisms involved in the immediate reactions to Amoxicillin.

Conclusions

To conclude, the patients with immediate reactions to amoxicillin have an early activation of T CD4$^+$ cells that significantly increase the expression of CD69. Also we found a late activation with the increase of expression HLA-DR and CD4$^+$ CD25$^+$ at 24 h. All of that is not observed in healthy controls.

References

1. Luque I, Leyva L, Jose Torres M, Rosal M, Mayorga C, Segura JM, Blanca M, Juarez C: In vitro T-cell responses to β-lactam drugs in immediate and nonimmediate allergic reactions. Allergy 2001; 56:611–618.
2. Gonzalez FJ, Leyva L, Posadas S, Luque I, Blanca M, Santamaría L, Juarez C: Participation of T lymphocytes in cutaneous allergic reactions to drugs. Clin Exp Allergy 1998; 28(Suppl. 4):3–6.
3. Padial A, Posadas S, Alvarez J, Torres MJ, Alvarez JA, Mayorga C, Blanca M: Nonimmediate reactions to systemic corticosteroids suggest an immunological mechanism. Allergy 2005; 60:665–670.
4. Torres MJ, Corzo JL, Leyva L, Mayorga C, Garcia-Martin FJ, Antunez C, Posadas S, Jurado A, Blanca M: Differences in the immunological responses in drug- and virus-induced cutaneous reactions in children. Blood Cells. Molecules and Diseases 2003; 30:124–131.
5. Werner J: Pichler. Direct T-cell stimulations by drug bypassing the innate immune system. Toxicology 2005; 209:95–100.
6. Pichler WJ: Pharmacological interaction of drugs with antigen-specific immune receptors: the p-i concept. Curr Opin Allergy Clin Immunol 2002; 2:301–305.
7. Geber BO, Picher WJ: Noncovalent interactions of drugs with immune receptors may mediate drug-induced hypersensitivity reactions. AAPS J 2006; 8:E160–165.
8. Sanz ML, Gamboa PM, Antépara I, Uasuf C, Vila L, García-Avilés C, Chazot M, de Weck AL: Flow cytometric basophil activation test by detection of CD63 expression in patients with immediate-type reactions to β-lactam antibiotics. Clin Exp Allergy 2002; 32:277–286.
9. Nyfeler B, Pichler WJ: The lymphocyte transformation test for the diagnosis of drug allergy: sensitivity and specificity. Clin Exp Allergy 1997; 27:175–181.
10. Werfel T, Boeker M, Kapp A: Rapid expression of the CD69 antigen on T-cells and natural killer cells upon antigenic stimulation of peripheral blood mononuclear cell suspensions. Allergy 1997; 52:465–469.
11. Godoy-Ramirez K, Franck K, Mahdavifar S, Anderson L, Gaines H: Optimum culture conditions for specific an nonspecific activation of whole blood an PBMC for intracellular cytokine assessment by flow cytometry. J Immunol Meth 2004; 292:1–15.
12. Sanz ML, Maselli JP, Gamboa PM, Oehling A, Diéguez I, de Weck AL: Flow cytometric basophil activation test: a review. J Investig Allergol Clin Immunol 2002; 12:143–154.

María L. Sanz

Department of Allergology and Clinical Immunology, University Clinic of Navarra, Apartado 4209, E-31080 Pamplona, Spain, E-mail mlsanzlar@unav.es

Integration of Regulatory T-Cells into the Th1/Th2 Paradigm

P.-Y. Mantel[1], H. Kuipers[2], O. Boyman[3], N. Ouaked[1], B. Rückert[1],
C. Karagiannidis[1], B.N. Lambrecht[2], R.W. Hendriks[4], K. Blaser[1],
and C.B. Schmidt-Weber[1]

[1]Swiss Institute of Allergy and Asthma Research Davos (SIAF), Switzerland, [2]Department of Pulmonary Medicine, Erasmus MC, Rotterdam, The Netherlands, [3]Division of Immunology and Allergy, Department of Medicine, CHUV, Lausanne, Switzerland, [4]Department of Immunology, Erasmus MC, Rotterdam, The Netherlands

Summary: *Background:* Allergy is characterized by allergen sensitization, driving T-cell differentiation toward Th2 phenotype. Regulatory T-cells (T_{regs}) can control the activity and expansion of T-cells. However, the origin of the T_{regs} is unclear and therefore also the concepts to integrate T_{regs} into the Th1/h2 paradigm of T-cell differentiation. The present study describes a mechanism repressing peripheral Treg induction on the basis of the FOXP3 promoter analysis. *Methods:* To understand the origin of T_{regs} we investigated the promoter of the FOXP3 transcription factor, which is decisive for T_{reg} differentiation as T-BET for Th1 and GATA-3 for Th2 cells. Following localization and confirmation of the FOXP3 promoter, using reporter-gene assays, we identified regulators of the FOXP3 gene. *Results:* We demonstrate that cytokines such as IL-4 and TGF-β present at the time of T-cell priming of the uncommitted cells are decisive not only in differentiating T-cells toward effector phenotypes, but also toward T_{regs}. Moreover, Th2-driving conditions that occur in allergic inflammation prevent the induction of T_{regs} by a GATA3-mediated inhibition of the FOXP3 promoter. It is demonstrated that GATA3 directly binds in the FOXP3 promoter and acts as repressor of gene transcription. *Conclusion:* It appears that T_{regs} require antigen-specific stimulation as Th1 or Th2 cells but differentiate only in the absence of Th1 and Th2 driving signals. T_{reg} differentiation pathways may therefore be considered as a default pathway occurring in the absence of Th1/Th2 polarizing danger signals. Thus, therapeutic establishment of allergen tolerance requires the control of inflammation to facilitate regulatory capacities of the immune system in allergic disease.

Keywords: allergen-tolerance, transcription factor, regulatory T-cells

Introduction

Allergen-specific immune reactions are characterized by Th2-skewed phenotype. A hallmark of Th1 and Th2 differentiation pathways is the exclusiveness of the individual mechanisms. IL-12 mediated STAT4-phosphorylation and T-bet expression are essential for Th1 differentiation. In contrast, IL-4-induced STAT6 and GATA3 inhibit differentiation into Th1 cells in the early phase of commitment.

GATA3 is sufficient to induce Th2 phenotypes and acts not only through induction of IL-4, IL-5, and IL-13, the Th2 cytokines, but also through inhibition of Th1 cell-specific factors. Recently it could be shown that T-bet directly modulates GATA3 function [1], suggesting that transcription factors compete in the early differentiation phase of T-cells to finally imprint the T-cell phenotype [2]. A GATA3 dominated immune response has been shown to be essential for airway hyperresponsiveness

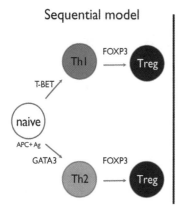

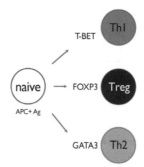

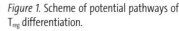

Figure 1. Scheme of potential pathways of T_reg differentiation.

[3, 4] and can break antigen-specific immune tolerance [5]. Overexpression of a dominant negative form of GATA3 [6] or treatment with antisense-mediated GATA3 blockade [7] decreased the severity of the allergic airway hyperresponsiveness.

The discovery of T_{regs} highlights another phenotype of T-cells, which is assumed to be critical for tolerance against allergens. However its integration in lineage development is not fully clear. Naturally-occurring T_{regs} (nT_{regs}) are generated in the thymus and are assumed to protect against the activity of autoreactive T-cells in the periphery. These cells express the forkhead transcription factor FOXP3 and constitutively express CD25 on their surface, but lack cytokine expression, which would set them in proximity of Th1 or Th2 lineages. Regarding allergen tolerance T_{regs} of the peripheral origin are potential targets for therapeutic intervention. These induced T_{regs} (iT_{reg}) were reported to express FOXP3, however expression may be transient [8] and the exact circumstances of iT_{reg} generation are unclear. TGF-β has been demonstrated to be important for the induction of these cells *in vitro* and *in vivo*, since animals lacking the TGF-βRII on T-cells are deficient in peripherally-iT_{regs} and suffer from a T-cell dependent multiorgan inflammatory disease [9–12]. Although the effect of TGF-β on T_{reg} induction is well documented, its molecular targets remain to be identified. Two different scenarios of T_{reg} induction can be hypothesized (Figure 1): one, in which T_{regs} can be induced in already committed effector cells,

which provides a scenario of an inherent shutdown mechanism of T-cell activation. The other suggests that T_{regs} differentiate from naïve T-cells as a separate lineage in a similar fashion as known for Th1 or Th2 commitment, a scenario providing a suppressive memory population. The current study provides evidence for the second model and focuses on GATA3 and FOXP3 which may play a similar role in T_{reg} commitment as T-bet and GATA3 for Th1 and Th2 differentiation respectively. This assumption is based on the observation that TCR activation is necessary to generate T_{regs} as well as the FOXP3 gene and that high and stable FOXP3 expression is sufficient to generate a regulatory phenotype. We show that GATA3 excludes FOXP3 expression and that IL-4, and thus Th2 cells inhibit FOXP3 expression both *in vitro* and *in vivo*.

Material and Methods

T-cells isolated by magnetic purification using the Miltenyi isolation system CD4CD45RA+ T-cells were driven along the Th1, Th2 and T_{reg} pathway and analyzed using westernblot analysis. Following localization and confirmation of the FOXP3 promoter, using reporter-gene assay [13], we identified regulators of the FOXP3 genes.

Results

In vitro differentiated Th1, Th2, or iT_{regs} were restimulated with plate-bound anti-CD3/

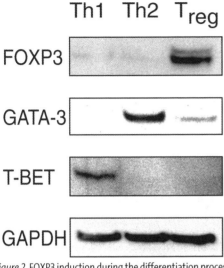

Figure 2. FOXP3 induction during the differentiation process of CD4CD45RA⁺ T-cells upon Th1, Th2 or T_{reg} driving conditions. Shown is a western blot analysis of FOXP3, GATA3 and T-bet; GAPDH served as internal control. Data are representative of three independent experiments.

CD28. Cells were harvested after 3 days for western blot analysis (Figure 2) of FOXP3, GATA3 and T-bet. The transcription factor were expressed in a lineage specific manner, specifically FOXP3 and GATA-3 expression where exclusive on a single cell level (data not shown). Since Il-4 inhibits dose-dependently the FOXP3 expression and the FOXP3 promoter was identified to carry a GATA-3 binding site, we investigated the potential molecular mechanism of GATA3 mediated repression of FOXP3. The GATA-binding site is located –400 bp upstream from the transcription start site, in a region which has already been described as important for the regulation of FOXP3 expression [13]. A site-specific mutation abolishing the GATA3-binding site of the human FOXP3 promoter increased luciferase activity by 2.5-fold in CD4⁺ T-cells, revealing a repressor activity of GATA3 on the FOXP3 promoter (Figure 3A). Overexpression of

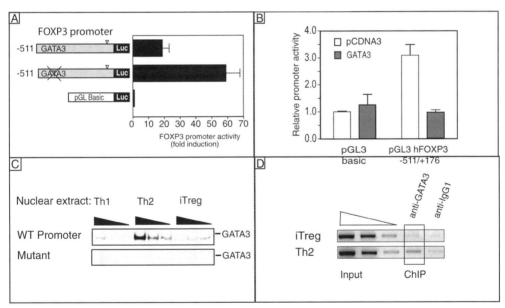

Figure 3. GATA3 binds to and represses the human FOXP3 promoter. (A) CD4 cells were transfected with wild-type or a GATA3 mutated FOXP3 promoter reporter construct. Bars show the mean ± SD of 3 independent experiments. (B) Overexpression of GATA3 in human CD4 cells with the 511 FOXP3 promoter construct decreases the luciferase activity of the FOXP3 promoter. Results shown are the mean ± SD of 3 different experiments performed in triplicate. (C) Biotinylated oligonucleotides were absorbed by streptavidin agarose beads and then incubated with nuclear extracts prepared from from Th1, Th2 and iT_{regs} T-cells. The amounts of GATA3 protein in the precipitates were assessed by immunoblotting with anti-GATA3 mAb. Total nuclear extracts were run as controls. These data are representative of 3 different experiments. (D) Th2 and iT_{regs} were analyzed by ChIP for GATA3 binding to the FOXP3 promoter. Shown is the PCR for the FOXP3 gene after reversing the cross-linking. The "input" represents PCR amplification of the total sample, which was not subjected to any precipitation. Results are representative of three independent experiments.

GATA3 diminished luciferase activity of the FOXP3 promoter compared to the control vector (pcDNA3; Figure 3A).

The ability of GATA3 to physically interact with the FOXP3 promoter was further investigated. Increasing amounts of lysates were incubated with oligonucleotides containing the GATA3-site of the FOXP3 promoter or a control oligonucleotide with a mutated GATA3 binding site. These oligonucleotides were precipitated and GATA3-specifically detected by western blot. GATA3-expressing Th2 cells and iTregs were subjected to this approach. Only Th2 cells (Figure 3C) showed GATA3-binding activity. This experiment proves that GATA3 can bind the FOXP3 promoter. In addition chromatin coimmunoprecipitation (ChIP) using a GATA3-specific antibody to precipitate chromatin of Th2 cells and iT$_{regs}$ was applied and confirmed GATA3 binding to the FOXP3 promoter in Th2 cells, but not in the iT$_{regs}$ (Figure 3D).

Discussion

The current study reveals that FOXP3-mediated T$_{reg}$ commitment is inhibited by GATA3, which is the key regulator for polarization toward Th2 cells. After differentiation the effector cells become refractory to conversion into a regulatory phenotype and particularly Th2 cells were unable to upregulate FOXP3. In this context we demonstrated that IL-4 was able to inhibit stable FOXP3 induction mediated by TGF-β and therefore prevented the conversion into the regulatory phenotype. Accordingly we investigated whether GATA3 overexpression affected FOXP3 induction and found that GATA3 overexpressing naïve human T-cells were characterized by a reduced capacity to express FOXP3. This inhibitory effect of GATA3 was further confirmed in transgenic mice, expressing GATA3 in T-cells (DO11.10: CD2GATA3 transgenic mice) [data not shown]. Thus GATA3 restrains the development of certain T$_{regs}$ subsets, presumably the inducible, peripheral population and not those of thymic origin. GATA3 represses FOXP3 expression directly by binding to the FOXP3

promoter region. Site-specific mutation of this site increased the activity of promoter constructs, thus revealing the repressive nature of this GATA element. This palindromic GATA element binds GATA3 protein as proven by pull-down experiments. Furthermore, it is shown by chromatin immune precipitation (ChIP) that GATA3 binds this element also in intact cells, indicating that this chromatin region is accessible for GATA3 binding. It is known that GATA3 can induce transcription by chromatin remodeling, by directly transactivating promoters [14] or, as shown in the current study, acts as a repressor of gene expression [1, 15, 16].

The molecular interactions enabling GATA3 to inhibit FOXP3 are not identified yet, but the GATA-binding site is located adjacent to positive, inducing sites, composed of AP-1-NFATc2 sites [13] and GATA3 may compete with the binding of AP-1/NFAT to the promoter (unpublished observations).

In summary, we demonstrated that GATA3 acts as an inhibitor of FOXP3 expression in early T-cell differentiation, by directly binding and repressing the FOXP3 promoter. These data support the idea that T$_{regs}$ evolve as a separate lineage apart from the Th1 and Th2. This interactive mechanism will give new perspectives in promoting allergen tolerance and the development of tolerogenic treatment strategies.

Acknowledgments

This work was supported by the Swiss National Foundation Grants Nr: 31–65436, 3100A0-100164 and 310000-112329, the Saurer Foundation Zurich and the Swiss Life Zurich.

References

1. Usui T, Nishikomori R, Kitani A, Strober W: GATA-3 suppresses Th1 development by down-regulation of Stat4 and not through effects on IL-12Rβ$_2$ chain or T-bet. Immunity 2003; 18:415–428.

2. Hwang ES, Szabo SJ, Schwartzberg PL, Glimcher LH: T helper cell fate specified by kinase-

mediated interaction of T-bet with GATA-3. Science 2005; 307:430–433.

3. Hasegawa A, Miki T, Hosokawa H, Hossain MB, Shimizu C,Hashimoto K, Kimura MY, Yamashita M, Nakayama T: Impaired GATA3-dependent chromatin remodeling and Th2 cell differentiation leading to attenuated allergic airway inflammation in aging mice. J Immunol 2006; 176:2546–2554.

4. Yamashita M, Hirahara K, Shinnakasu R, Hosokawa H, Norikane S,Kimura MY, Hasegawa A, Nakayama T: Crucial role of MLL for the maintenance of memory T helper type 2 cell responses. Immunity 2006; 24:611–622.

5. Oriss TB, Ostroukhova M, Seguin-Devaux C, Dixon-McCarthy B, Stolz DB, Watkins SC, Pillemer B, Ray P, Ray A: Dynamics of dendritic cell phenotype and interactions with CD4+ T-cells in airway inflammation and tolerance. J Immunol 2005; 174:854–863.

6. Zhang DH, Yang L, Cohn L, Parkyn L, Homer R, Ray P, Ray A: Inhibition of allergic inflammation in a murine model of asthma by expression of a dominant-negative mutant of GATA-3. Immunity 1999; 11:473–482.

7. Finotto S, De Sanctis GT, Lehr HA, Herz U, Buerke M, Schipp M, Bartsch B, Atreya R, Schmitt E, Galle PR, Renz H, Neurath MF: Treatment of allergic airway inflammation and hyperresponsiveness by antisense-induced local blockade of GATA-3 expression. J Exp Med 2001; 193:1247–1260.

8. Gavin MA, Torgerson TR, Houston E, DeRoos P, Ho WY, Stray-Pedersen A, Ocheltree EL, Greenberg PD, Ochs HD, Rudensky AY: Single-cell analysis of normal and FOXP3-mutant human T-cells: FOXP3 expression without regulatory T-cell development. Proc Natl Acad Sci USA 2006; 103:6659–6664.

9. Chen W, Jin W, Hardegen N, Lei KJ, Li L, Marinos N, McGrady G, Wahl SM: Conversion of peripheral CD4+ CD25− naive T-cells to CD4+ CD25+ regulatory T-cells by TGF-β induction of transcription factor Foxp3. J Exp Med 2003; 198:1875–1886.

10. Fantini MC, Becker C, Monteleone G, Pallone F, Galle PR, Neurath MF: Cutting edge: TGF-β induces a regulatory phenotype in CD4+ CD25− T-cells through Foxp3 induction and down-regulation of Smad7. J Immunol 2004; 172:5149–5153.

11. Ostroukhova M, Ray A: CD25+ T-cells and regulation of allergen-induced responses. Curr Allergy Asthma Rep 2005; 5:35–41.

12. Ostroukhova M, Seguin-Devaux C, Oriss TB, Dixon-McCarthy B, Yang L, Ameredes BT, Corcoran TE, Ray A: Tolerance induced by inhaled antigen involves CD4(+) T-cells expressing membrane-bound TGF-β and FOXP3. J Clin Invest 2004; 114:28–38.

13. Mantel PY, Ouaked N, Ruckert B, Karagiannidis C, Welz R, Blaser K, Schmidt-Weber CB: Molecular mechanisms underlying FOXP3 induction in human T-cells. J Immunol 2006; 176:3593–3602.

14. Zheng W, Flavell RA: The transcription factor GATA-3 is necessary and sufficient for Th2 cytokine gene expression in CD4 T-cells. Cell 1997; 89:587–596.

15. Sadat MA, Kumatori A, Suzuki S, Yamaguchi Y, Tsuji Y, Nakamura M: GATA-3 represses gp91phox gene expression in eosinophil-committed HL-60-C15 cells. FEBS Lett 1998; 436:390–394.

16. Schwenger GT, Fournier R, Kok CC, Mordvinov VA, Yeoman D, Sanderson CJ: GATA-3 has dual regulatory functions in human interleukin-5 transcription. J Biol Chem 2001; 276:48502–48509.

Carsten B. Schmidt-Weber

Allergy and Clinical Immunology, Imperial College London, South Kensington Campus, Sir Alexander Fleming Building, Room 365, Exhibition Road, London SW7 2AZ, UK, tel. +44 20 7594-9276, e-mail c.schmidt-weber@imperial.ac.uk

Association Between Epidermal Caspase-3 Cleavage and Dermal Interferon-γ Expressing Cells in Atopic Dermatitis

D. Simon[1], R.L.P. Lindberg[2], E. Kozlowski[3], L.R. Braathen[1], and H.-U. Simon[3]

[1]Department of Dermatology, University of Bern, Bern, Switzerland, [2]Clinical Neuroimmunology Laboratory, Departments of Research and Neurology, University Hospitals Basel, Basel, Switzerland, [3]Department of Pharmacology, University of Bern, Bern, Switzerland

Summary: *Background:* Keratinocyte apoptosis mediated by Fas/Fas ligand molecular interactions is believed to play an important role in the formation of spongiosis in atopic dermatitis (AD) lesions. We investigated the cleavage of caspase-3 that is indicative for its activation, in the epidermis of AD skin under *in vivo* conditions. Furthermore, Fas expression on keratinocytes as well as IFN-γ expression known to by involved in regulating keratinocyte apoptosis were analyzed. *Methods:* Immunofluorescence staining was undertaken on sections of skin biopsies taken from 15 patients with AD before and after topical therapy with calcineurin inhibitors, and on normal skin. *Results:* In normal skin, caspase-3 cleavage was detected in single cells of the basal layer. In contrast, in acute lesional AD skin, we obtained evidence for increased expression of cleaved caspase-3 in keratinocytes of the basal layer, but also of the spinous cell layer, in particular in spongiotic areas. Short-term topical treatment of the skin lesions with tacrolimus or pimecrolimus abolished the expression of cleaved caspase-3 in the spinous layer. Epidermal caspase-3 cleavage correlated with the numbers of dermal interferon (IFN)-γ expressing CD4+ and CD8+ lymphocytes in skin lesions of AD patients. The increased Fas expression on keratinocytes in acute AD lesions was markedly reduced upon treatment. *Conclusion:* These data suggest that caspase-3 cleavage in the spinous layer of the epidermis is a pathologic event contributing to spongiosis formation in AD. Moreover, these data support the view that IFN-γ is important for the activation of proapoptotic pathways in keratinocytes by upregulating surface Fas expression.

Keywords: apoptosis, atopic dermatitis, caspase, interferon, keratinocytes

Acute AD lesions present typical histopathologic features characterized by epidermal spongiosis, sometimes leading to vesicle formation, and a perivascular inflammatory infiltrate in the dermis [1, 2]. This infiltrate consists mainly of T lymphocytes [3], but eosinophils, mast cells, as well as B-cells are also present [4,5]. Although a predominance of T helper (Th)2 cells has been observed in acute AD lesions [6, 7], considerable numbers of CD4+ and CD8+ lymphocytes expressing interferon (IFN)-γ appear to be also present [5, 8].

Apoptosis of keratinocytes has recently been implicated as a key mechanism of spongiosis in atopic dermatitis [9]. In this process, caspases may play a role. Since caspase-3 is expressed in keratinocytes [10], we investigated the cleavage of caspase-3 that is indicative for its activation in the epidermis of acute AD lesions under *in vivo* conditions. Because IFN-γ was demonstrated to induce keratinocyte apoptosis by upregulating the Fas receptor on the surface of these cells [9], we also analyzed dermal expression of IFN-γ and epidermal expression of Fas. Moreover, we monitored the effects of topical calcineurin inhibitor therapy.

To investigate the expression of cleaved caspase-3, we performed immunofluorescence analysis on skin sections using an antibody, which recognized cleaved but not full-length caspase-3 [11]. Cleaved caspase-3 was detectable in keratinocytes of the basal layer of all skin specimens taken from lesional AD skin before and after treatment as well as normal skin. In the spinous cell layer, cleaved caspase-3 was observed in all specimens taken from lesional AD skin. Strongest positive staining was noticed in areas of spongiosis. In contrast, in both normal and nonlesional AD skin, no cleaved caspase-3 staining was detectable above the basal layer. A marked decrease of cleaved caspase-3 expression was observed after treatment, which was also associated with clinical improvement.

Since IFN-γ was reported to regulate keratinocyte apoptosis [9,12], we investigated the IFN-γ expression in the skin. In acute AD lesions, a considerable number of IFN-γ expressing CD4+ and CD8+ lymphocytes were detected in the dermal infiltrate. Upon treatment with topical calcineurin inhibitors, reduced numbers of IFN-γ expressing CD4+ and CD8+ lymphocytes were found. In three patients, we additionally analyzed IFN-γ mRNA expression in the dermis of AD skin before and after therapy with topical tacrolimus and pimecrolimus, respectively. In all three patients, IFN-γ mRNA expression declined parallel to the clinical improvement upon immunomodulatory therapy. Next, we investigated whether there is an association between the numbers of IFN-γ expressing lymphocytes and the numbers of epidermal cells exhibiting caspase-3 cleavage in AD. Indeed, expression of cleaved caspase-3 throughout the suprabasal cell layer and above was only observed, if the numbers of IFN-γ expressing lymphocytes in the dermis

exceeded approximately 25 cells per mm². Following treatment with calcineurin inhibitors, the fewer numbers of IFN-γ expressing lymphocytes correlated with less expression of cleaved caspase-3.

It has previously been shown that IFN-γ enhances Fas receptor expression on keratinocytes [9], a mechanism, which may contribute to apoptosis induction in AD lesions [12]. We observed strong Fas expression of keratinocytes in lesional AD skin. In contrast, Fas expression on keratinocytes was almost undetectable in AD skin after topical calcineurin inhibitor therapy and in normal skin.

Taken together, we demonstrate cleavage of caspase-3 in the spinous cell layer especially in spongiotic areas of acute lesional AD skin. Increased epidermal caspase-3 cleavage was associated with increased numbers of infiltrating lymphocytes expressing IFN-γ. Treatment with calcineurin inhibitors resulted in reduced dermal infiltration of IFN-γ expressing lymphocytes, reduced epidermal Fas expression and caspase-3 cleavage. IFN-γ is suggested to be involved in spongiosis formation by mediating cleavage of caspace-3 via Fas receptor activation in acute AD lesions.

Acknowledgments

We are grateful to Inès Schmid and Francine Hoffmann for excellent technical assistance. This study was supported by the Swiss National Science Foundation (310000–107526), OPO-Foundation, Zurich, and Novartis-Foundation, Basel.

References

1. Leung DYM, Bieber T: Atopic dermatitis. Lancet 2003; 361:151–160.
2. Mihm MC, Soter NA, Dvorak HF, Austen KF: The structure of normal skin and the morphology of atopic eczema. J Invest Dermatol 1976; 67:305–312.
3. Braathen LR, Förre O, Natvig JB, Eeg-Larsen T: Predominance of T lymphocytes in the dermal infiltrate of atopic dermatitis. Br J Dermatol 1979; 100:511–519.
4. Akdis CA, Akdis M, Simon D, Dibbert B, Weber

M, Gratzl S, Kreyden O, Disch R, Wuethrich B, Blaser K, Simon H-U: T-cells and T-cell-derived cytokines as pathogenic factors in the nonallergic form of atopic dermatitis. J Invest Dermatol 1999; 113:628–634.

5. Simon D, Vassina E, Yousefi S, Kozlowski E, Braathen LR, Simon HU: Reduced numbers of cytokine-expressing cells in atopic dermatitis after topical tacrolimus treatment. J Allergy Clin Immunol 2004; 114:887–895.

6. Hamid Q, Boguniewicz M, Leung DYM: Differential in situ cytokine expression in acute versus chronic atopic dermatitis. J Clin Invest 1994; 94:870–876.

7. Hamid Q, Naseer T, Minshall EM, Song YL, Boguniewicz M, Leung DYM: *In vivo* expression of IL-12 and IL-13 in atopic dermatitis. J Allergy Clin Immunol 1996; 98:225–231.

8. Simon D, Vassina E, Yousefi S, Braathen LR, Simon HU: Inflammatory cell numbers and cytokine expression in atopic dermatitis after topical pimecrolimus treatment. Allergy 2005; 60:944–951.

9. Trautmann A, Akdis M, Kleemann D, Altznauer F, Simon H-U, Graeve T, Noll M, Bröcker E-B, Blaser K, Akdis CA: T-cell-mediared Fas-induced keratinocyte apoptosis plays a key role in eczematous dermatitis. J Clin Invest 2000; 106:25–35.

10. Takahashi T, Ogo M, Hibino T: Partial purification and characterization of two distinct types of caspases from human epidermis. J Invest Dermatol 1998; 111:367–372.

11. Hague A, Eveson JW, MacFarlane M, Huntley S, Janghra N, Thavaraj S: Caspase-3 expression is reduced, in the absence of cleavage, in terminally differentiated normal oral epithelium but is increased in oral squamous cell carcinomas and correlates with tumor stage. J Pathol 2004; 204:175–182.

12. Arnold R, Seifert M, Asadullah K, Volk HD: Crosstalk between keratinocytes and T lymphocytes via Fas/Fas ligand interaction: modulation by cytokines. J Immunol 1999; 162:7140–7147.

Dagmar Simon

Department of Dermatology, University of Bern, Inselspital, CH-3010 Bern, Switzerland, Tel. +41 31 632-2278, Fax +41 31 381-5815, E-mail dagmar.simon@insel.ch

Plasticity of Histamine H$_1$ Receptor Expression in Human Mononuclear Phagocytes

M. Triggiani[1], A. Petraroli[1], S. Loffredo[1], R.I. Staiano[2], F. Granata[1], G. Giannattasio[1], and G. Marone[1]

[1]Division of Clinical Immunology and Allergy and Center for Basic and Clinical Immunology Research (CISI), University of Naples Federico II, Italy, [2]Division of Pharmacology, Department of Neuroscience, University of Naples Federico II, Italy

Summary: *Background:* Histamine plays a pivotal role in allergic inflammation by inducing proinflammatory and immunoregulatory effects which are primarily mediated by activation of the H$_1$ receptor. The responses elicited by histamine in human inflammatory cells are quite different, suggesting that the expression of H$_1$ receptors can be differently regulated. *Methods and Results:* To examine the expression of the H$_1$ receptor in human mononuclear phagocytes, we explored accumulation of mRNA for the H$_1$ receptor in a model of macrophages developed *in vitro* by incubation of blood monocytes for 10 days in the presence of 20% FCS. Quantitative RT-PCR experiments showed that the mRNA for the H$_1$ receptor increased 15-fold in differentiated macrophages as compared to blood monocytes. Incubation of differentiating macrophages with budesonide (0.1–1 µM) for 24 h resulted in approximately 50 percent inhibition of H$_1$ receptor expression. The receptor upregulated was functionally active since incubation of macrophages with histamine (1 µM) induced a significant increase in intracellular Ca^{2+} that was blocked by the H$_1$ antagonist levocetirizine. Histamine induced a concentration-dependent production of IL-8 in macrophages, whereas this response was not detectable in the precursor monocytes. *Conclusions:* These data indicate that differentiation of monocytes into macrophages, either *in vivo* in the lung or *in vitro*, is associated with upregulation of the histamine H$_1$ receptor.

Keywords: histamine, H$_1$ receptor, macrophage, monocyte, budesonide

Introduction

Histamine may play an important role in allergic inflammation by inducing immunoregulatory effects on several cells including T-cells, dendritic cells, monocytes and macrophages [1]. The biological effects of histamine are mediated by the activation of four distinct receptors named H$_1$, H$_2$, H$_3$, and H$_4$ [1, 2]. However, most of the histamine-induced immunoregulatory responses are due to the activation of H$_1$ and H$_2$ receptors [3]. Indeed, the interaction of histamine with these two receptors elicits responses that are of-

ten divergent with H$_1$ activation being predominantly stimulatory and H$_2$ being inhibitory in most cases [2]. Thus, the expression of histamine receptors may be a potential mechanism to regulate cell responsiveness to this mediator and to explain the heterogeneity of histamine's effects on inflammatory and immune cells. The observation that the level of expression of the H$_1$ receptor may be significantly different between various human cells [4] led to the hypothesis that plasticity of this receptor could be a factor modulating the intensity of responses to histamine in peripheral tissues.

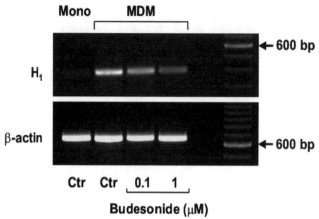

Figure 1. Effects of budesonide on histamine H_1 receptor mRNA expression in monocyte-derived macrophages. H_1 receptor (upper gel) RT-PCR amplification products from a representative experiment in which monocytes (Mono) were differentiated into monocyte-derived macrophages (MDM) in the presence of medium alone (Ctr) or Budesonide (0.1–1 µM) added during the last 24 h of culture. A 100 bp DNA ladder was used as standard. Adequate normalization of RNA for each sample was confirmed by the equality of RT-PCR amplification products for β-actin mRNA expression at subsaturating cycle number (lower gel).

Monocytes, macrophages and dendritic cells are components of the mononuclear phagocyte system (MPS), a cellular network widely distributed within organs and tissues that plays a primary role in innate immunity [5]. Monocytes are the predominant MPS cells in the blood and they differentiate into macrophages or dendritic cells as they migrate within peripheral tissues [6].

In this study we compared the expression of the H_1 receptor in blood monocytes and macrophages either purified from human lung tissue (HLM) or differentiated *in vitro* (MDM).

Material and Methods

Monocytes were purified from buffy coats of normal donors by negative immunomagnetic selection [7]. Monocyte-derived macrophages (MDM) were obtained by culturing purified monocytes for 10 days in RPMI containing 20% fetal calf serum (FCS) [8]. In selected experiments MDM differentiated for 10 days were incubated during the last 24 h of culture with budesonide (0.1–1 µM) or medium alone. Monocyte-derived DC were generated as previously reported [9]. Lung macrophages (HLM) were purified from the parenchyma of patients undergoing thoracic surgery by centrifugation over density gradients and adherence to plastic dishes [10]. Expression of mRNA for H_1 histamine receptor was evaluated by real-time quantitative PCR. Intracellular calcium changes induced by histamine in monocytes and MDM were monitored by a

single cell microfluorimetric technique in cells loaded with Fura2 [10]. In the experiments on IL-8 production, monocytes and MDM cultured for 10 days were incubated (18 h, 37 °C) with histamine. At the end of the incubation IL-8 release was measured by ELISA.

Results

In previous experiments we compared the expression of the H_1 receptor gene in blood monocytes, HLM and monocyte-derived dendritic cells (DC) and we found that HLM and DC contained larger quantities of mRNA for H_1 receptor than monocytes (HLM: 3.9 ± 0.7 fold *vs.* monocytes; DC: 4.5 ± 0.5 fold *vs.* monocytes; $n = 4$). Since blood monocytes are the circulating precursors of macrophages and DC, these data suggested that differentiation of macrophages or DC could be associated with an enhancement of H_1 gene transcription. We therefore examined the expression of the H_1 receptor in a model of macrophages developed *in vitro* (MDM). Experiments of quantitative real time-PCR revealed that the expression of H_1 receptor increased 15.0 ± 2.9 fold in MDM after 10 days of culture as compared to monocytes ($p < .01$) (Figure 1). In a second group of experiments we examined whether glucocorticoids influence the upregulation of the H_1 receptor in differentiating MDM. Figure 1 shows the results of a PCR experiment showing that the amount of mRNA for the H_1 receptor is greatly increased in MDM as compared to monocytes. Addition of budesonide to the differentiating MDM during the last 24 h of culture reduced in a concentration-dependent fashion the accumulation of mRNA for the H$_1$ receptor. Maximal inhibition ($\geq 50\%$) of H$_1$ receptor expression was achieved at 1 µM concentration of budesonide.

To test the functional activity of the H$_1$ receptor overexpressed in MDM, we examined the changes in intracellular calcium induced by histamine at a single-cell level by a microfluorimetric technique. Histamine (1 µM) induced a significant increase in the intracellular calcium concentration ($[Ca^{2+}]_i$) in MDM (126.0 ± 2.8 nM before histamine *vs.* 173.8 ± 4.7 nM after histamine; $p < .01$), whereas it failed to induce changes in $[Ca^{2+}]_i$ in monocytes (121.5 ± 10.0 nM before histamine *vs.* 121.5 ± 12.0 nM after histamine). The selective H$_1$ antagonist levocetirizine (10 µM) completely blocked the $[Ca^{2+}]_i$ induced by histamine in MDM.

In the last group of experiments we investigated histamine-induced IL-8 production in monocytes and macrophages to examine whether upregulation of the H$_1$ receptor induced an increased responsiveness to histamine. In four different experiments histamine induced a concentration-dependent production of IL-8 in MDM (3.85 ± 1.9 ng/mg of protein *vs.* control: 1.06 ± 0.8 ng/mg of protein). Histamine-induced IL-8 production in MDM was significant at 0.01 µM histamine and was maximal at 1 µM. In contrast, histamine did not increase basal IL-8 production in precursor monocytes (2,19 ± 1,69 ng/mg of protein *vs.* control: 1.90 ± 1.59 ng/mg of protein).

Discussion

Histamine H$_1$ receptor expression is increased in human lung macrophages and dendritic cells as compared to their blood precursor monocytes. The overexpression of the H$_1$ receptor confers to mature macrophages the capacity to generate Ca^{2+} signals and to produce IL-8 upon stimulation with histamine indicating that the inducible receptor is functionally active. Macrophages purified *ex vivo* from the human lung have an expression profile of the H$_1$ receptor comparable to that of MDM and show similar responsiveness to histamine in terms of cytokine production [10]. The ability of tissue macrophages to respond to H$_1$ receptor activation by releasing proinflammatory cytokines and chemokines reinforce the potential role of these cells in bronchial asthma [11]. A novel observation in this work is that upregulation of the H$_1$ receptor in macrophages is inhibited by approximately 50% by incubation with budesonide. Further studies are required to understand the mechanism by which glucocorticoids modulate histamine receptor expression.

The observation that H$_1$ receptor expression can be modulated raises the hypothesis that its overexpression could be involved in the pathogenesis of allergic disorders such as rhinitis, asthma, urticaria and anaphylaxis. An increased number of H$_1$ receptors may cause exaggerated responses to histamine in the skin or in the airways in patients with urticaria or asthma, respectively. Our study supports the hypothesis that the up- or down-regulation of H$_1$ receptor may be a general phenomenon occurring in several cells which are targets of histamine *in vivo* and may thus be relevant to the pathogenesis of allergic diseases.

References

1. Akdis CA, Blaser K: Histamine in the immune regulation of allergic inflammation. J Allergy Clin Immunol 2003; 112:15–22.
2. Hill SJ, Ganellin CR, Timmerman H, Schwartz JC, Shankley NP, Young JM, Schunack W, Levi R, Haas HL: International Union of Pharmacology. XIII. Classification of histamine receptors. Pharmacol Rev 1997; 49:253–278.
3. Jutel M, Watanabe T, Akdis M, Blaser K, Akdis CA: Immune regulation by histamine. Curr Opin Immunol 2002; 14:735–740.
4. Togias A: H$_1$-receptors: localization and role in airway physiology and in immune functions. J Allergy Clin Immunol 2003; 112:60–68.
5. Hume DA, Ross IL, Himes SR, Sasmono RT, Wells CA, Ravasi T: The mononuclear phagocyte system revisited. J Leukoc Biol 2002; 72:621–627.
6. Takahashi K, Naito M, Takeya M: Development and heterogeneity of macrophages and their re-

lated cells through their differentiation pathways. Pathol Int 1996; 46:473–485.

7. Triggiani M, Granata F, Oriente A, Gentile M, Petraroli A, Balestrieri B, Marone G: Secretory phospholipases A_2 induce cytokine release from blood and synovial fluid monocytes. Eur J Immunol 2002; 32:67–76.

8. Servillo L, Balestrieri C, Giovane A, Pari P, Palma D, Giannattasio G, Triggiani M, Balestrieri ML: Lysophospholipid transacetylase in the regulation of PAF levels in human monocytes and macrophages. Faseb J 2006; 20:1015–1017.

9. Sallusto F, Lanzavecchia A: Efficient presentation of soluble antigen by cultured human dendritic cells is maintained by granulocyte/macrophage colony-stimulating factor plus interleukin 4 and downregulated by tumor necrosis factor α. J Exp Med 1994; 179:1109–1118.

10. Triggiani M, Gentile M, Secondo A, Granata F, Oriente A, Taglialatela M, Annunziato L, Marone G: Histamine induces exocytosis and IL-6 production from human lung macrophages through interaction with H_1 receptors. J Immunol 2001; 166:4083–4091.

11. Viksman MY, Liu MC, Bickel CA, Schleimer RP, Bochner BS: Phenotypic analysis of alveolar macrophages and monocytes in allergic airway inflammation. I. Evidence for activation of alveolar macrophages, but not peripheral blood monocytes, in subjects with allergic rhinitis and asthma. Am J Respir Crit Care Med 1997; 155:858–863.

Massimo Triggiani

Division of Clinical Immunology and Allergy, Center for Basic and Clinical Immunology Research (CISI), University of Naples Federico II, Via S. Pansini 5, I-80131 Naples, Italy, Tel. +39 081 7462218, Fax +39 081 3722607, E-mail triggian@unina.it

The Role of NKT-Cells in the Development of Asthma

D.T. Umetsu, O. Akbari, E.H. Meyer, and R.H. DeKruyff

Children's Hospital, Harvard Medical School, Boston, MA

Summary: Asthma is a common pulmonary disease, characterized increased mucus in the airways and by an inflammatory process in the peribronchial space, consisting of eosinophils and a large numbers of CD4+ T-cells producing IL-4 and IL-13. The CD4+ T-cells include class II MHC restricted CD4+ T-cells as well as a newly identified subset of T-cells called natural killer T (NKT)-cells. The NKT-cells express a conserved (invariant) T-cell receptor (TCR), have potent immunoregulatory function, and have been shown to required for the development of allergen-induced airway hyperreactivity (AHR), a cardinal feature of asthma. NKT-cells do not respond to peptide antigens, but rather to glycolipids, and direct activation of NKT-cells by NKT-cell-activating glycolipids results in the development of AHR and airway inflammation, independent of class II MHC restricted CD4+ T-cells and adaptive immunity. Moreover, NKT-cells are present in the lungs of patients with persistent asthma, but not in the lungs of patients with pulmonary sarcoidosis or normal healthy individuals. These studies strongly suggest that NKT-cells play a very prominent role in the pathogenesis of asthma.

Keywords: asthma, airway hyperreactivity, allergy, NKT-cells, Th2 cells

Asthma is characterized by airway inflammation dominated by the presence of eosinophils and CD4+ T lymphocytes. The CD4+ T-cells secreting IL-4 and IL-13 are thought to play a critical and obligatory role in orchestrating the inflammation in of asthma. The precise characteristics of the CD4+ T-cells involved in asthma is not completely clear, particularly because the CD4 antigen is expressed both by conventional class II MHC restricted T-cells as well as by natural killer (NK) T-cells.

NKT-cells constitute a small subset of lymphocytes that express characteristics of both Natural Killer cells and conventional T-cells. NKT-cells are either CD4+ or double negative, and in humans a small subset express CD8. NKT-cells express TCRs, and most NKT-cells express a conserved or invariant (*i*) TCR, called Vα14 in mice and Vα24 in humans. Unlike the TCRs of conventional CD4 T-cells, which recognize peptides of proteins in the context of MHC class II molecules on APC,

the TCR of *i*NKT-cells recognize glycolipid antigens, in the context of the nonpolymorphic, class I-like protein called CD1d on APCs. Moreover, when *i*NKT-cells are activated through this invariant TCR, *i*NKT-cells rapidly produce large amounts of IL-4 and IFN-γ, and they produce these cytokines much more rapidly than do conventional T-cells. This rapid production of IFN-γ and IL-4 by *i*NKT-cells is a manifestation of innate-like immunity, and endows *i*NKT-cells with the capacity to critically amplify adaptive immune responses.

Because *i*NKT-cells produce large amounts of IL-4 and IL-13, several groups suspected that they might play and important role in the development of asthma. The role of *i*NKT-cells was first examined in a mouse model of asthma, using CD1d−/− mice, which lack the restriction element of *i*NKT-cells, and therefore lack NKT-cells. In this mouse model of asthma, WT BALB/c mice, when sensitized and challenged with OVA, were shown to develop severe AHR. Surprisingly, CD1d$^{-/-}$ mice failed to develop AHR when sensitized and challenged in the same way. This was quite striking, and therefore we tried to induce AHR with different protocols and different antigens, but in all cases, the CD1d$^{-/-}$ mice failed to develop AHR. We also examined another iNKT-cell deficient mouse strain, Jα18$^{-/-}$ mice [1], and these also failed to develop AHR. These studies indicate that iNKT-cells are required for the development of AHR measured in several different ways, in several different mouse strains.

Now in these studies, OVA and other protein antigens were used to induce AHR. But iNKT-cells do not recognize proteins, but respond rather to glycolipid antigens. So we believe that in these studies the iNKT-cells were activated by endogenous glycolipids that are expressed in the inflammatory environment induced with protein antigens. But we asked, if you could directly activate iNKT-cells with glycolipids, could the iNKT-cells alone induce AHR? Therefore, we activated the iNKT-cells with the glycolipid α-GalactocylCeramide (α-GalCer), which has been shown to be very specific in activating iNKT-cells. We found that when α-GalCer was given to BALB/c mice, within 2 h a measurable increase in AHR developed, which peaked at 24 h, at levels of AHR comparable to that seen with OVA as allergen. Moreover, the AHR induced with α-GalCer was associated with a significant inflammatory response in the airways with infiltrates in the peribronchial space. This inflammation and AHR did not occur in CD1d $-/-$ mice treated with α-GalCer, or in the control vehicle treated mice [2]. Therefore, direct activation of iNKT-cells by α-GalCer induced all of the features that typify the hyperreactivity and inflammation induced by protein allergens, indicating that the activation of iNKT-cells is sufficient for the development of AHR.

iNKT-cells did not evolve to respond to α-GalCer, which is derived from a marine sponge. So we have searched for environmental antigens that might activate iNKT-cells. So far we have found that a bacterial glycolipid from Sphingomonas bacteria can activate iNKT-cells, and induce AHR. Thus when mice are challenged with Sphingomonas glycolipid they develop AHR, and this requires iNKT-cells since it does not occur in iNKT-cell deficient mice. Sphingomonas bacteria do not appear to infect humans. However, these studies suggest that glycolipids from other pathogens might be able to activate pulmonary iNKT-cells and cause wheezing. In addition, a recent report showed that iNKT-cells can recognize lipids from cypress pollen [3], suggesting that iNKT-cells could play an important role in human asthma.

To directly examine the role of iNKT-cells in human asthma, we studied 14 patients with moderate to severe persistent asthma. 10 of the asthma patients were on corticosteroids to control their symptoms, while 4 had not received corticosteroids for more than 3 months prior to enrollment, not because they did not need steroids, but because they were noncompliant. The mean age of the asthmatic patients was 44 years. The mean FEV1 of the 10 patients on steroids was 84% predicted, which is normal, indicating that their corticosteroid therapy was effective in controlling their disease. The 4 patients not on steroids had an FEV1 was 71%predicted, indicating the presence of significant disease. The mean total serum IgE for all 14 patients was 325 u/ml, and 73% of the patients were allergic as defined by + skin tests to common allergens, indicating that many but not all of our patients had the most common form of asthma, allergic asthma. We also studied 6 normal healthy subjects, and obtained BAL fluid from these subjects, as well as biopsies of the bronchial epithelium.

About 15% of the BAL fluid cells from the patients with asthma were lymphocytes, and the majority of these cells were CD4$^+$. We stained the cells in BAL fluid with CD1d tetramers loaded with α-GalCer, which are known to bind to the invariant TCR of iNKT-cells, and with an antibody 6B11 and which recognizes the CDR3 region of the α-chain of the invariant TCR of human iNKT-cells. A large fraction of double positive cells were present in the BAL fluid, indicating that iNKT-cells were present in the BAL fluid, as defined by expression of the invariant TCR of NKT-cells.

To quantitate the number of *i*NKT-cells, we stained for and gated on CD3+ cells in the BAL fluid because in some of the patients, many of the negative events were due to RBC that contaminated the lymphocyte gate. Of the CD3+ cells, we focused on CD4+ cells, since many investigators have shown that large numbers of CD4+ Th2 cells are present in the lungs of patients with asthma. Surprisingly, we found that a large fraction of the CD4 T-cells in the BAL fluid of patients with asthma stained with CD1d tetramers, indicating that they were *i*NKT-cells. In this subject, 65% of the CD4 cells stained with tetramers. In the 14 patients with asthma, we found that 45–85% of the CD4 T-cells were actually *i*NKT-cells, as defined by expression of the invariant TCR of *i*NKT-cells [4].

To confirm the results with flow cytometry, we examined biopsy specimens from patients with asthma, using confocal laser scanning microscopy. On confocal microscopy, many cells stained for *i*NKT-cells in blue, and many cell stained for CD4 in red. The merged image was pink, indicating that most of the CD4 cells were *i*NKT-cells. Because the healthy adults had virtually no *i*NKT-cells in BAL fluid, as control, we examined patients with sarcoidosis. These patients have large numbers of CD4 T-cells in the lungs, which are thought to be Th1 cells since they secrete IFN-γ. In the biopsy section from patients with sarcoidosis there were essentially no *i*NKT-cells, but large numbers of CD4 T-cells. The merged image is red, indicating that very few if any of the CD4 T-cells are *i*NKT-cells.

In the patients with asthma, 55–85% of the CD3+ cells in BAL fluid were *i*NKT-cells. In contrast, in patients with sarcoidosis, less than 3% of the CD3+ cells in BAL fluid were *i*NKT-cells. In the four patients who did not received corticosteroids for more than 3 months prior to bronchoscopy, the percent of CD3+ cells that were *i*NKT-cells was not reduced, suggesting that steroids did not affect the percentage of *i*NKT-cells in BAL fluid. These results suggest that the presence of *i*NKT-cells in the lungs is very specific for asthma, and this is not affected by corticosteroids, perhaps explaining steroid resistant asthma. However,

*i*NKT-cells appear to play no role in sarcoidosis [4].

In the peripheral blood of patients with asthma, about half of the *i*NKT-cells were CD4+ and half were double negative, and a small population was CD8+. This was also true for the normal nonasthmatic individuals, and for the patients with sarcoidosis. However in BAL fluid of patients with asthma, >90% of the *i*NKT were CD4+. This suggested that a CD4+ subset of NKT-cells was preferential recruited or expanded in the lungs in patients with asthma.

The cytokines produced by the *i*NKT-cells from the BAL fluid of asthma patients was also examined. The *i*NKT-cells were stimulated with PMA and ionomycin or with α-Gal-Cer, which specifically activates *i*NKT-cells. The BAL *i*NKT-cells produced IL-4, IL-13, but very little IFN-γ, which is a typical Th2 profile. In contrast, *i*NKT-cells from the peripheral blood of asthma patients produced an unrestricted cytokine profile. This suggests that there is a preferential recruitment or expansion of a subset of *i*NKT-cells in the lungs of patients with asthma (this subset is CD4+ and produces Th2 cytokines), and that a Th2-like subset of *i*NKT-cells is present in the lungs of patients with asthma.

In summary, we showed that *i*NKT-cells producing IL-4 and IL-13 are required for the development of AHR in mice, and that the activation of *i*NKT-cells is sufficient for the development of AHR. In human patients with moderate to severe persistent asthma, the majority of CD4+ T-cells in the lungs of asthmatic patients but not sarcoidosis patients were *i*NKT-cells. The *i*NKT-cells in the lungs of asthmatic individuals produced IL-4, and IL-13, but not IFN-γ, and thus had characteristics of Th2 cells.

We believe that the role of *i*NKT-cells in asthma has been underappreciated in the past, presumably because the technology for identifying these cells was not available until recently. Nevertheless, much more work needs to be done to understand the relationship between *i*NKT-cells and conventional CD4+ T-cells, how *i*NKT-cells get into the lung, and how *i*NKT-cells become activated. We do believe however, that the best treatment for asthma will require reduction in the function of *i*NKT-cells or that they be eliminated from the airways.

References

1. Akbari O, Stock P, Meyer E, Kronenberg M, Sidobre S, Nakayama T, Taniguchi M, Grusby MJ, DeKruyff RH, Umetsu DT: Essential role of NKT-cells producing IL-4 and IL-13 in the development of allergen-induced airway hyperreactivity. Nature Medicine 2003; 9:582–588.
2. Meyer EH, Goya S, Akbari O, Berry GJ, Savage PB, Kronenberg M, Nakayama T, DeKruyff RH, Umetsu DT: Glycolipid activation of invariant T-cell receptor + NK T-cells is sufficient to induce airway hyperreactivity independent of conventional CD4$^+$ T-cells. Proc Natl Acad Sci USA 2006; 103:2782–2787.
3. Agea E, Russano A, Bistoni O, Mannucci R, Nicoletti I, Corazzi L, Postle A, De Libero G, Porcelli S, Spinozzi F: Human CD1-restricted T-cell recognition of lipids from pollens. J Exp Med 2005; 202:295–308.
4. Akbari O, Faul JL, Hoyte EG, Berry GJ, Wahlstrom J, Kronenberg M, DeKruyff RH, Umetsu DT: CD4$^+$ invariant T-cell-receptor + natural killer T-cells in bronchial asthma. N Engl J Med 2006; 354:1117–1129.

Dale T. Umetsu

Karp Laboratories, Rm 10127, One Blackfan Circle, Boston, MA 02115, USA, E-mail dale.umetsu@childrens.harvard.edu

Ten Years' Experience in Epidermal Dendritic Cell Phenotyping (EDCP) as a Diagnostic Tool

A. Wollenberg, H.C. Rerinck, and S. Kamann

Department of Dermatology and Allergy, Ludwig-Maximilians-University of Munich, Germany

Summary: *Background:* The differential diagnosis of atopic dermatitis (AD) is largely based on clinical features. Epidermal dendritic cell phenotyping (EDCP) describes flow cytometric analysis of dendritic cells (DC) in epidermal cell suspensions prepared from lesional skin biopsies. The underlying concept is that the immunophenotype and distribution of the dendritic cell subsets reflect the disease specific microenvironment of the clinically defined skin diseases and that EDCP may help in differential diagnosis of inflammatory skin diseases on the level of single lesions. *Methods:* Epidermal singe cell suspensions were prepared from 952 skin biopsies of numerous skin diseases. The immunophenotype of epidermal DC was quantitatively determined by EDCP, correlated with the clinical and histological data from the patient's charts and analyzed statistically to re-evaluate and improve our initially proposed diagnostic criteria. *Results:* Myeloid DC accumulated in skin lesions of intrinsic AD and lichen planus, whereas lupus erythematodes showed highest plasmacytoid DC numbers. Extrinsic AD could be identified by an expression ratio of FcεRI/CD32 on myeloid DC exceeding 1.5 with a sensitivity of 75% and a specificity of 91%. Psoriasis was identified by an expression ratio of CD64/CD11b on IDEC exceeding 0.3 with a sensitivity of 81% and a specificity of 89%. Netherton syndrome and persistent light reaction fulfil the EDCP criteria for AD, whereas ichthyosis congenita, eosinophilic cellulitis, chronic hand dermatitis and Dorfman-Chanarin-syndrome do not. *Conclusion:* EDCP may be a helpful procedure for differential diagnosis of inflammatory skin diseases, as well as an experimental procedure for the investigation of skin immunobiology.

Keywords: epidermal dendritic cell phenotyping, Langerhans cells, inflammatory dendritic epidermal cells, flow cytometry, atopic dermatitis, differential diagnosis

The differential diagnosis of atopic dermatitis (AD) is largely based on clinical features [1]. Skin prick and patch tests may indicate the sensitization state of an individual, but does not assess single lesions. Histological analysis, in contrast, shows a limited diagnostic power to differentiate between the various eczematous skin diseases [2]. Therefore, in 1995, we proposed epidermal dendritic cell phenotyping (EDCP) as a diagnostic tool [3]. This method is based on multi parameter flow cytometric analysis of myeloid and plasmacytoid dendrit-

ic cells (DC) in epidermal cell suspensions prepared from lesional skin biopsies [4–6]. The underlying concept is that the immunophenotype and distribution of the dendritic cell subsets reflect the disease specific microenvironment of the clinically defined skin diseases and that EDCP may help in differential diagnosis of inflammatory skin diseases on the level of single lesions.

During the last 10 years, we have performed EPDC from epidermal singe cell suspensions in a standardized technique [7]. This resulted in an

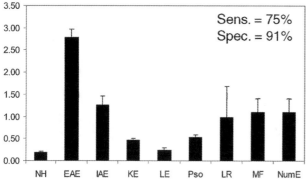

Figure 1. The FcεRI/CD32 expression ratio – a marker for extrinsic atopic dermatitis.

EPDC database of a total of 952 skin biopsies from extrinsic and intrinsic atopic dermatitis, psoriasis, contact dermatitis, eczema herpeticum and numerous other skin diseases. In addition, skin lesions were induced by patch test with haptens and atopy patch test procedure as described [8, 9]. The expression of Fc-receptors, adhesion molecules and MHC complexes were quantitatively determined, correlated with the clinical and histological data from the patient's charts and analyzed statistically to re-evaluate and possibly improve our initially proposed diagnostic criteria [7].

Myeloid IDEC accumulated in skin lesions of intrinsic AD and lichen planus, whereas lupus erythematosus showed highest plasmacytoid DC numbers. The correlation between the expression of FcεRI on myeloid DC and the serum-IgE level could be confirmed in a larger data set. Extrinsic AD was identified by an expression ratio of FcεRI/CD32 on myeloid DC exceeding 1.5 with a sensitivity of 75% and a specificity of 91% (Figure 1). Psoriasis was identified by an expression ratio of CD64/CD11b on IDEC exceeding 0.3 with a sensitivity of 81% and a specificity of 89%. This nicely confirmed our published algorithms derived from a smaller data set [7]. Cases of Netherton syndrome and persistent light reaction fulfil the EDCP criteria for AD, whereas ichthyosis congenita, eosinophilic cellulitis, chronic hand dermatitis and Dorfman-Chanarin-syndrome do not.

We conclude that immunophenotyping of epidermal dendritic cells may be a helpful pro-cedure for differential diagnosis of inflammatory skin diseases, and an experimental procedure for the investigation of skin immunobiology.

References

1. Leung DY, Bieber T: Atopic dermatitis. Lancet 2003; 361:151–160.
2. Eckert F: Histopathological and immunohistological aspects of atopic dermatitis. In T Ruzicka, J Ring, B Przybilla (Eds.), Handbook of atopic dermatitis (p. 127–131). Berlin: Springer 1991.
3. Wollenberg A, Wen S, Bieber T: Langerhans cell phenotyping: a new tool for differential diagnosis of inflammatory skin diseases. Lancet 1995; 346:1626–1627.
4. Wollenberg A, Kraft S, Hanau D, Bieber T: Immunomorphological and ultrastructural characterization of Langerhans cells and a novel, inflammatory dendritic epidermal cell (IDEC) population in lesional skin of atopic eczema. J Invest Dermatol 1996; 106:446–453.
5. Farkas L, Beiske K, Lund-Johansen F, Brandtzaeg P, Jahnsen FL: Plasmacytoid dendritic cells (natural interferon-α/β-producing cells) accumulate in cutaneous lupus erythematosus lesions. Am J Pathol 2001; 159:237–243.
6. Wollenberg A, Wagner M, Gunther S, Towarowski A, Tuma E, Moderer M et al.: Plasmacytoid dendritic cells: a new cutaneous dendritic cell subset with distinct role in inflammatory skin diseases. J Invest Dermatol 2002; 119:1096–1102.
7. Wollenberg A, Wen S, Bieber T: Phenotyping of epidermal dendritic cells: clinical applications of a flow cytometric micromethod. Cytometry 1999; 37:147–155.
8. Darsow U, Laifaoui J, Kerschenlohr K, Wollen-

berg A, Przybilla B, Wüthrich B et al.: The prevalence of positive reactions in the atopy patch test with aeroallergens and food allergens in subjects with atopic eczema: a European multicenter study. Allergy 2004; 59:1318–1325.

9. Kerschenlohr K, Decard S, Przybilla B, Wollenberg A: Atopy patch test reactions show a rapid influx of inflammatory dendritic epidermal cells (IDEC) in extrinsic and intrinsic atopic dermatitis patients. J Allergy Clin Immunol 2003; 111:869–874.

Andreas Wollenberg

Department of Dermatology and Allergy, Ludwig-Maximilians-University of Munich, Frauenlobstr. 9–11, D-80337 Munich, Germany, Tel. +49 89 5160-6251, Fax +49 89 5160-6252, E-mail wollenberg@lrz.uni-muenchen.de

Probability of Hospital Admission with Acute Asthma Exacerbation Increases with Increasing Specific IgE Antibody Levels

C.S. Murray[1], G. Poletti[1], S. Ahlstedt[3,4], L. Soderstrom[3], S.L. Johnston[2], and A. Custovic[1]

[1]*University of Manchester, North West Lung Centre, Manchester, UK*
[2]*Department of Respiratory Medicine, NHLI, Faculty of Medicine, Imperial College London, UK*
[3]*Phadia AB, Uppsala, Sweden,* [4]*Center for Allergy Research, National Institute Environmental Medicine, Karolinska Institute, Stockholm, Sweden*

Summary: *Background:* Asthma exacerbation is a common cause of hospital admission in children. We aimed to investigate whether the level of IgE antibodies to inhalant allergens is associated with an increased risk of asthma hospitalization in childhood. *Methods:* Children ($n = 84$; age 3–17 years) hospitalized with an acute asthma exacerbation (AA) were matched (age, sex) with 2 controls: stable asthmatics (SA) and children hospitalized with nonrespiratory conditions (IC). Subjects underwent measurement of specific IgE (mite, cat, dog; ImmunoCAP™) and nasal lavage for common respiratory pathogens (PCR). *Results:* A significantly higher proportion of AA had a respiratory pathogen detected (44%) compared to SA (18%) and IC (17%; $p < .001$). Sensitization (IgE > 0.35 kU$_A$/l) was significantly more common amongst AA than SA and IC groups (90% vs. 65% vs. 33% respectively; $p < .001$). Further analysis of risk factors for hospital admission was carried out within the two groups of asthmatic patients (AA, SA) using logistic regression. The risk of admission increased significantly with increasing IgE to mite (OR 1.18, 95% CI 1.05–1.34, $p = .005$). When specific IgE levels to mite, cat and dog were summed, the probability of hospitalization increased 1.3-fold (95% CI 1.1–1.4, $p < .001$) per logarithmic unit increase in IgE. In the multivariate analysis, the sum of mite, cat and dog specific IgE remained a significant, independent associate of hospital admission (OR 1.33, 1.12–1.57, $p = .001$). In addition, there was a significant interaction between the sum of IgEs and virus infection in increasing the risk of admission (OR 1.45, 1.03–2.06, $p = .035$). *Conclusions:* Increasing specific IgE antibody levels interact with natural virus infection in increasing the probability of hospitalization amongst childhood asthmatics.

Keywords: asthma, childhood, sensitization, IgE, viruses

Introduction

Asthma is one of the commonest causes of acute admission to hospital in children. Several studies have reported the association of viral infection and asthma exacerbations [1, 2] with recent studies in children detecting viruses in around 80% of exacerbations in children [3]. Reports have also shown increased emergency room visits and hospital admissions with asthma attacks in children who are both sensitized and exposed to allergens [4]. Most studies which have investigated the relationship between allergy and respiratory symptoms, have considered IgE-mediated sensitization only as a dichotomous variable, i.e., individuals are either sensitized or not (often based on differing cut-off points) [5]. In food allergy the level of specific IgE is frequently used as a predictor of likelihood of reaction [6]. However, there is much less data to suggest that IgE values may help to predict symptoms in respiratory allergy [7, 8].

We have recently demonstrated a synergism between allergen sensitization, exposure to sensitizing allergen and respiratory virus infection in increasing the risk of hospital admission amongst children [9]. In a further analysis of the data from this study, we investigated whether the level of IgE antibodies to inhalant allergens is associated with an increased risk of asthma hospitalization in childhood and examined whether there was an interaction between the specific IgE levels and viral infection.

Methods

Children aged 3–17 years admitted to hospital with acute asthma over a one-year period (asthma admission; AA) were matched for age (+/–2 years) and sex with stable asthmatic patients recruited from the outpatient department (SA) [9]. Controls were enrolled within three weeks of recruitment of the index case. The study was approved by the local ethics committee, and informed consent was obtained from parents.

Outcomes

We ascertained the following information:
- Specific serum IgE (mite, cat, dog, ryegrass; ImmunoCAP™, Phadia, Sweden).
- Virus detection: Nasal lavage was collected within 24 h of recruitment. Samples were analyzed by PCR for picornaviruses (rhinoviruses and enteroviruses), coronaviruses, respiratory syncytial virus, influenza A and

B, parainfluenza 1–3, adenoviruses, *Chlamydia* and *Mycoplasma pneumoniae* [9].

Statistical Analysis

Comparisons of the groups with respect to individual risk factors were carried out using logistic regression with STATA version 6.0 (STATA Corp, College Station, TX). Subsequently multiple conditional logistic regression analysis was used to assess the significance of various factors adjusting for the influence of other variables shown to be significant associates of AA group in the univariate analysis. Results are presented as ORs and 95% confidence intervals (95% CI).

Results

Eighty-four of 125 children (55 [65.5%] male, mean age 7.04 years) admitted to hospital for asthma exacerbation between 1st February 2000 and 31st January 2001 were recruited into the study with matched controls. A significantly higher proportion of AA had a respiratory pathogen detected (44%) compared to SA (18%) and IC (17%; $p < .001$). Similarly, sensitization was significantly more common amongst AA than SA and IC groups (90% vs. 65% vs. 33%, respectively; $p < .001$) [9].

Table 1. Odds Ratios and 95% CI for hospital admission for specific IgEs and at given values for Sum of mite, cat and dog specific IgE.

IgE (kU/L)	OR (95% CI)
Specific IgE Mite	1.18 (1.05–1.34)
Specific IgE Cat	1.13 (0.96–1.33)
Specific IgE Dog	1.15 (0.99–1.35)
Specific IgE Rye	1.09 (0.95–1.24)
Sum of mite/cat/dog IgE in kU/L	OR (95% CI)
1.0	1.43 (1.17, 1.75)
3.0	1.82 (1.29, 2.55)
10.0	2.37 (1.45, 3.88)
30.0	3.02 (1.61, 5.67)
100.0	3.94 (1.81, 8.60)

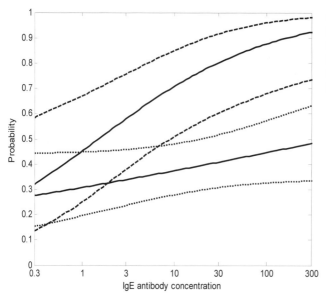

Figure 1. Fitted predicted probability curve (and 95% CIs) for hospital admission at given IgE antibody concentrations (sum of mite, cat and dog specific IgE) alone (. . . .) and with virus detected (- - - -) derived from multivariate logistic regression analysis.

Further analysis of risk factors for hospital admission was carried out within the two groups of asthmatic patients (AA and SA) using logistic regression. Using specific IgE levels as a continuous variable, the risk of admission increased significantly only with increasing IgE to mite (OR 1.18, 95% CI 1.05–1.34, p = .005), Table 1.

When specific IgE levels to mite, cat and dog were summed, the probability of hospitalization increased 1.3-fold (95% CI 1.1–1.4, p < .001) per logarithmic unit increase in IgE, such that a sum of 3 kU/L increased the risk almost 2 fold and a sum of 30 kU/L increased the risk more than 3 fold (Table 1). This corresponds to about a 35% and 50% probability of being admitted to hospital, respectively (see Figure 1). Among sensitized children, the association between sum of mite, cat and dog specific IgE and the risk of hospitalization just failed to reach statistical significance (1.22, 0.98–1.53, p = .08).

In the multivariate regression analysis, adjusting for the presence of contemporaneous viral infection, the use of inhaled corticosteroids and previous hospital admissions, the sum of specific IgE to mite, cat and dog remained a significant independent associate of admission to hospital with an asthma exacerbation (OR 1.33, 1.12–1.57, p = .001).

In addition there was a significant interaction between the sum of specific IgE to mite, cat and dog and virus infection increasing the risk for hospital admission over and above that of the specific IgE antibodies alone (OR 1.45, 1.03–2.06, p = .035). Thus, a sum of 3 kU/L of IgE antibodies with a virus infection correspond to almost a 60% probability of hospital admission compared with approximately 35% risk without virus infection, Figure 1).

Discussion

Both viruses and sensitization have been highlighted previously as risk factors for acute exacerbations with asthma. In this study we demonstrated that quantification of specific IgE to common inhalant allergens can give a more accurate prediction than using IgE as a dichotomous variable. Within this context, the sum of specific IgE to mite, cat and dog of 3, 30 and 300 kU/L give a predicted probability of hospital admission in an asthmatic child of 35%, 50% and 65%, respectively. In addition we have shown that the presence of virus interacts significantly with the IgE concentration, such that with increasing sum of specific IgE to mite, cat and dog from 3, 30 and 300 kU/L risk of admission increases to 60%, 80% and 95% respectively.

References

1. Horn ME, Brain EA, Gregg I, Inglis JM, Yealland SJ, Taylor P: Respiratory viral infection and wheezy bronchitis in childhood. Thorax 1979; 34:23–28.
2. Johnston SL, Pattemore PK, Sanderson G, Smith S, Campbell MJ, Josephs LK, Cunningham A, Robinson BS, Myint SH, Ward ME, Tyrrell DA, Holgate ST: The relationship between upper respiratory infections and hospital admissions for asthma: a time-trend analysis. Am J Respir Crit Care Med 1996; 154: 654–660.
3. Johnston SL, Pattemore PK, Sanderson G, Smith S, Lampe F, Josephs L, Symington P, O'Toole S, Myint SH, Tyrrell DA, Holgate ST: Community study of role of viral infections in exacerbations of asthma in 9–11 year old children. BMJ 1995; 310:1225–1229.
4. Rosenstreich DL, Eggleston P, Kattan M, Baker D, Slavin RG, Gergen P, Mitchell H, McNiff-Mortimer K, Lynn H, Ownby D, Malveaux F: The role of cockroach allergy and exposure to cockroach allergen in causing morbidity among inner-city children with asthma. N Engl J Med 1997; 336:1356–1363.
5. Sears MR, Herbison GP, Holdaway MD, Hewitt CJ, Flannery EM, Silva PA: The relative risks of sensitivity to grass pollen, house dust mite and cat dander in the development of childhood asthma. Clin Exp Allergy 1989; 19:419–424.
6. Sampson HA: Utility of food-specific IgE concentrations in predicting symptomatic food allergy. J Allergy Clin Immunol 2001; 107(5):891–896.
7. Simpson A, Soderstrom L, Ahlstedt S, Murray CS, Woodcock A, Custovic A: IgE antibody quantification and the probability of wheeze in preschool children. J Allergy Clin Immunol 2005; 116(4): 744–749.
8. Wickman M, Lilja G, Soderstrom L, van Hage-Hamsten M, Ahlstedt S: Quantitative analysis of IgE antibodies to food and inhalant allergens in 4-year-old children reflects their likelihood of allergic disease. Allergy 2005; 60(5):650–657.
9. Murray CS, Poletti G, Kebadze T, Morris J, Woodcock A, Johnston SL, Custovic A: Study of modifiable risk factors for asthma exacerbations: virus infection and allergen exposure increase the risk of asthma hospital admissions in children. Thorax 2006; 61(5):376–382.

Adnan Custovic

University of Manchester, Wythenshawe Hospital, Second Floor, Education and Research Centre, Manchester M23 9LT, UK, Tel. +44 161 291 5869, Fax +44 161 291 5730, E-mail adnan.custovic@manchester.ac.uk

IgE-Dependent Cytokine Release from Human Lung Tissue

L.R.C. Barnicott, T.-L. Hackett, and J.A. Warner

School of Biological Sciences, University of Southampton, UK

Summary: *Background:* The IgE dependent release of cytokines in the airways leads to a complex and protean inflammatory environment that is difficult to study *in vivo*. We have used a simple human lung tissue explant model to investigate the release of cytokines following IgE-crosslinking. *Methods:* Human lung tissue explants ($n = 19$) were stimulated with a range of different concentrations of anti-IgE or buffer control for 24 h at 37 °C and cytokine release assayed by ELISA. Four patients gave a history of allergic disease and were analyzed separately. *Results:* The release of the proinflammatory cytokine, TNFα, was maximal at 1000 µg/ml anti-IgE. A similar pattern of release was seen with the anti-inflammatory cytokine IL-10 giving maximum release at 1000 µg/ml. In contrast, the release of the Th2 cytokines IL-5 and IL-13 was maximal at 1 µg/ml anti-IgE and both cytokines showed a bell shaped dose response curve. The allergic status of the patients did not affect the release of any of the cytokines. *Conclusions:* Crosslinking of IgE leads to the release of cytokines from human lung tissue without any requirement for additional sensitization with IgE. We noted distinct patterns of cytokine release with the proinflammatory cytokine, TNFα and the anti-inflammatory cytokine, IL-10 showing dose dependent release that was maximal at 1000 µg/ml. In contrast, the release of the Th2 cytokines, IL-5 and IL-13, was maximal at 1 µg/ml and both cytokines showed a bell-shaped dose response curve. The allergic status of the patients did not significantly affect either the cytokine profile or the magnitude of the response.

Keywords: cytokine, lung tissue, IgE, TNFα, IL-10, IL-5, IL-13

Introduction

IgE crosslinking is known to be important in the pathogenesis of allergic inflammation in the airways and contributes to airway remodelling. The IgE dependent release of cytokines in the airways leads to a complex and protean inflammatory environment. These cytokines are responsible for maintaining airways inflammation, recruiting leukocytes to the tissues and activating inappropriate repair mechanisms. Studying the complex interactions between different cells and cytokines is not possible *in vivo* and so we have examined the release of cytokines by human lung tissue in response to anti-IgE and assessed the effects of patients' allergic history on the magnitude of the response.

Methods

Normal margin of resected human lung tissue was obtained from 19 patients (12M:7F) undergoing lung tumour resection at Guy's Hospital, London, UK, see Table 1. All patients gave informed consent. Four patients had a history of allergic disease and were analyzed separately.

Lung tissue fragments (approximately 2 mm^3 in size) were incubated with goat anti human IgE (Sigma, Poole UK) or a buffer control at 37 °C for 24 h [1]. The supernatant was then recovered and stored at –70 °C and the tissue weighed.

Levels of the cytokines TNFα and IL-13 were assayed using commercially available

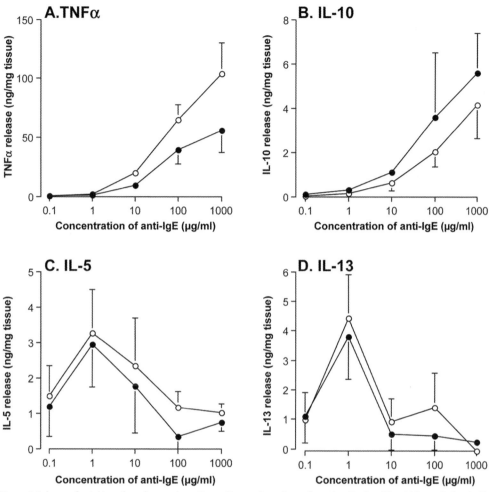

Figure 1. Release of cytokines from human lung tissue. Human lung tissue from 4 patients with a history of allergic disease(filled circles) and 15 control patients (open circles) was stimulated with a range of different concentrations of anti-IgE for 24 h at 37 °C. The supernatant was harvested and cytokines measured by ELISA.

ELISAs (R&D Systems Abingdon, UK.) while levels of IL-5 and IL-10 were analyzed using ELISA kits from Biosource Europe (Nivelles, Belgium.) Cytokine levels were corrected for tissue weight. Nonparametric statistics were used throughout and a value of $p < .05$ was accepted as a significant result.

Table 1. Patient characteristics.

	"Allergic"	Nonallergic
Age	72.3 ± 1.6	66.3 ± 3.4
Gender	3M/1F	9M/6F
Lung function (FEV$_1$/FVC)	0.75 ± 0.05	0.66 ± 0.03
Smoking status	3 exsmokers 1 nonsmoker	6 smokers, 7 exsmokers and 2 nonsmokers

Results

Human lung tissue released substantial amounts of the proinflammatory cytokine TNFα following stimulation with anti-IgE, see Figure 1A. Release was dose dependent with maximum release at 1000 µg/ml. The allergic status of the patients did not affect the magnitude of the release. There was a similar dose response dependent release of the anti-inflammatory cytokine IL-10 with maximum release at 1000 µg/ml anti-IgE, see Figure 1B. While there was a trend for the allergic patients to release slightly higher levels of IL-10 this did not reach statistical significance. In contrast to both TNFα and IL-10 the maximum release of the Th2 cytokine, IL-5, occurred at 1 µg/ml anti-IgE with evidence of a bell shaped dose response curve, see figure 1C. A second Th2 cytokine, IL-13, had a similar profile with maximum release at 1 µg/ml, see figure 1D. The allergic status of patients did not affect the magnitude of the release of either IL-5 or IL-13.

Intriguingly, the maximum levels of TNFα were approximately 10-fold higher than the levels of IL-10, IL-5 and IL-13 when the data was corrected for tissue weight.

Discussion

The tissue environment is an important determinant of cell function and cytokines are important components of that environment. While *in vivo* studies provide an invaluable snapshot of cytokine profiles they are not amenable to extended kinetic investigations or comparing the effects of more than one pharmacological agent. We have adapted a simple model of human tissue explants to study the effects of crosslinking IgE on the release of cytokines and investigated the kinetics and dose dependence of the release [2]. Substantial amounts of cytokines could be detected without the need for additional sensitization with IgE. The release of TNFα and IL-10 were found to be dose dependent with a maximum release at 1000 µg/ml anti-IgE. In contrast, the

release of the Th2 cytokines IL-5 and IL-13 were maximal at 1 µg/ml and gave a bell shaped dose response curve. Recent studies have highlighted a potential role for TNFα [3] in severe asthma we have found that the levels of TNFα released are approximately 10 fold higher than either IL-10, IL-5 or IL-13.

Acknowledgments

We would like to thank Prof Tom Treasure and the cardiothoracic team at Guy's Hospital for generously supplying the lung tissue also Dr Stuart Hirst and Dr Varsha Kanabar for their assistance in retrieving the tissue. Study funded by the University of Southampton.

References

1. Bochner BS, Landy SD, Plaut M, Dinarello CA, Schleimer RP: Interleukin 1 production by human lung tissue. I. Identification and characterization. J Immunol 1987; 139:2297–2302.
2. Barnicott, LRC, Hackett, TL, Warner JA: The role of cytokines in allergic inflammation in human lung tissue. J Allergy Clin Immunol 2006; 117:254.
3. Howarth PH, Babu KS, Arshad HS, Lau L, Buckley M, McConnell W, Beckett P, Al Ali M, Chauhan A, Wilson SJ, Reynolds A, Davies DE, Holgate ST: Tumour necrosis factor (TNFα) as a novel therapeutic target in symptomatic corticosteroid dependent asthma. Thorax 2005; 60:1012–1018.

Jane A Warner

Mail point 825, School of Medicine, University of Southampton, Southampton General Hospital, Southampton SO16 6YD, UK, Tel. +44 23 8059-4363, Fax +44 23 8059-4419, E-mail jawarner@soton.ac.uk

Detailed Sequence and Haplotype Analysis of the β2 Adrenergic Receptor Gene in Caucasians and African Americans

G.A. Hawkins, V. Ortega, and E.R. Bleecker

Center for Human Genomics, Wake Forest University School of Medicine, Winston-Salem, NC, USA

Summary: β agonists are the most prescribed medication for the treatment of chronic airway obstructive disease. The primary target of β agonists is the β-2 adrenergic receptor. The gene for the receptor, ADRβ2, is small, however considerable genetic variation, including the common coding variants Gly^{16}Arg and Gln^{27}Glu, have been identified in the gene. In addition, there are considerable differences in ADRβ2 genetic variations between ethnic groups, which contribute to a complex ADRβ2 haplotype structure that also differs considerably between ethnic groups. While the common coding variants Gly^{16}Arg and Gln^{27}Glu have been extensively studied for their affects on β agonist response, it is now believed that other genetic variants identified in ADRβ2 may contribute significantly to the wide variations observed in β agonist therapy and may also provide additional insight into the risks observed in treating specific individuals with β-agonists.

Keywords: β-2 adrenergic receptor, DNA sequencing, polymorphism, haplotype, β-agonist, asthma, pharmacogenetics

Introduction

β-agonists, such as albuterol and salmeterol, are the most commonly prescribed bronchodilator medications for treating chronic airway obstructive disease. Responses to β-agonists are known to vary considerably between patients and appear to be influenced by several factors such as the degree of airway obstruction, disease severity, age, and the concurrent use of other medications. Years of research has also shown that genetic variation in the β-2 adrenergic receptor gene (ADRβ2) plays a critical role in receptor expression and function [1–11]. These genetic variations may affect the inter-personal response to β-agonists [10, 12–29] and also play a critical role in predicting rare adverse affects of β-agonist therapy that may be ethnic group specific [10, 12, 13, 19, 23, 30–36]. In addition, because ADRβ2 is located at 5q31, a chromosomal region genetically linked to asthma and its related phenotypes, there have been numerous studies to determine if ADRβ2 is a genetic contributor to asthma risk [6, 8, 11, 14, 32, 37–61]. In order to fully understand how genetic variations contribute to asthma risk and β-agonist response, detailed sequence analysis of ADRβ2 has been necessary to characterize not only the common genetic variants, but also to identify rare genetic variations that may make significant contributions to differences in recep-

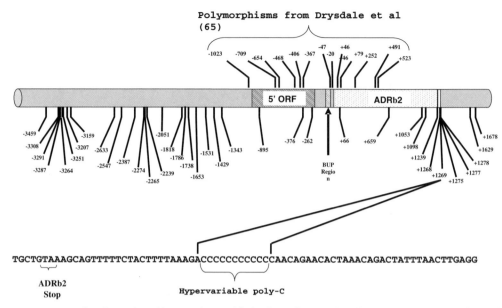

Figure 1. Diagram of *ADRβ2* as adapted from Hawkins et al. [32]. Polymorphisms are listed by number as previously referenced [32, 65].

tor expression and function between ethnic groups.

There is a long history of genetic characterization of the β-2 adrenergic receptor gene (ADRβ2) [51, 62–64]. ADRβ2 was first cloned and sequenced nearly 20 years ago [63, 64]. ADRβ2 is a small, one exon gene (Figure 1) with a single opening reading frame (ORF) that encodes a 413 amino acid G-protein coupled receptor. Two additional ORFs are located 5' of the ADRβ2 start codon and within the putative promoter region of the gene. The largest 5' open reading frame is 753 bases and extends from positions –987 to –235 5' of the start codon and has the potential to produce a 251 amino acid peptide. To date, it is not known whether this ORF is expressed or what functional effects this ORF could have on ADRβ2 expression. This ORF, however, does not exist in species other than human. A second 56 base ORF, called the Leader Cistron (LC) region, extends from positions –101 to –44 and encodes a 19 amino acid peptide called the β2-adrenergic receptor *u*pstream *p*eptide (BUP). The BUP is functional, and has been show to affect the expression of ADRβ2 by modulating the rate of ADRβ2 mRNA translation [9].

The first detailed mutational analysis of ADRβ2 was reported in 1992 by Reihaus [51]. In this report, nine genetic variations were identified in the coding region of ADRβ2, four of which, located at bases +46, +79, +100, and +491 (relative to the start codon), create the non-synonymous amino acid changes Gly[16]Arg, Gln[27]Glu, Val[34]Met, and Thr[164]Ile, respectively. The mutations Gly[16]Arg and Gln[27]Glu have been identified in every ethnicity screened thus far; however the frequencies of Gly[16]Arg and Gln[27]Glu can vary considerably between ethnic groups, as is the case for Caucasians and African Americans. *In vitro* expression studies have shown that both Gly[16]Arg and Gln[27]Glu have effects on receptor regulation, with receptors containing Gly[16]/Gln[27] or Arg[16]/Gln[27] haplotypes being down regulated by as much as 41% and 26%, respectively, while Gly[16]/Glu[27] receptors are down regulated as much as 39% [2]. Receptors containing Arg[16]/Glu[27] haplotype were not found to cause receptor down regulation. The mutation Val[34]Met is very rare (frequency < 1%) and appears to have no affect on receptor function [51]. The mutation Thr[164]Ile is also not common, however receptors containing [164]Ile have been found to exhibit a 2- to 3-fold lower β-agonist binding affinity [2]. So far, no individuals homozygous for Thr[164]Ile have been identified, leading to speculation that this mutation may be lethal. More recently, a new coding variation at +659, creating the mutation, Ser[220]Cys, was identified in African Americans [32] and Mexican Hispanics (unpublished observation). The functional effects of this coding change have not been characterized.

Additional polymorphisms have been identified in the promoter, 5' LC region, and the 3' untranslated region (UTR) of ADRβ2. One 5' polymorphism, located –47 bases 5' of the start codon, has been found to have an important affect on regulation of ADRβ2 expression. This polymorphism, which occurs in the LC region, changes Cys[19] to Arg[19] in the BUP. Functional studies have shown that the –47 T allele (BUP Cys[19]) increases the level of translation of the β-2 receptor even though the levels of ADRβ2 mRNA remained unchanged [9]. This polymorphism is in strong linkage disequilibrium with the Glu[27]Glu mutation (position +79), with the –47 T allele (BUP Cys[19]) always being inherited with the +79 C allele (Gln[27] in the receptor) [32, 65]. The co-inheritance of the Gly[16]Arg mutation and the –47 allele varies, with the –47 T allele (BUP Cys[19]) co-inherited with either the +46 A allele (Arg[16] in the receptor) or the +46 G allele (Gly[16] in the receptor), while only the –47 C allele (BUP Arg[19]) is coinherited with the +46 G allele (Gly[16] in the receptor). This coinheritance of the –47 allele and the +46 allele is further complicated by the fact that the frequency of the +46 G allele (Arg[16]) is approximately 3 to 4 times higher in Caucasians than in African Americans, suggesting that regulation of ADRβ2 expression may be associated with the haplotypes formed between the three polymorphisms at –47, +46, and +79, and that the expression levels of ADRβ2 in Caucasian and African American may correlate with differences in β-agonist response.

Drysdale et al. [65] explored the possibility of ADRβ2 haplotype effects by sequencing a subset of Caucasians, African Americans, Asians, and Hispanic-Latinos, defining the most common haplotypes in each ethnic group, and then comparing ADRβ2 haplo-

type pairs with β-agonist response in 121 Caucasians. Twelve ADRβ2 haplotypes were identified, five of which represented >95% of haplotypes in these populations. ADRβ2 haplotypes 2, 4, and 6 (48.3%, 33.0%, and 13.2%, respectively) comprised 94.5% of the haplotypic variation in Caucasians while ADRβ2 haplotypes 1, 2, 4, and 6 (25%, 6.3%, 29.7%, and 31.3%, respectively) comprised 92.3% of the haplotypic variation in African American. ADRβ2 haplotype frequencies for Asians and Hispanic-Latinos were more similar to Caucasians than African Americans. A comparison of ADRβ2 haplotypes pairs with β-agonist response in Caucasians showed that individuals with a 4/4 haplotype pair (Arg[16]/Arg[16] and Gln[27]/Gln[27]) had the lowest response to albuterol (change in%Fev1) while individuals with a 2/2 haplotype pair (Gly[16]/Gly[16] and Glu[27]/Glu[27]) showed a significantly higher response. Individuals with a 2/4 haplotype pair had a β-agonist response between that of the 2/2 and 4/4 haplotype pairs, as would be expected if responses are directly correlated to haplotypes. However, individuals with the 4/6 haplotype pair (Arg[16]/Gly[16] and Gln[27]/Gln[27]) were observed to have the highest β-agonist response, contradicting what might be expected if responses were correlated to the amino acids Gly and Gln at positions 16 and 27 of the receptor, both of which have been associated with receptor down regulation *in vitro* [2]. In addition, this data showing that Arg[16]/Arg[16] individuals (4/4 haplotype pair) (Arg[16]/Arg[16]) have decreased β-agonist response compared to Gly[16]/Gly[16] (2/2 haplotype pair) contradicts previous studies [8, 29, 56]. A recent report by Taylor also tested the effects of haplotype pairs on acute bronchodilator responses in Caucasians, however, they found no significant relationship between haplotype pairs and the use of albuterol [26]. Because both of these studies concentrated on responses in Caucasians, little is still known about the β-agonist response profile of ADRβ2 haplotype pairs in African Americans and other ethnicities.

Recently, a highly detailed sequence and haplotype analysis of a 5.3 kb region of

ADRβ$_2$ was reported for 669 Caucasians and 240 African Americans [32]. Forty-nine polymorphisms were identified, twenty-one of which had not been previously reported (Figure 1). Four of the new polymorphisms were unique to African Americans, including a nonsynonymous coding change at +659 (Ser^{220}Cys, MAF = 0.03) and a 25 base duplication in the putative promoter region at −376 (MAF = 0.02). This 25 base duplication has also been identified in Puerto Ricans with asthma (unpublished observation). Five of the polymorphisms, all with MAF ≤ 0.01, were unique to Caucasians. One potentially important DNA sequence located 23 bases after the stop codon in the 3' UTR was a hypervariable poly-cytosine (poly-C) repeat that varied in length from 9 Cs to 15 Cs (Figure 1). This hypervariable poly-C repeat is interrupted by two additional polymorphisms at +1268 and +1277 (relative to the start codon). Detailed analysis revealed that distribution of the poly-C lengths varied by ethnicity, with Caucasians having a bimodal distribution of 11 Cs (frequency = 0.40) and 13 Cs (frequency = 0.34), and African Americans having predominantly 13 Cs (frequency = 0.64). Using thirty-one polymorphisms with MAF > 0.03, including the hypervariable poly-C repeat, 24 ADRβ$_2$ haplotypes were identified and subcategorized according to shorter ADRβ$_2$ haplotypes identified by Drysdale [65]. Of the original twelve Drysdale haplotypes, only haplotypes 2, 4, 6, and 9 were observed in Caucasians while haplotypes 1, 2, 4, 6, 7, and 10 were observed in African Americans [32]. As found previously [65], Drysdale haplotype 1 was only observed in African Americans. When additional polymorphisms were considered, significant subdivision of the Drysdale haplotypes was observed for Caucasians and African Americans. For example, Drysdale haplotype 1, present only in African Americans, was divided into three subhaplotypes. Drysdale haplotypes 2, 4, and 6, present in both Caucasians and African Americans, were divided into seven, eight, and five subhaplotypes, respectively [32]. Most of these subhaplotypes were differentiated by poly-

morphisms in the 3' portion of ADRβ$_2$, which includes the poly-C repeat region. There was no correlation between acute bronchodilator response and haplotype pairs in this study, but a trend in poly-C length did correlate with FEV$_1$% predicted FVC, and (FEV$_1$/FVC)^2, but only in African Americans. This latter observation suggests that the hypervariable poly-C repeat may have a functional role in ADRβ$_2$ expression, or the repeat may be in linkage disequilibrium with another genetic variant that affects gene expression. Based on the distribution of poly-C lengths in Caucasian (bimodal distribution of 11 and 12 Cs) and African Americans (primarily 13 Cs), this data also suggests the hypervariable poly-C repeat could be an important marker for differentiation of ADRβ$_2$ haplotypes between Caucasians and African Americans, and possibly other ethnicities.

In spite of the genetic and functional studies performed on ADRβ$_2$, the exact roles that ADRβ$_2$ polymorphisms and haplotypes play in predicting receptor response to β-agonist and/or asthma risk are still not fully understood. ADRβ$_2$ is a small gene. However the amount of genetic variation in ADRβ$_2$ is quite high and is further complicated by differences in polymorphism frequencies between different ethnicities. Population stratification and genetic admixture also complicate data analysis since the racial/ethnic effects on inheritance are hard to measure on an inter-personal basis, as is probably the case in populations such as the Puerto Ricans [12, 13]. In addition, rare genetic variations, some of which are ethnic group specific, may make a significant contribution to ADRβ$_2$ expression or receptor function, but are difficult to detect without intensive DNA sequencing. Such rare genetic variants may be the source of rare adverse effects of β-agonist therapy that occur more frequently within specific ethnic groups [30, 35]. Respective of all these factors, delineation of ADRβ$_2$ expression and effects on β-agonist therapy will not be simple, and may require not only genetic analysis of ADRβ$_2$ but also other genetic factors that influence regulation of ADRβ$_2$.

References

1. Green SA, Cole G, Jacinto M, Innis M, Liggett SB: A polymorphism of the human β₂-adrenergic receptor within the fourth transmembrane domain alters ligand binding and functional properties of the receptor. J Biol Chem 1993; 23116–23121.

2. Green SA, Turki J, Innis M, Liggett SB: Amino-terminal polymorphisms of the human β₂-adrenergic receptor impart distinct agonist-promoted regulatory properties. Biochemistry 1994; 9414–9419.

3. Green SA, Turki J, Bejarano P, Hall I.P, Liggett SB: Influence of β₂-adrenergic receptor genotypes on signal transduction in human airway smooth muscle cells. Am J Respir Cell Mol Biol 1995; 25–33.

4. Green SA, Turki J, Hall IP, Liggett SB: Implications of genetic variability of human β₂-adrenergic receptor structure. Pulm Pharmacol 1995; 1–10.

5. Green SA, Rathz DA, Schuster AJ, Liggett SB: The Ile164 β(2)-adrenoceptor polymorphism alters salmeterol exosite binding and conventional agonist coupling to G(s). Eur J Pharmacol 2001; 141–147.

6. Joos L, Pare PD, Sandford AJ: β(2)-Adrenergic receptor polymorphisms and asthma. Curr Opin Pulm Med 2001; 69–74.

7. Liggett SB, Bouvier M, O'Dowd BF, Caron MG, Lefkowitz RJ, DeBlasi A: Substitution of an extracellular cysteine in the β₂-adrenergic receptor enhances agonist-promoted phosphorylation and receptor desensitization. Biochem. Biophys Res Commun 1989; 257–263.

8. Lipworth BJ, Hall IP, Tan S, Aziz I, Coutie W: Effects of genetic polymorphism on ex vivo and in vivo function of β₂-adrenoceptors in asthmatic patients. Chest 1999; 324–328.

9. McGraw DW, Forbes SL, Kramer LA, Liggett SB: Polymorphisms of the 5' leader cistron of the human β₂-adrenergic receptor regulate receptor expression. J Clin Invest 1998; 1927–1932.

10. Taylor DR, Hancox RJ, McRae W, Cowan JO, Flannery EM, McLachlan CR, Herbison GP: The influence of polymorphism at position 16 of the β2-adrenoceptor on the development of tolerance to β-agonist. J Asthma 2000; 691–700.

11. Taylor DR, Kennedy MA: Genetic variation of the β(2)-adrenoceptor: its functional and clinical importance in bronchial asthma. Am J Pharmacogenomics 2001; 165–174.

12. Burchard EG, Avila PC, Nazario S, Casal J, Torres A, Rodriguez-Santana JR, Toscano M, Sylvia JS, Alioto M, Salazar M, Gomez I, Fagan JK, Salas J, Lilly C, Matallana H, Ziv E, Castro R, Selman M, Chapela R, Sheppard D, Weiss ST, Ford JG, Boushey HA, Rodriguez-Cintron W, Drazen JM, Silverman EK: Lower bronchodilator responsiveness in Puerto Rican than in Mexican subjects with asthma. Am J Respir Crit Care Med 2004; 386–392.

13. Choudhry S, Ung N, Avila PC, Ziv E, Nazario S, Casal J, Torres A, Gorman JD, Salari K, Rodriguez-Santana JR, Toscano M, Sylvia JS, Alioto M, Castro RA, Salazar M, Gomez I, Fagan JK, Salas J, Clark S, Lilly C, Matallana H, Selman M, Chapela R, Sheppard D, Weiss ST, Ford JG, Boushey HA, Drazen JM, Rodriguez-Cintron W, Silverman EK, Burchard EG: Pharmacogenetic differences in response to albuterol between Puerto Ricans and Mexicans with asthma. Am J Respir Crit Care Med 2005; 563–570.

14. Fenech A, Hall IP: Pharmacogenetics of asthma. Br J Clin Pharmacol 2002; 3–15.

15. Hall IP: Pharmacogenetics of asthma. Eur Respir J 2000; 449–451.

16. Hancox RJ, Aldridge RE, Cowan JO, Flannery EM, Herbison GP, McLachlan CR, Town GI, Taylor DR: Tolerance to β-agonists during acute bronchoconstriction. Eur Respir J 1999; 283–287.

17. Israel E, Drazen JM, Liggett SB, Boushey HA, Cherniack RM, Chinchilli VM, Cooper DM, Fahy JV, Fish JE, Ford JG, Kraft M, Kunselman S, Lazarus SC, Lemanske RF, Martin RJ, McLean DE, Peters SP, Silverman EK, Sorkness CA, Szefler SJ, Weiss ST, Yandava CN: The effect of polymorphisms of the β(2)-adrenergic receptor on the response to regular use of albuterol in asthma. Am J Respir Crit Care Med 2000; 75–80.

18. Israel E, Drazen JM, Liggett SB, Boushey HA, Cherniack RM, Chinchilli VM, Cooper DM, Fahy JV, Fish JE, Ford JG, Kraft M, Kunselman S, Lazarus SC, Lemanske RF Jr, Martin RJ, McLean DE, Peters SP, Silverman EK, Sorkness CA, Szefler SJ, Weiss ST, Yandava CN: Effect of polymorphism of the β(2)-adrenergic receptor on response to regular use of albuterol in asthma. Int Arch Allergy Immunol 2001; 183–186.

19. Israel E, Chinchilli VM, Ford JG, Boushey HA, Cherniack R, Craig TJ, Deykin A, Fagan JK, Fahy JV, Fish J, Kraft M, Kunselman SJ, Lazarus SC, Lemanske RF Jr, Liggett SB, Martin RJ, Mitra N, Peters SP, Silverman E, Sorkness CA, Szefler SJ, Wechsler ME, Weiss ST, Drazen JM: Use of regularly scheduled albuterol treatment in asthma: genotype-stratified, randomized, place-

bo-controlled cross-over trial. Lancet 2004;
1505–1512.

20. Joos L, Weir TD, Connett JE, Anthonisen NR,
Woods R, Pare PD, Sandford, AJ: Polymorphisms in the β_2 adrenergic receptor and
bronchodilator response, bronchial hyperresponsiveness, and rate of decline in lung function in
smokers. Thorax 2003; 703–707.

21. Lazarus SC, Boushey HA, Fahy JV, Chinchilli
VM, Lemanske RF Jr, Sorkness CA, Kraft M,
Fish JE, Peters SP, Craig T, Drazen JM, Ford JG,
Israel E, Martin RJ, Mauger EA, Nachman SA,
Spahn JD, Szefler SJ: Long-acting β_2-agonist
monotherapy vs continued therapy with inhaled
corticosteroids in patients with persistent asthma: a randomized controlled trial. JAMA 2001;
2583–2593.

22. Lee DK, Currie GP, Hall IP, Lima JJ, Lipworth
BJ: The arginine-16 β_2-adrenoceptor polymorphism predisposes to bronchoprotective subsen-
sitivity in patients treated with formoterol and
salmeterol. Br J Clin Pharmacol 2004; 68–75.

23. Lima JJ, Mohamed MH, Self TH, Eberle LV,
Johnson JA: Importance of $\beta(2)$adrenergic receptor genotype, gender and race on albuterol-
evoked bronchodilation in asthmatics. Pulm
Pharmacol Ther 2000; 127–134.

24. Sears MR, Taylor DR: Regular inhaled β-adren-
ergic agonists in the treatment of bronchial asthma. Am Rev Respir Dis 1992; 734–735.

25. Taylor DR, Sears MR: Regular β-adrenergic
agonists. Evidence, not reassurance, is what is
needed. Chest 1994; 552–559.

26. Taylor DR, Epton MJ, Kennedy MA, Smith AD,
Iles S, Miller AL, Littlejohn MD, Cowan JO,
Hewitt T, Swanney MP, Brassett KP, Herbison
GP: Bronchodilator response in relation to β_2-ad-
renoceptor haplotype in patients with asthma.
Am J Respir Crit Care Med 2005; 700–703.

27. Wechsler ME, Lehman E, Lazarus SC, Lemanske RF Jr, Boushey HA, Deykin A, Fahy JV,
Sorkness CA, Chinchilli VM, Craig TJ, Diman-
go E, Kraft M, Leone F, Martin RJ, Peters SP,
Szefler SJ, Liu W, Israel E: β-Adrenergic receptor polymorphisms and response to salmeterol.
Am J Respir Crit Care Med 2006; 519–526.

28. Hancox RJ, Sears MR, Taylor, DR: Polymorphism of the β_2-adrenoceptor and the response to
long-term β_2-agonist therapy in asthma. Eur Respir J 1998; 589–593.

29. Martinez FD, Graves PE, Baldini M, Solomon S,
Erickson R: Association between genetic polymorphisms of the β_2-adrenoceptor and response
to albuterol in children with and without a history
of wheezing. J Clin Invest 1997; 3184–3188.

30. Food and Drug Administration Pulmonary-Al-
lergy Drugs Advisory Committee. Ref Type: Report 2005.

31. Belfer I, Buzas B, Evans C, Hipp H, Phillips G,
Taubman J, Lorincz I, Lipsky RH, Enoch MA,
Max MB, Goldman D: Haplotype structure of
the β-adrenergic receptor genes in US Caucasians and African Americans. Eur J Hum Genet
2005; 341–351.

32. Hawkins GA, Tantisira K, Meyers DA, Ample-
ford EJ, Klanderman B, Liggett SB, Peters SP,
Weiss ST, Bleecker ER: Sequence, haplotype
and association analysis of $ADR\beta_2$ in multi-eth-
nic asthma case/control subjects. Am J Respir
Crit Care Med 2006.

33. Liggett SB: β_2-adrenergic receptor polymorphisms and sudden cardiac death: a signal to follow. Circulation 2006; 1818–1820.

34. Lima JJ, Thomason DB, Mohamed MH, Eberle
LV, Self TH, Johnson JA: Impact of genetic polymorphisms of the β_2-adrenergic receptor on albuterol bronchodilator pharmacodynamics. Clin
Pharmacol Ther 1999; 519–525.

35. Sears MR, Taylor, DR: Bronchodilator treatment
in asthma. Increase in deaths during salmeterol
treatment unexplained. BMJ 1993; 1610–1611.

36. Wraight JM, Smith AD, Cowan JO, Flannery
EM, Herbison GP, Taylor DR: Adverse effects of
short-acting β-agonists: potential impact when
anti-inflammatory therapy is inadequate. Respirology 2004; 215–221.

37. Dai LM, Wang ZL, Zhang YP, Liu L, Fang LZ,
Zhang JQ: [Relationship between the locus 16
genotype of β_6 $_{52}$ adrenergic receptor and the
nocturnal asthma phenotype]. Sichuan Da Xue
Xue Bao Yi Xue Ban 2004; 32–34.

38. Dewar J, Wheatley A, Wilkinson J, Holgate ST,
Thomas NS, Lio P, Morton NE, Hall IP: Association of the Gln 27 β_6 $_{52}$-adrenoceptor polymorphism and IgE variability in asthmatic families.
Chest 1997; 78–79.

39. Dewar JC, Wilkinson J, Wheatley A, Thomas
NS, Doull I, Morton N, Lio P, Harvey JF, Liggett
SB, Holgate ST, Hall IP: The glutamine 27 β_2-
adrenoceptor polymorphism is associated with
elevated IgE levels in asthmatic families. J Allergy Clin Immunol 1997; 261–265.

40. Dewar JC, Wheatley AP, Venn A, Morrison JF,
Britton J, Hall IP: β_2-adrenoceptor polymorphisms are in linkage disequilibrium, but are not
associated with asthma in an adult population.
Clin Exp Allergy 1998; 442–448.

41. Gao JM, Lin YG, Qiu CC, Gao J, Ma Y, Liu YW,
Liu, Y: [Association of polymorphism of human
β_6 $_{52}$-adrenergic receptor gene and bronchial

asthma]. Zhongguo Yi Xue Ke Xue Yuan Xue Bao 2002; 626–631.

42. Hall IP, Wheatley A, Wilding P, Liggett SB: Association of Glu 27 $\beta_{6\,52}$-adrenoceptor polymorphism with lower airway reactivity in asthmatic subjects. Lancet 1995; 1213–1214.

43. Hall IP: β_2-adrenoceptor polymorphisms and asthma. Monogr Allergy 1996; 153–167.

44. Hancox RJ, Stevens DA, Adcock IM, Barnes PJ, Taylor DR: Effects of inhaled β-agonist and corticosteroid treatment on nuclear transcription factors in bronchial mucosa in asthma. Thorax 1999; 488–492.

45. Holloway JW, Dunbar PR, Riley GA, Sawyer GM, Fitzharris PF, Pearce N, Le Gros GS, Beasley R: Association of β_2-adrenergic receptor polymorphisms with severe asthma. Clin Exp Allergy 2000; 1097–1103.

46. Holloway JW, Yang, IA: β_2-Adrenergic receptor polymorphism and asthma: true or false? J Allergy Clin Immunol 2005; 960–962.

47. Hopes E, McDougall C, Christie G, Dewar J, Wheatley A, Hall IP, Helms PJ: Association of glutamine 27 polymorphism of $\beta_{6\,52}$ adrenoceptor with reported childhood asthma: population based study. BMJ 1998; 664.

48. Liggett SB: Genetics of $\beta_{6\,52}$-adrenergic receptor variants in asthma. Clin Exp Allergy 1995; 89–94.

49. Ramsay CE, Hayden CM, Tiller KJ, Burton PR, Goldblatt J, Lesouef, PN: Polymorphisms in the β_2-adrenoreceptor gene are associated with decreased airway responsiveness. Clin Exp Allergy 1999; 1195–1203.

50. Rasmussen F, Taylor DR, Flannery EM, Cowan JO, Greene JM, Herbison GP, Sears MR: Risk factors for airway remodeling in asthma manifested by a low postbronchodilator FEV1/vital capacity ratio: a longitudinal population study from childhood to adulthood. Am J Respir Crit Care Med 2002; 1480–1488.

51. Reihsaus E, Innis M, MacIntyre N, Liggett, SB: Mutations in the gene encoding for the $\beta_{6\,52}$-adrenergic receptor in normal and asthmatic subjects. Am J Respir Cell Mol Biol 1993; 334–339.

52. Santillan AA, Camargo CA Jr, Ramirez-Rivera A, gado-Enciso I, Rojas-Martinez A, Cantu-Diaz F, Barrera-Saldana HA: Association between β_2-adrenoceptor polymorphisms and asthma diagnosis among Mexican adults. J Allergy Clin Immunol 2003; 1095–1100.

53. Sears MR, Taylor DR: The $\beta_{6\,52}$-agonist controversy. Observations, explanations and relationship to asthma epidemiology. Drug Saf 1994; 259–283.

54. Silverman EK, Kwiatkowski DJ, Sylvia JS, Lazarus R, Drazen JM, Lange C, Laird NM, Weiss ST: Family-based association analysis of β_2-adrenergic receptor polymorphisms in the childhood asthma management program. J Allergy Clin Immunol 2003; 870–876.

55. Summerhill E, Leavitt SA, Gidley H, Parry R, Solway J, Ober C: β(2)-adrenergic receptor Arg16/Arg16 genotype is associated with reduced lung function, but not with asthma, in the Hutterites. Am J Respir Crit Care Med 2000; 599–602.

56. Tan S, Hall IP, Dewar J, Dow E, Lipworth B: Association between $\beta_{6\,52}$-adrenoceptor polymorphism and susceptibility to bronchodilator desensitization in moderately severe stable asthmatics. Lancet 1997; 995–999.

57. Turki J, Liggett SB: Receptor-specific functional properties of $\beta_{6\,52}$-adrenergic receptor autoantibodies in asthma. Am J Respir Cell Mol Biol 1995; 531–539.

58. Turki J, Pak J, Green SA, Martin RJ, Liggett SB: Genetic polymorphisms of the $\beta_{6\,52}$-adrenergic receptor in nocturnal and nonnocturnal asthma. Evidence that Gly16 correlates with the nocturnal phenotype. J Clin Invest 1995; 635–1641.

59. Turner SW, Khoo SK, Laing IA, Palmer LJ, Gibson NA, Rye P, Landau LI, Goldblatt J, Le Souef PN: β_2 adrenoceptor Arg16Gly polymorphism, airway responsiveness, lung function and asthma in infants and children. Clin Exp Allergy 2004; 1043–1048.

60. Weir TD, Mallek N, Sandford AJ, Bai TR, Awadh N, Fitzgerald JM, Cockcroft D, James A, Liggett SB, Pare PD: β_2-Adrenergic receptor haplotypes in mild, moderate and fatal/near fatal asthma. Am J Respir Crit Care Med 1998; 787–791.

61. Wilson AM, Gray RD, Hall IP, Lipworth, BJ: The effect of β_2-adrenoceptor haplotypes on bronchial hyper-responsiveness in patients with asthma. Allergy 2006; 254–259.

62. Caron MG, Kobilka BK, Frielle T, Bolanowski MA, Benovic JL, Lefkowitz RJ: Cloning of the cDNA and genes for the hamster and human β_6 $_{52}$-adrenergic receptors. J Recept Res 1988; 7–21.

63. Kobilka BK, Frielle T, Dohlman HG, Bolanowski MA, Dixon RA, Keller P, Caron MG, Lefkowitz, RJ: Delineation of the intronless nature of the genes for the human and hamster $\beta_{6\,52}$-adrenergic receptor and their putative promoter regions. J Biol Chem 1987; 7321–7327.

64. Kobilka BK, Dixon RA, Frielle T, Dohlman HG, Bolanowski MA, Sigal IS, Yang-Feng TL, Fran-

cke U, Caron MG, Lefkowitz RJ: cDNA for the human β$_6$ $_{52}$-adrenergic receptor: a protein with multiple membrane-spanning domains and encoded by a gene whose chromosomal location is shared with that of the receptor for platelet-derived growth factor. Proc Natl Acad Sci USA 1987; 46–50.

65. Drysdale CM, McGraw DW, Stack CB, Stephens JC, Judson RS, Nandabalan K, Arnold K, Ruano G, Liggett SB: Complex promoter and coding region β$_6$ $_{52}$-adrenergic receptor haplotypes alter receptor expression and predict in vivo responsiveness. Proc Natl Acad Sci USA 2000; 10483–10488.

Gregory A. Hawkins

Section of Pulmonary, Critical Care, Allergy and Immunologic Diseases, Center for Human Genomics, Wake Forest University Health Sciences, Winston-Salem, NC 27157, USA, Tel. +1 336 713-7511, Fax +1 336 713-7566, E-mail ghawkins@wfubmc.edu

Atheroma – Another "Modern Disease" Explained by the Hygiene Hypothesis

R. Clancy[1,2], Z. Ren[2], G. Pang[2], P. Fletcher[3], and C. D'Este[4]

[1]Immunology Unit, Hunter Area Pathology Service, John Hunter Hospital, Newcastle, NSW, Australia, [2]Discipline of Immunology and Microbiology, University of Newcastle, Newcastle, NSW, Australia, [3]Discipline of Medicine – Cardiovascular, University of Newcastle, John Hunter Hospital, Newcastle, NSW, Australia, [4]Centre for Clinical Epidemiology and Biostatistics, University of Newcastle, Newcastle, NSW, Australia

Summary: The demonstration that the amount of secreted IL-4, but not secreted INF-γ, correlated with the extent of angiographically defined coronary artery disease ($p = .006$) and that *Chlamydia pneumoniae* (*C.pn*) seropositive subjects at every level secreted more IL-4 than did seronegative subjects, has been interpreted to support the concept that atheroma fits a framework outlined by the "hygiene hypothesis." These observations provide the first evidence of a mechanism linking the presence of *C.pn* with atheroma growth.

Keywords: atherosclerosis, IL-4, IFN-γ, *Chlamydia pneumoniae*, Helicobacter pylori

Introduction, Methods, Results, Discussion

Asthma has been a model where changing epidemiological patterns have been linked with a shift in cytokine balance, which in turn reflects a particular environmental experience at critical periods of development. This phenomenon has been termed "the hygiene hypothesis." Two key immunological factors involved in pathogenesis within the "hygiene hypothesis" framework are (i) dominant IL-4-dependent mechanisms and (ii) extrinsic antigens to drive this response. A candidate is atheroma. Several pathogens, notably *Chlamydia pneumoniae* (C.pn) [1], have been associated with coronary artery disease. This study examined the hypothesis that a C.pn-driven Th2 cytokine response was present in coronary artery disease.

The host response to C.pn infection in 139 subjects having angiography to investigate stable chest pain was assessed in terms of cytokine secretion using a whole blood culture method, with or without added C.pn antigen [2]. *Helicobacter pylori* infection status was used as an infection control. For analysis mild disease was defined as "normal or one-vessel disease"; moderate disease as "two vessel disease"; severe as "three vessel disease."

C.pn-seropositive subjects secreted significantly more IL-4 than did those who were seronegative ($p = .02$) (Table 1) in all disease groups. No significant difference was noted for secreted IFN-γ. The amount of secreted IL-4, but not of secreted IFN-γ (Table 2), posi-

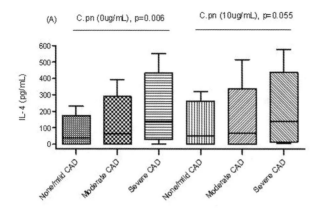

Figure 1. Secretion of INF-γ in whole blood culture in relation to extent of atheroma.

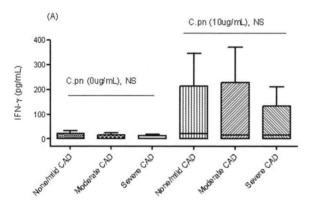

Figure 2. Secretion of IL-4 in whole blood culture in relation to extent of atheroma.

tively correlated with the extent of coronary artery disease, albeit in a nonlinear fashion ($p = .006$) (Table 1). A similar correlation with secreted IL-4 was not identified with *H.pylori* infection (data not shown). These data are the first evidence in man that IL-4 linked mechanisms contribute to the growth of atheroma and that C.pn infection contributes to the pathogenesis of atheroma by augmenting IL-4 secretion, supporting evidence in murine models (3). The whole blood cytokine secretion assay depends on ligation of CD40L on committed CD4$^+$ T-cells by CD40 on platelets (2), reflecting a possible *in-vivo* mechanism. IL-4 secretion was not increased in *H.pylori* seropositive subjects, indicating specificity with respect to infection with C.pn. These results suggest that the mechanism whereby C.pn infection contributes to coronary artery disease is through promotion of atheroma growth, rather than the enhancement of plaque rupture.

Clinical events due to plaque rupture have been the sole endpoint of antibiotic intervention studies, most of which have been negative. The present results indicate that atheroma load may be a more appropriate endpoint of such trials.

Acknowledgments

We wish to thank the cardiologists of the John Hunter Hospital for their cooperation. The study was funded in part by the National Heart Foundation.

References

1. Saikku P, Leinonen M, Mattila K, Ekman MR, Nieminen MS, Makela PH: Serological evidence of an association of a novel Chlamydia, TWAR, with chronic coronary heart disease and acute myocardial infarction. Lancet 1988; 8618:983–986.

2. Ren Z, Pang G, Lee R, Batey R, Dunkley M, Borody T, Clancy R: Circulating T-cell response to *Helicobacter pylori* infection in chronic gastritis. Helicobacter 2000; 5(3):135–141.
3. King VL, Szilvassy SJ, Daugherty A: Interleukin-4 deficiency decreases atherosclerotic lesion formation in site-specific manner in female LDL receptor –/– mice. Arterioscler Thromb Vasc Biol 2002; 22:456–461.

Robert Clancy

Level 4, David Maddison Clinical Sciences Building, University of Newcastle, Newcastle NSW 2308, Australia, E-mail robert.clancy@newcastle.edu.au

Systemic Corticosteroid Treatment

Reduces Bronchial Mucosal Activation of Activator Protein-1 (AP-1) Components in Corticosteroid Sensitive, but Not Resistant Asthmatics

T.-K. Loke, K.H. Mallett, J. Ratoff, B.J. O'Connor, S. Ying,
Q. Meng, C. Soh, T.H. Lee, and C.J. Corrigan

*King's College London School of Medicine and MRC & Asthma UK Centre
in Allergic Mechanisms of Asthma, London, UK*

Summary: *Background:* Over expression of the transcriptional regulatory factor activator protein-1 (AP-1) may contribute to T-cell corticosteroid refractoriness in corticosteroid resistant asthma. We hypothesized that clinically corticosteroid resistant asthma is accompanied by failure of systemic corticosteroid to inhibit phosphorylation of c-jun and c-jun N-terminal kinase (JNK) in bronchial mucosal cells. *Methods*: Enumeration of total (CD45$^+$) leukocytes and cells expressing c-fos and total and phosphorylated c-jun and JNK in bronchial biopsy sections from 9 corticosteroid sensitive and 17 resistant asthmatics taken before and after oral prednisolone (40 mg/1.72 m^2 body surface area daily for 14 days) using specific antibodies, immunohistochemistry and image analysis. *Results*: At baseline, mean total (CD45$^+$) mucosal leukocytes, total cells expressing phosphorylated c-jun and JNK and mean percentages of cells in which these molecules were phosphorylated were similar in both groups, whereas mean total numbers of c-fos immunoreactive cells were elevated in the corticosteroid resistant asthmatics ($p = .04$). Following prednisolone, the mean total cells expressing phosphorylated c-jun and JNK, as well as mean percentages of cells in which these molecules were phosphorylated were significantly reduced in the corticosteroid sensitive ($p < .02$), but not the resistant asthmatics. Mean total CD45$^+$ leukocytes and c-fos immunoreactive cells were not significantly altered in either group. *Conclusions:* Clinical corticosteroid responsiveness in asthma is accompanied by reduced phosphorylation of bronchial mucosal c-jun and JNK, a phenomenon not seen in resistant patients. Dysregulation of AP-1 activation leading to clinical corticosteroid resistance may reflect identifiable environmental influences and is a target for future therapy.

Keywords: asthma, corticosteroid, activator protein-1, therapy, resistance

Introduction

Some asthmatics do not improve their FEV$_1$ following administration of CS therapy at therapeutic dosages. Our previous studies [1, 2] suggested that blood mononuclear cells from CS resistant asthmatics inappropriately over-express the transcriptional regulatory protein AP-1, which sequesters and inactivates the ligand-bound CS receptor.

The most stable AP-1 complex in activated cells is the c-fos/c-jun heterodimer [3], which trans-activates a number of asthma-relevant cytokine genes including IL-5 and GM-CSF [4, 5]. AP-1 is activated through the transcriptional regulation of c-fos [6] and the phos-

Table 1. Demographic and clinical characteristics of CS sensitive and resistant asthmatics.

	CS sensitive	CS resistant	*p* value*
N (males)	9(8)	17(11)	
Age (yr)	48 ± 3	53 ± 3	.31
Atopy (% total)	6 (67%)	9 (53%)	
Daily inhaled CS dosage (BDP equivalent μg)	1430 ± 487	1048 ± 153	.35
Pretrial inhaled LABA therapy (% total)	5 (56%)	7 (41%)	
Baseline FEV_1 (liter)	1.94 ± 0.20	1.89 ± 0.16	
Baseline FEV_1 (% predicted)	58.9 ± 5.1	58.7 ± 4.6	.97
β_2-agonist reversibility (%)	33.3 ± 6.2	23.6 ± 2.9	.12
Oral CS FEV_1 reversibility (liter)	0.62 ± 0.10	0.001 ± 0.04	.001**
Oral CS FEV_1 reversibility (%)	39.4 ± 13.4	0.38 ± 2.51	.02**
Serum [ACTH] day 0 (ng/l)	18.3 ± 2.31	17.2 ± 1.9	
Serum [ACTH] day 14 (ng/l)	5.7 ± 0.63	5.4 ± 0.59	.77**

Oral CS FEV_1 reversibility (%) = $(FEV_{1day14} - FEV_{1day0}) / FEV_{1day0} \times 100\%$. CS resistant asthma is defined as oral CS reversibility $\leq 15\%$. Data are expressed as the mean $\pm$ SEM. BDP = beclometasone dipropionate; LABA = long-acting β_2-agonist. *Student's two sample t-test comparing absolute values at baseline or **changes in each group following oral prednisolone.

phorylation of c-jun, which is the end result of the action of a cascade of kinases [7] including jun N-terminal kinase (JNK), which is in turn activated by phosphorylation by JNK kinase.

Since CS have been reported to diminish AP-1 activity by inhibiting JNK phosphorylation [8], we hypothesized that clinically CS resistant asthma is accompanied by failure of CS to inhibit phosphorylation of c-jun and JNK within cells of the bronchial mucosa. We measured the expression of c-fos and total and phosphorylated c-jun and JNK in bronchial mucosal cells in groups of CS sensitive and resistant asthmatics before and after a course of systemic CS therapy.

Methods

Patients

With written, informed consent, we recruited adult, nonsmoking asthmatics (defined by ATS criteria [9]) with $\geq 15\%$ reversibility of the FEV_1 in response to inhaled β_2-agonist (Table 1).

Trial of Oral Corticosteroid Therapy

Subjects took oral prednisolone (40 mg/ 1.73 m^2) as a single dosage at 8.00 am daily for 2 weeks (days 1–14) and discontinued any long-acting $\beta_2$2-agonist 48 hr prior to, and throughout the study. Spirometry was performed on days 0 and 14. Subjects were classified as CS resistant if the change in FEV_1 between days 0 and 14, expressed as a percentage of the baseline value, was $\leq 15\%$, and sensitive if $> 15\%$ [10].

Fiberoptic Bronchoscopy

Fiberoptic bronchoscopy was performed on days 0 and 14 according to ATS guidelines. Up to 10 endobronchial biopsies were taken from segmental and subsegmental bronchi in the right lower lobe. Biopsies were snap frozen, sectioned (5 μm), fixed in acetone (15 min) and stored at –70 °C.

Immunohistochemistry and Image Analysis

Primary antibodies for immunostaining were used at preoptimized dilutions as follows:

murine monoclonal anti-CD45 (pan leukocyte marker, 200 µg/ml, 1:100 dilution); rabbit polyclonal anti-c-fos (H-125, 200 µg/ml, 1:50); rabbit polyclonal anti-c-jun (H-79, 200 µg/ml, 1:200); murine monoclonal anti-phosphorylated c-jun (KM-1, 200 µg/ml, 1:50); murine monoclonal anti-JNK (F-3, 200 µg/ml, 1:50); murine monoclonal anti-phosphorylated JNK (G-7, 200 µg/ml, 1:50). All antibodies were from Santa Cruz Biotechnology (Autogen Bionuclear, Wiltshire, UK) except anti-CD45 which was from Dako (High Wycombe, UK). Biotinylated secondary antibodies (swine anti-rabbit, 1:200 and rabbit anti-mouse, 1:400) were from Dako.

The staining procedure was as previously described [11,12]. The signal was developed with Fast DAB (Sigma-Aldrich, Dorset, UK). The sections were counterstained with Mayer's hematoxylin (Sigma). Positive (brown) cells were enumerated per unit area of the entire submucosal areas of the biopsies (excluding epithelium, glands and muscle). Statistical analysis was parametric throughout using Student's paired and two-sample t-tests as appropriate.

Results

The CS sensitive and resistant asthmatics so defined were well matched in terms of age, gender, atopic status, pretrial medication, pretrial lung function and β_2-agonist reversibility (Table 1). By definition they showed highly significant differences in their FEV_1 responses to the trial of oral prednisolone (Table 1). Serum ACTH concentrations were suppressed in all patients following oral prednisolone, consistent with compliance with the therapy (Table 1).

Total (CD45+) Leukocytes

Mean (SEM) total numbers of mucosal CD45+ leukocytes were similar in the CS sensitive and resistant asthmatics and did not change significantly following oral prednisolone therapy (sensitive: 605 ± 85 to 593 ± 92 cells/mm²,

$p = .83$; resistant: 748 ± 81 to 693 ± 85 cells/mm², $p = .53$).

C-fos Immunoreactivity

Mean total numbers of mucosal c-fos immunoreactive cells did not significantly change in either the CS sensitive or the resistant asthmatics following oral prednisolone (sensitive: 248 ± 44 to 275 ± 41 cells/mm², $p = .62$; resistant: 380 ± 42 to 390 ± 59 cells/mm², $p = .80$). The CS resistant patients did however have significantly greater numbers of cells expressing c-fos at baseline than the sensitive patients ($p = .04$).

Total and Phosphorylated c-jun

Mean total numbers of mucosal cells expressing immunoreactivity for phosphorylated c-jun did not significantly differ in the CS sensitive and resistant asthmatics at baseline. In association with oral prednisolone therapy, however, there was a significant fall in the mean numbers of cells expressing phosphorylated c-jun in the sensitive, but not the resistant patients (sensitive: 117 ± 30 to 54 ± 15 cells/mm², $p = .02$; resistant: 148 ± 27 to 173 ± 35 cells/mm², $p = .29$). The mean total numbers of mucosal cells expressing immunoreactivity for c-jun did not significantly change in both the CS sensitive and resistant asthmatics following prednisolone. Consequently, the mean percentage of the total c-jun immunoreactive cells in which the c-jun was phosphorylated was significantly reduced in the sensitive, but not the resistant patients (sensitive: 61 ± 7 to $37 \pm 5\%$, $p = .002$; resistant: 46 ± 5 to $56 \pm 6\%$, $p = .09$).

Total and Phosphorylated JNK

Mean total numbers of mucosal cells expressing immunoreactivity for phosphorylated JNK did not significantly differ in the CS sensitive and resistant asthmatics at baseline. In association with oral prednisolone therapy, however, there was a significant fall in the mean numbers of cells expressing phosphorylated JNK in the sensitive, but not the resistant patients (sensitive: 58 ± 10 to 31 ± 2 cells/mm^2, $p = .01$; resistant: 76 ± 14 to 68 ± 19 cells/mm^2, $p = .55$). The mean total numbers of mucosal cells expressing immunoreactivity for JNK did not significantly change in the CS sensitive asthmatics, but showed a significant fall in the CS resistant patients following prednisolone. Consequently, the mean percentage of the total JNK immunoreactive cells in which the JNK was phosphorylated was significantly reduced in the sensitive, but not the resistant patients (sensitive: 58 ± 7 to $40 \pm 4\%$, $p = .01$; resistant: 46 ± 3 to $58 \pm 5\%$, $p = .09$).

Discussion

The data lend further support to the hypothesis that clinically CS resistant asthma is associated with altered regulation of the expression and activation of the components of AP-1 within bronchial mucosal cells. CS resistant, as compared with sensitive asthmatics showed elevated baseline bronchial mucosal cellular expression of c-fos, and evidence of impaired down regulation of the MEK/JNK/c-jun phosphorylation cascade after systemic CS therapy.

Although the mechanism by which these biochemical abnormalities regulate airways caliber in asthma is unclear, it is possible to speculate that increased activation of c-jun and expression of c-fos might increase AP-1 activity within mucosal inflammatory cells, increasing the transcription of asthma-relevant cytokines such as IL-4 and IL-5, while sequestering and inactivating the ligand-bound CS receptor.

The relationship between expression of AP-1 components and the inhibitory effects of CS in asthma is likely complex and in dynamic equilibrium. On the one hand, CS inhibits phosphorylation of c-jun and JNK. On the other hand, c-jun has been shown to down regulate transcription of the CS receptor gene by acting on its promoter [13], whereas AP-1 binds to the CS receptor directly, with mutual inhibition of the activities of both moieties. Whereas in most asthmatics systemic CS exerts a net anti-inflammatory effect, this equilibrium appears to be destabilized in favour of

excessive production of AP-1 components in CS resistant patients, with consequent CS hyporesponsiveness in inflammatory cells. We hypothesize that external, environmental influences, particularly oxidative stress [14] (for example from infection, smoking or poor dietary anti-oxidant intake) may contribute to this phenomenon.

Acknowledgment

The authors would like to thank Kheem Jones and Cherilyn Mitchell, and Marianne Morgan and Steve Greenaway and their staff for excellent clinical and technical assistance.

References

1. Adcock IM, Lane SJ, Brown CR et al.: Defective binding of corticosteroid receptor to DNA in steroid-resistant asthma. J Immunol 1995; 154:3500–3505.
2. Adcock IM, Lane SJ, Brown CR et al.: Abnormal corticosteroid receptor-activator protein 1 interaction in steroid-resistant asthma. J Exp Med 1995; 182:1951–1958.
3. Halazonetis TD, Georgopoulos K, Greenberg ME, Leder P: c-jun dimerizes with itself and with c-fos, forming complexes of different DNA binding affinities. Cell 1988; 55:917–924.
4. Wang CY, Bassuk AG, Boise LH, Thompson CB, Bravo R, Leiden JM: Activation of the granulocyte-macrophage colony-stimulating factor promoter in T-cells requires cooperative binding of Elf-1 and AP-1 transcription factors. Mol Cell Biol 1994; 14:1153–1159.
5. de Groot RP, van Dijk TB, Caldenhoven E et al.: Activation of 12-O-tetradecanoylphorbol-13-acetate response element- and dyad symmetry element-dependent transcription by interleukin-5 is mediated by jun N-terminal kinase/stress-activated protein kinase kinases. J Biol Chem 1997; 272:2319–2325.
6. Curran T, Bravo R, Muller R: Transient induction of c-fos and c-myc is an immediate consequence of growth factor stimulation. Cancer Surv 1985; 4:655–681.
7. English JM, Cobb MH: Pharmacological inhibitors of MAPK pathways. Trends in Pharmacological Sciences 2002; 23:40–45.
8. Gonzalez MV, Jimenez B, Berciano MT et al.: Corticosteroids antagonize AP-1 by inhibiting

the activation/phosphorylation of JNK without affecting its subcellular distribution. J Cell Biol 2000; 150:1199–1208.

9. Standards for the diagnosis and care of patients with chronic obstructive pulmonary disease (COPD) and asthma. This official statement of the American Thoracic Society was adopted by the ATS Board of Directors, November 1986. Am Rev Respir Dis 1987; 136:225–224.

10. Lee TH, Brattsand R, Leung D: Corticosteroid action and resistance in asthma. Am J Respir Crit Care Med 1996; 154:51.

11. Sousa AR, Parikh A, Scadding G, Corrigan CJ, Lee TH: Leukotriene-receptor expression on nasal mucosal inflammatory cells in aspirin-sensitive rhinosinusitis. N Engl J Med 2002; 347:1493–1499.

12. Corrigan C, Mallett K, Ying S, Roberts D, Parikh A, Scadding G, Lee T: Expression of the cysteinyl leukotriene receptors cysLT1 and cysLT2 in aspirin-sensitive and aspirin-tolerant chronic rhinosinusitis. J Allergy Clin Immunol 2005; 115:316–322.

13. Cabral AL, Hays AN, Housley PR, Brentani MM, Martins VR: Repression of corticosteroid receptor gene transcription by c-jun. Mol Cell Endocrinol 2001; 175:67–79.

14. Ichijo H, Nishida E, Irie K et al.: Induction of apoptosis by ASK1, a mammalian MAPKKK that activates SAPK/JNK and p38 signalling pathways. Science 1997; 275:90–94.

Chris Corrigan

Department of Asthma, Allergy & Respiratory Science, 5th Floor, Thomas Guy House, Guy's Hospital, London SE1 9RT, UK, Tel. +44 207 188 0599, Fax +44 207 403 8640, E-mail chris.corrigan@kcl.ac.uk

Biphasic Itch Stimulus Model for Investigations Using Functional Magnetic Resonance Tomography

F. Pfab[1,2], M. Valet[3], T. Sprenger[3], T.R. Tölle[3], G.I. Athanasiadis[1], H. Behrendt[2], J. Ring[1], and U. Darsow[1,2]

[1]*Department of Dermatology and Allergy,* [2]*Division of Environmental Dermatology and Allergy GSF/TUM,* [3]*Department of Neurology, all Technische Universität München, Munich, Germany*

Summary: *Background:* Itch is a crucial symptom of allergic skin disease with difficult objective measurement. Functional magnetic resonance tomography (fMRI) studies on itch have been hampered by the lack of a phasic stimulus. We present a short-term temperature-modulated human itch model with subsequent exemplary use in fMRI. *Methods:* In 9 healthy right-handed volunteers (age 29 ± 2.6 years), 1% histamine dihydrochloride was used as validated itch stimulus in the skin prick test on the right forearm with subsequent modulation of the target skin area temperature by a Medoc TSA thermode in 14 cycles (32 °C to 25 °C) in boxcar design. Subjective scales were recorded using a computerized visual analog scale (VAS). Exemplary fMRI using the biphasic stimulus model was performed with EPI sequence technique. *Results:* All subjects reported localized itch without pain. In each cycle itch intensity was generally perceived as higher during cold blocks than during warm blocks. Mean itch intensity during the first (49.5% ± 4.1%) as well as second half (52.2% ± 4.1%) of the cold block was significantly higher ($p < .001$) as during the first (34.5% ± 3.5%) as well as second half (32.7% ± 3.7%) of the warm block. The fMRI activation patterns showed involvement of different brain structures involved in sensory processing corresponding to the multidimensional aspects of itch. *Conclusions:* A significant enhancement of histamine induced itch by short term cooling was shown serving as phasic fMRI stimulus paradigm.

Keywords: itch, histamine, biphasic, model, alternating, temperature, modulation, supra-threshold, physiology

Introduction

Itch is a complex and unpleasant sensory experience that induces the urge to scratch [1]. It is the most prevalent symptom of inflammatory skin diseases [2, 3] and difficult to be measured objectively. Its pathophysiology remains poorly understood in spite of numerous studies [2]. Itch can easily be elicited experimentally – most effectively via a histamine stimulus [4]. With its mainly subjective characteristics itch has some psycho-physiological similarity to pain. Although some degree of overlap is present, recent neurophysiological studies have confirmed that itch pathways are clearly distinct from pain pathways [5, 6]. In contrast to pain, so far no method has been described to elicit and stop the sensation of itch within seconds. We investigated the itch sensation using a methodology with short term temperature changes for modulation of histamine-induced itch. As proof of principle the paradigm was subsequently investigated using fMRI in a healthy volunteer.

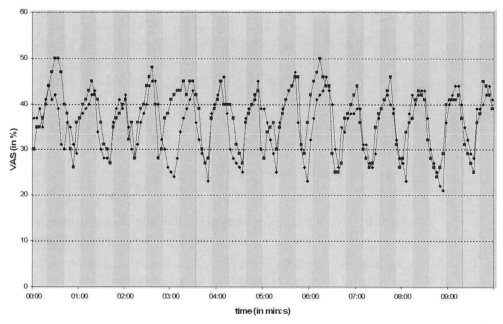

Figure 1. Typical itch intensity (VAS) scores of the two sessions (black and violet) in one volunteer: 14 cycles each lasting 43s, beginning with a 21.5 s warm block (32 °C; red background) and ending with a 21.5 s cold block (25 °C; blue background). The yellow line represents the scratch threshold (33% itch-intensity).

Material and Methods

In 9 healthy right-handed male volunteers, 1% histamine dihydrochloride was used as evaluated itch stimulus [4] in the skin prick test on the right forearm with subsequent modulation of the target skin area temperature by a Medoc TSA thermode. The latter is capable of heating or cooling the skin as needed and was placed exactly above the stimulus area. Using a boxcar design 14 equal cycles were applied: Each cycle started with a warm block producing a constant skin temperature of 32 °C for 20 s then changing within 1.5 s (ramp 5 °C/s) to a cold block of 25 °C also lasting for 20 s. The used temperature range was the result of extensive pilot trials. When the subject reported no further itching, a second session of histamine stimulation was performed on a different skin area followed by alternating temperature modulation.

Subjective scales were recorded using a computerized visual analog scale (VAS) ranging from 0 to 100 at 4 s intervals. At one-third of the VAS (33/100) the intervention point of the

"scratch threshold" was installed. Above this threshold each individual felt the clear-cut desire to scratch; this, however, was not permitted nor done. Itch intensity was quantitatively expressed in percent of the maximum VAS value.

Functional neuroimaging was performed on a Siemens Symphony 1.5 Tesla MR scanner with EPI sequence technique (155 images, first 5 images discarded because of T1 equilibration effects, matrix: 64×64; TE: 50 ms; TR: 3000 ms; α: 90 °; FOV: 192 mm, 28 axial slices; resulting voxel size: $3 \times 3 \times 5$ mm)

Statistical Analysis

Temperature blocks were compared with respect to VAS using a two sample t-test for dependent variables. In case of significance bivariate posthoc t-tests were performed using Bonferroni correction for multiple testing. p values less than .05 were considered as statistically significant. All tests were performed two-tailed.

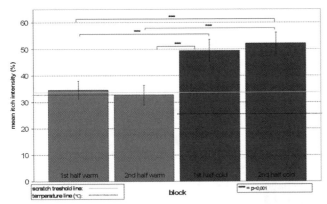

Figure 2. Mean itch intensity of averaged warm and cold sessions at the temperature blocks (*n* = 9). The red columns indicate the first and second half of the warm block, whereas the blue columns mark the first and second half of the cold block, each block lasting 20 s. The yellow line represents the scratch threshold (33% itch-intensity). Asterisks indicate significant differences between intervals. ***p < .001.

Results

All subjects reported itch without pain within 40 seconds after histamine application. None of the volunteers ever felt sensation of pain during the whole experiment.

In each individual subject as well as in the total group, significant differences between VAS rating intervals concerning itch intensity were noted. In each cycle itch intensity was generally perceived as higher during cold blocks than during warm blocks (Figure 1). Mean itch intensity during the first (49.5% ± 4.1%) as well as second half (52.2% ± 4.1%) of the cold block was significantly higher (*p* < .001) than during the first (34.5% ± 3.5%) as well as second half (32.7% ± 3.7%) of the warm block (Figure 2).

Alternating changes in mean itch perception comparing warm and cold blocks were remarkably reproducible (Figure 1).

fMRI using the biphasic stimulus model exemplarily in one volunteer showed activation in numerous brain areas (prefrontal cortex, cerebellum, insular cortex, brainstem, supplementary motor cortex, parietal cortex) (Figure 3).

Discussion

In spite of the common knowledge that intensive cold inhibits itch sensation, a reproducible, significant enhancement of histamine-induced itch by short term cooling was shown. This effect might be explained by peripheral

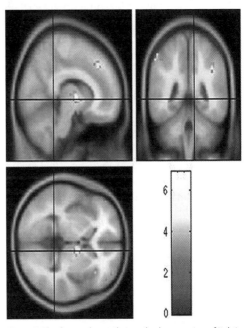

Figure 3. The figure shows the cerebral processing of itch in a healthy human volunteer, who was investigated with functional magnetic resonance imaging using the short term alternating temperature modulation of histamine induced itch. The functional activation map is superimposed on his structural T1 image. Right side of the image corresponds to the right side of the brain. Activations are found in numerous brain areas (prefrontal cortex, cerebellum, insular cortex, brainstem, supplementary motor cortex, parietal cortex).

and central adaptation processes triggered by abnormal afferent activity patterns.

Paradoxical phenomena in this context have already been described: e.g., "paradoxical heat" where perception of heat is reported when the skin temperature is innocuously cooled [7] or "hyperknesis" which describes the experience that the stimulation of A-delta-fibers by cooling or punctuate stimulation leads to an increase of itch sensation [8].

The biphasic stimulus model was finally studied in fMRI. The results confirm previous imaging studies showing that itch is processed via various brain structures contributing to the encoding of multidimensional aspects of itch [9].

In conclusion the presented method allows controlled and rapid modulation of itch. Short term cooling enhances histamine-induced itch, providing the possibility of further and more detailed investigations of itch by functional imaging methods such as fMRI.

Acknowledgments

The authors thank Dr. Regina Hollweck (Institut für Medizinische Statistik und Epidemiologie, Technische Universität München, Germany) for her support regarding statistical evaluation.

F. Pfab and M. Valet made an equal contribution to this work.

References

1. Hafenreffer S: Nosodochium, in quo cutis, eique adaerentium partium, affectus omnes, singulari methodo, et cognoscendi e curandi fidelisime traduntur. Ulm, Kuhnen 1660: 98–102.
2. Charlesworth EN, Beltrani VS: Pruritic dermatoses: overview of etiology and therapy. Am J Med 2002; 113(9A):25–33.
3. Behrendt H, Krämer U, Schäfer T, Kasche A, Eberlein-König B, Darsow U, Ring J: Allergotoxicology – a research concept to study the role of environmental pollutants in allergy. ACI International 2001; 13:122–128.
4. Darsow U, Ring J, Scharein E, Bromm B: Correlations between histamine-induced wheal, flare and itch. Arch Dermatol Res 1996; 288:436–441.
5. Yosipovitch G, Greaves MW, Schmelz M: Itch. The Lancet 2003; 361:690–694.
6. Darsow U, Drzezga A, Frisch M, Munz F, Weilke F, Bartenstein P, Schwaiger M, Ring J: Processing of histamine-induced itch in the human cerebral cortex: a correlation analysis with dermal reactions. J Invest Dermatol 2000; 115:1029–1333.
7. Davis KD, Pope GE, Crawley AP, Mikulis DJ: Perceptual illusion of "paradoxical heat" engages the insular cortex. J Neurophysiol 2004; 92:1248–1251.
8. Atanassoff PG, Brull SJ, Zhang J, Greenquist K, Silverman DG, Lamotte RH: Enhancement of experimental pruritus and mechanically evoked dysesthesiae with local anesthesia. Somatosens Mot Res 1999; 16:291–298.
9. Darsow U, Drzezga A, Frisch M et al.: Processing of histamine-induced itch in the human cerebral cortex: a correlation analysis with dermal reactions. J Invest Dermatol 2000; 115:1029–1333.

Ulf Darsow

Klinik und Poliklinik für Dermatologie und Allergologie am Biederstein, TU München, Biedersteiner Strasse 29, D-80802 München, Germany, Tel. +49 89 4140-3463, Fax +49 89 4140-3171, E-mail ulf.darsow@lrz.tum.de

Further Considerations on the Mechanisms of NSAID Hypersensitivity

A.L. de Weck[1], M.L. Sanz[1], and P. Gamboa[2]

[1]*Department of Allergology and Clinical Immunology, University of Navarra, Pamploba, Spain*
[2]*Allergy Division, Hospital Basurto, Bilbao, Spain*

Summary: In a multicentric study sponsored by the European Network for Drug Allergy (ENDA), 150 patients hypersensitive to NSAIDs and 163 controls have been investigated with the flow cytometric basophil activation test (BAT) and the sulfidoleukotriene release assay (CAST). While positive results have been obtained in 70–75% of the patients, it has been found that a variable number of NSAID-tolerant controls,may also show some degree of dose-dependent activation, depending upon the conditions of the test. It appears that basophil activation by NSAID is a dose-dependent pharmacological effect, with a shift of the dose-curve response in clinically hypersensitive patients.

Keywords: NSAID, hypersensitivity, basophil activation test, CAST

The hypersensitivity syndrome to nonsteroidal anti-inflammatory drugs (NSAIDs) is characterized clinically by airway symptoms, such as asthma, sinusitis and nasal polyposis (the aspirin triad) or by cutaneous symptoms such as urticaria and angiedema. Both are seldom associated. It is presumed that the pathophysiological mechanism is linked to the pharmacological cyclooxygenase 1 (COX-1) inhibiting effect of the various NSAIDs which cause it and that increased release of LTC4 plays an important role in the symptoms. Up to recently, however, it was consistently stated that no in vitro tests enable to detect that condition, which may only be confirmed by provocation tests.

Previous studies on the participation of blood basophils to the NSAID hypersensitivity syndrome, manifested by CD63 expression detected by flowcytometry (FLOW CAST) and the release of sulfido leukotrienes (sLTs) (CAST) have been reported before [1–4]. These results suggested that NSAID hypersensitivity is due to the joint effect of several factors, such as a local tissue inflammatory background raising cellular hyperreactivity and expression of a pharmacogenetic abnormality.

We may now report the results of a multicentric study sponsored by the European Network for Drug Allergy (ENDA) involving 12 European groups, with 150 validated NSAID-hypersensitive sensitive patients and 163 NSAID-tolerant controls [5]. Patients were investigated with FLOW CAST and CAST in parallel with two concentrations each of 5 NSAIDs (Aspirin, 1 and 0.2 mg/ml; Diclofenac, 0.3 and 0.06 mg/ml; Paracetamol, 1 and 0.2 mg/ml; Naproxen 1 and 0.2 mg/ml; Metamizol, 5 and 1 mg/ml). Technical details are described elsewhere [1, 2].This study has confirmed the high sensitivity (75% for FLOW CAST; 84% for FLOW CAST and CAST combined). which may be obtained under appropriate technical conditions. This multicentric study was performed with isolated leukocytes, like the original Sanz reports- On the other hand, other groups have reported lower sensitivities of 25% [6] and 30% [7] when performing the test in whole blood, a fact confirmed by a direct comparative study [8].

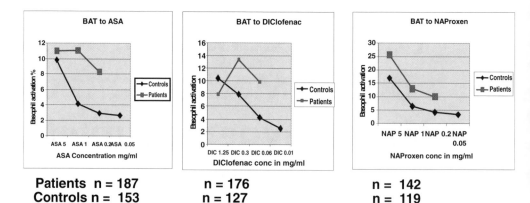

Patients n = 187   n = 176   n = 142
Controls n = 153   n = 127   n = 119

Figure 1. Doses response curves to three NSAIDs, aspirin (ASA), diclofenac (DIC), and naproxen (NAP) for basophil activation (expression of CD63) in groups of NSAID-hypersensitive and NSAID-tolerant patients.

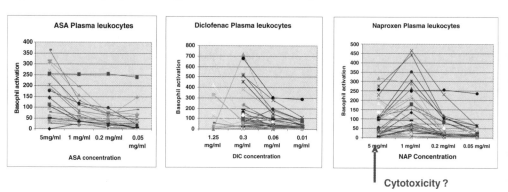

Figure 2. Individual dose-response curves to ASA, DIC, and NAP in NSAID-tolerant controls.

ASA	Leuko				Buffy coat				
5mg /ml	1 mg/ml	0.2 mg/ml	0.05 mg/ml		5 mg/ml	1 mg/ml	0.2 mg/ml	0.05 mg/ml	Patient No
60	52	26	23		88	16	11	9	15
190	100	89	65		94	19	13	14	16
364	130	73	89		317	82	39	28	17
316	194	78	67		300	59	29	25	18
305	155	54	147		303	29	13	4	19
92	41	62	30		237	43	408	357	20
31	45	39	70		28	147	153	23	21
103	34	24	24		185	34	10	10	22
203	81	64	57		133	39	23	14	23
40	18	20	7		35	18	13	8	24
105	35	23	5		50	13	5	10	25
78	60	27	8		28	13	5	5	26
50	34	23	7		83	15	0	0	27
143	35	15	18		125	28	23	18	28
255	251	255	238		200	178	220	213	29

Ex:

Positive :

Figure 3. Individual dose response results to ASA (basophil activation in% × 10) for NSAID-tolerant controls tested with plasma leukocytes (left panel) and buffy coat leukocytes (right panel).

Examples

NAP c2	ASA c2	DilC C2
135	23	165
182	53	140
320	131	441
222	84	379
443	114	519
352	119	67
153	72	235
25	17	0
181	39	94
75	43	140
6	12	6
0	0	14
3	3	6
8	0	12
24	73	75
21	13	51
9	13	19
41	7	74
94	0	31
23	115	65
289	42	721
4	97	6

Figure 4. The same NSAID-tolerant patients react with basophil activation (CD63 activation ub% × 10) to ASA, DIC and

The importance of the cellular environment in assessing flowcytometric basophil activation by NSAIDs became obvious when comparing the results obtained in various groups in NSAID-tolerant controls. While some groups obtained few positive controls and hence a high specificity around 90%, as originally reported [1, 2], other groups reported many positive controls with the specificity dropping accordingly below 50%. Further enquiry among the participating laboratories revealed that the ones obtaining few positive controls were using buffy coat cells (first hard centrifugation at 500 g for 10 min) while the others obtaining many positive controls were using plasma leukocytes (first low centrifugation at 200 g for 5 min) and specificity of the flowcytometric basophil activation test FLOW-CAST test. This differential was then confirmed in a series of direct comparative experiments on the same blood samples.

The results may be summarized as follows:

a) Both NSAID-hypersensitive and NSAID-tolerant individuals may respond by basophil activation (CD63 expression) in a dose-dependent manner. Clinical hypersensitivity is associated with a shift of the dose-response curves toward lower NSAID concentrations (Figure 1)

b) Basophil reactivity toward NSAIDs varies greatly among NSAID-tolerant individuals (Figure 2). This reactivity is better revealed among plasma leukocytes than among buffy coat cells; however, it is the same individuals who react (Figure 3)

c) It is also the same NSAID tolerant individuals who react to aspirin, diclofenac and naproxen (Figure 4); the correlation seems not only qualitative but quantitative (Figure 5). Paracetamol and metamizol only seldom cause reactions. These reactions seem there-

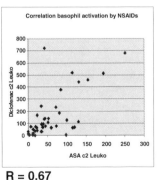
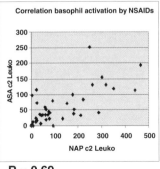
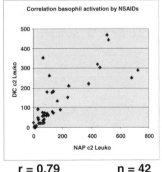

| R = 0.67 | R = 0.69 | r = 0.79 | n = 42 |

Figure 5. Basophil activation to ASA, DIC, and NAP in NSAID-tolerant patients is quantitatively correlated.

fore to be linked to the COX-1 inhibiting pharmacological effect of the drugs.

These observations seems to be the first documenting a differential cellular reactivity to NSAIDs in normal blood cells. However, retrospective analysis show well a great individual variability in the inhibiting effect of NSAIDs on PGE2 synthesis of blood cells [9]. The possible clinical significance of this finding is not yet clear. Is the pharmacological dose-response curve to NSAID a fluctuating variable, influenced by chronic inflammation and/or viral events, leading at the most extreme to clinical NSAID hypersensitivity? And is it possible that reported cases of IgE-mediated reactions considerably increased by aspirin occur precisely in those individuals who have not yet reached clinical NSAID hypersensitivity but who do show a higher basophil reactivity to NSAID [10]?

References

1. Gamboa P, Sanz ML, Caballero MR, Urrutia I, Antepara I, Esparza I, de Weck AL: The flor-cytometric determination of basophil activation induced by aspirin and other nonsteroidal anti-inflammatory drugs (NSAIDs) is useful for in vitro diagnosis of the NSAID hypersensitivity syndrome. Clin Exp Allergy 2004; 34:1448–1457.
2. Sanz ML, Gamboa P, de Weck AL: A new combined test with flowcytometric basophil activation and determination of sulfidoleukotrienes Is useful for in vitro diagnosis of hypersensitivity to aspirin and other nonsteroidal anti-inflammatory drugs Int Arch Allergy 2005; 36:58–72.
3. De Weck AL, Sanz ML: Cellular Allergen Stimulation Test (CAST) 2003, a review. J Investig Allergy Clin Immunol 2004; 14:253–273.
4. De Weck AL, Sanz ML, Gamboa P: [New pathophysiological concepts on aspirin hypersensitivity (Widal syndrome); diagnostic and therapeutic consequences]. Bull Acad Narl Me 2005; 189:1201–1218.
5. De Weck AL, Sanz ML, Gamboa PM, Aberer W, Sturm G, Blanca M, Torres M, Mayorga L, Correia S, Kowalski M, Medrala W, Sczeklik A, ENDA group: Diagnosis of hypersensitivity to nonsteroidal anti-inflammatory drugs (NSAIDs) in vitro by flowcytometry (Flow-CAST) and sulfidoleukotriene assay. A multicentric study. EAACI Vienna 2006; (Abtsr 654).
6. Kvedariene V, Arnoux B, Rongier M, Bousquet PF, Demoly P: Benefit of the basophil activation test for the diagnosis of immediate drug hypersensitivity reaction. Allergy Clin Immunol Int; J World Allergy Org 2005; Suppl. 1, 128, (Abstr 371).
7. Erdmann SM, Ventocilla S, Moll-Slodowy S, Sauer L, Merk HF: Basophil activation tests in the diagnosis of drug reactions. Hautarzt 2005; 56:38–43.
8. De Weck AL, Gamboa P, Sanz ML: Comparison of two commercial basophil activation cytofluorometric tests for the diagnosis of allergies and pseudoallergies. EAACI Paris 2003, pp. 369–370 (Abstr 1299).
9. Dallob A, Hawkey CJ, Greenberg H, Wight N, De Schepper P, Waldmann S, Wong P, De Tora L, Gertz B, Agrawal N, Wagner J, Gottesdiener K: Characterization of etoricoxib, a novel, selective COX-2 inhibitor. J Clin Pharmacol 2003; 43:573–585.
10. Aihara M, Miyazawa M, Osuna H, Tsubaki K, Ikebe T, Aihara Y, Ikezawa Z: Food-dependent exercise-induced anaphylaxis: influence of concurrent aspirin administration on skin testing and provocation. Br J Dermatol 2002; 146:466–472.

AL de Weck

Beaumont 18, 1700 Fribourg, Switzerland, E-mail alain.dew@bluewin.ch

Mechanotransduction of uPA-uPAR in Airway Epithelial Cells

E.K. Chu[1,2], K.J. Haley[1], D.J. Tschumperlin[2], and J.M. Drazen[1,2]

[1]*Department of Pulmonary and Critical Care Medicine, Brigham and Women's Hospital and*
[2]*Harvard School of Public Health, Physiology Program, all Boston, MA, USA*

Summary: Asthma has classically been considered as an inflammatory disease of the airways. In this construct both the events initiating and perpetuating the micro-environment of the airway are considered primarily inflammatory in nature. We have previously shown that airway epithelial cells in air-liquid interface culture respond to a trans-cellular pneumatic pressure gradient by manifesting an inflammatory phenotype even though there are no inflammatory cells present in the culture system. Here we review evidence that mechanical compression activates the urokinase plasminogen activator and the urokinase plasminogen activator receptor system in these cells and in human airways recovered from children dying with status asthmaticus.

Keywords: plasminogen, airway remodeling

During normal breathing the mechanical forces acting on the airway epithelium are minimal. However, there are significant forces on the airway epithelium that arise as result of bronchoconstriction. When we first approached this problem over a decade ago, we estimated the effects of bronchoconstriction on the airway using finite element analysis [1]. When the airway narrows, the epithelium buckles and a normal (in the geometric sense) stress is exerted on the cells of the epithelium [1] on the order of 20–40 cm H_2O [2].

We devised a simple system to study the effects of mechanical stress on airway epithelial cells, which used human epithelial cells grown in air-liquid interface (ALI) cultures and differentiated to achieve a mixed population of surface secretory (goblet) and pseudostratified columnar epithelial cells. These cells are grown in Transwells® (Costar) which are short open-ended plastic cylinders covered on one side with a porus membrane. The cylinders are immersed in tissue culture medium, the cells seeded on the membrane and then cultured submerged, for about 7–10 days, until confluent. The liquid is then removed from the upper well and the cells exposed to a fully humidified atmosphere of 5% CO_2 in air. After a few days the cells differentiate until "an epithelium" is formed. Mechanical stress is applied to the cells by capping the Transwell® with a plug and increasing the pressure of the air/CO_2 mixture applied to the cells. We used cells grown in this system to examine the panel of genes expressed as a result of mechanical compression. Full details of the experimental methods and detailed results have been previously published [3].

Aliquots of RNA from 4 experiments in which there were replicable results were combined by time of exposure and used to hybridize an Affymetrix HU-133A genechip at each time point. Hybridization and processing of the samples to Affymetrix genechips was performed by the Harvard Medical School – Partners Healthcare Center for Genetics and Genomics. The resultant gene expression image files were processed using Robust Multi-array Average

(RMA) [4]. Validity of the gene expression data from chip to chip was confirmed by examining several housekeeping genes (representing 18 different probe sets) that we had previously determined did not change with compressive stress, as well as several "positive-control" genes that are known to be regulated by compression (HB-EGF, c-fos, Egr-1).

The 22,284 probe sets (representing over 14,000 genes) were then ranked from most differentially regulated to least differentially regulated by compression using Significant Analysis of Microarrays [5]. The 3000 most differentially regulated genes were selected and categorized with hierarchical clustering using Cluster 3.0 for further analysis [6]. Examination of the cluster of 1024 most differentially regulated genes identified several ligands of the epidermal growth factor receptor (EGFR) as differentially regulated. This was reassuring since we knew from our prior work that HB-EGF was regulated by compressive stress.

Further analysis with gene ontology using the Database for Annotation, Visualization and Integrated Discovery (DAVID) [7] identified several groups of significantly over-represented ontological categories in the gene clusters. In particular, several plasminogen-related genes were noted, including urokinase plasminogen activator (uPA), urokinase plasminogen activator receptor (uPAR), plasminogen activator inhibitor-1 (PAI-1) and tissue plasminogen activator (tPA). Analysis by a second independent method, principal component analysis, also showed that these genes were coordinately regulated. The chip results have subsequently been confirmed using the same approach with cells obtained from a second donor.

Follow-up experiments were performed to validate the expression and function of these genes. Quantitative real-time PCR confirmed that compression coordinately increased expression of the plasminogen-related genes. These were validated in both the original samples used for gene expression profiling as well as additional compression stimulated NHBE cells.

Protein expression of uPA, uPAR, and PAI-1 was examined in the cell lysates and media of compressed NHBE cells and unstimulated time-matched controls after 8 h and 24 h. Compres-

sive stress increased protein levels of uPA in cell lysates. In the cell culture media compressive stress increased uPAR protein levels at 8 and 24 h after the onset of compression ($1.04 \pm$ vs 0.14 vs 0.64 ± 0.09 ng/mL $p = .053$ and 1.3 ± 0.08 vs 0.86 ± 0.07 ng/mL, $p = .007$, respectively). uPA and PAI-1 protein secretion into the media was increased 24 h after the onset of compressive stress (4.7 ± 1.1 vs 3.3 ± 0.86 ng/mL, $p = .02$; 50 ± 13 vs 36 ± 10 ng/mL, $p = .006$, respectively).

In addition to RNA and protein product we demonstrated that there was increased plasminogen activator activity in response to compressive stress (0.0113 vs 0.0079 Optical Density units (OD)/min, $p = .06$ and 0.008965 vs 0.003325 OD/min, $p = .033$) after 8 h and 24 h of stimulation. The plasmin generation activity of the compressed cell lysates was specific for urokinase as demonstrated by anti-uPA antibodies that inhibited plasmin generation ($p = .00039$ and $p = .0058$ for $25 \mu g/mL$ and $2.5 \mu g/mL$ of anti-uPA respectively).

We next asked whether our finding derived from airway epithelial cells in culture were informative with respect to human asthma. In order to address this problem we obtained lung tissue from two patients who had died as a result of status asthmaticus and tissue for comparison from lungs that had been donated to lung transplant programs but had not been implanted in a recipient within the allotted time. Standard immunohistochemical techniques were used to visualize uPA and uPAR, Figure 1 [3].

We observed prominent immunostaining for both uPA and uPAR in the airways of the two status asthmaticus patients, but little or no immunopositivity in the six lung donor samples (Figure 1, A–D). At higher magnification notable immunostaining could be seen on the surface of airway epithelial cells in the status asthmaticus samples; again, little staining was observed in the airway epithelium of lung donor tissue (Figure 1, E–H). To verify the specificity of the observed immunostaining, we replaced the uPA and uPAR antibodies with a nonspecific isotype control, and found little staining in the status asthmaticus or lung donor tissues (Figure 1, I–J).

These data provided a direct demonstration

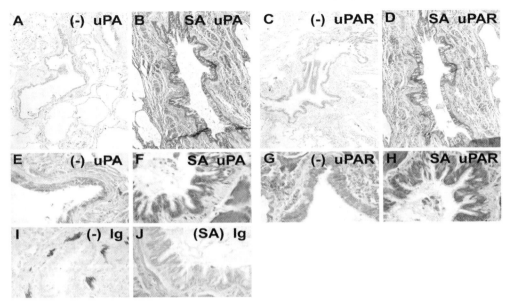

Figure 1. Immunostaining for uPA and uPAR in human lung tissue. Representative images are shown from one of six lung donors, and one of two patients who died in status asthmaticus. Low-power fields (*original magnification*: ×10) for uPA (*A, B*) and uPAR (*C, D*) reveal increased staining in status asthmaticus (*B, D*) relative to lung donor (*A, C*) tissue. Higher-power fields (*original magnification*: ×40) highlight the increased epithelial staining for uPA (*E, F*) and uPAR (*G, H*) in status asthmaticus (*F, H*) relative to lung donor (*E, G*) airways. A relative absence of epithelial staining was found with a nonspecific isotype control antibody in both lung donor (*I*) and status asthmaticus (*J*) airway epithelium, although some nonspecific reactivity was seen in airway smooth muscle.

that uPA and uPAR could be upregulated in the absence of an inflammatory response and by airway epithelial cells alone.

Acknowledgments

Eric Chu is supported by a fellowship grant from the Canadian Institutes of Health Research. D.J. Tschumperlin is a Parker B. Francis Fellow in Pulmonary Research. Funding sources include NIH HL-33009 and an American Lung Association Research Grant.

References

1. Wiggs BR, Hrousis CA, Drazen JM, Kamm RD: On the mechanism of mucosal folding in normal and asthmatic airways. J Appl Physiol 1997; 83(6):1814–1821.
2. Hrousis CA, Wiggs BJR, Drazen JM, Parks DM, Kamm RD: Mucosal folding in biologic vessels. J Biomech Eng 2002; 124(4):334–341.
3. Eric K, Chu JC, Foley JS, Mecham BH, Owen CA, Haley KJ, Mariani TJ, Kohane IS, Tschum-perlin DJ, Drazen, JM: induction of the plasminogen activator system by mechanical stimulation of human bronchial epithelial cells. Am J Respir Cell Mol Biol 2006; 35:628–638.
4. Irizarry RA, Bolstad BM, Collin F, Cope LM, Hobbs B, Speed TP: Summaries of affymetrix genechip probe level data. Nucleic Acids Res 2003; 31(4):15.
5. Tusher VG, Tibshirani R, Chu G: Significance analysis of microarrays applied to the ionizing radiation response. Proceedings of the National Academy of Sciences 2001; 98(9):5116–5121.
6. Eisen MB, Spellman PT, Brown PO, Botstein D: Cluster analysis and display of genome-wide expression patterns. Proc Natl Acad Sci 1998; 95(25):14863–14868.
7. Dennis G, Sherman B, Hosack D et al.: DAVID: Database for annotation, visualization, and integrated discovery. Genome Biology 2003; 4(5):3.

Jeffrey M. Drazen

Harvard School of Public Health, Physiology Program, 665 Huntington Ave, Boston, MA 02115, USA, Tel. +1 617 432-4561, Fax +1 617 432-3468, E-mail jdrazen@nejm.org

Eosinophilic Esophagitis: Escalating Epidemiology?

A. Straumann[1], P. Heer[1], H. Spichtin[2], and H.-U. Simon[3]

[1]Department of Gastroenterology, Kantonsspital Olten, Switzerland, [2]Institute for Clinical Pathology Viollier, Basel, Switzerland, [3]Department of Pharmacology, University of Bern, Switzerland

Summary: *Background*: Eosinophilic esophagitis (EE), a chronic inflammatory disorder of the esophagus, was originally considered rare, but is now increasingly recognized. Some demographic data exist for pediatric patients, but not for adults, the primary target population of this study. *Methods*: We report on 27 adult cases selected from a continuing database commenced in 1989 that prospectively enrolls EE patients. All patients presented here lived in Olten County, Switzerland, an area having only one gastroenterology and pathology center, approximately 100,000 inhabitants, and having undergone no relevant demographic changes within recent decades. Diagnostic criteria as well as database inclusion criteria remained unchanged throughout the whole study period. *Results*: Throughout an almost 17-year observation period, an average annual incidence of 1.59/100,000 inhabitants was noted (range 0–6) with a marked increase in newly-diagnosed cases during the last years, leading to a current prevalence of 27/100,000 inhabitants. *Conclusions*: Given the stability of demographic and recording conditions, it is very likely that this remarkable trend reflects a real increase in EE and not just enhanced awareness. Today, EE may be one of the leading causes of dysphagia in adults and, once believed to be a rare anomaly, occurs at a considerable frequency and may soon reach that of chronic inflammatory bowel diseases.

Keywords: eosinophilic esophagitis, demography, incidence, prevalence

Introduction

Eosinophilic esophagitis (EE) is a chronic [1, 2], IL-5 driven [3], inflammatory disorder of the esophagus. The leading symptom in adults is dysphagia for solids with the imminent risk of food impaction [4, 5]. EE is defined as a clinicopathological disease characterized by (1) symptoms of an impaired esophageal function and (2) a dense esophageal eosinophilia, both of which persistent despite treatment with proton pump inhibitors. Furthermore, eosinophilic inflammation is absent in the stomach, small intestine and colon. The ongoing inflammation may induce esophageal tissue damage and subsequent fibrosis with ensuing narrowing and stricture [6].

Previously considered obscure, the startling prevalence of EE has reached epidemic proportions. Today, EE may be even one of the leading causes of dysphagia, particularly in younger patients [7]. But whether this worrying trend is due to a true rise in the incidence or simply to an increased awareness of the disease is still unclear. Noel *et al.* provided the first pediatric demographic data for EE when they reported a 4-fold increase in the EE-prevalence among children from the USA between 2000–2003 [8].

The purpose of this study was to determine reliable demographic data on an adult population, analyzing a prospectively conducted database.

Methods

We report on 27 adult cases selected from a continuing national database commenced in 1989 that prospectively enrolls EE patients.

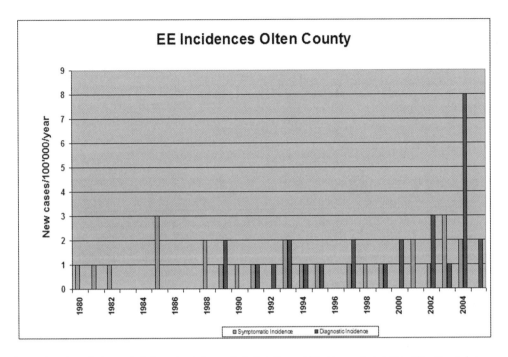

Figure 1. Symptomatic (≅ onset of disease) and diagnostic (= first diagnosis) Incidence of adult EE in Olten County between 1989 and 2005. (Newly diagnosed cases per year per 100,000 population.)

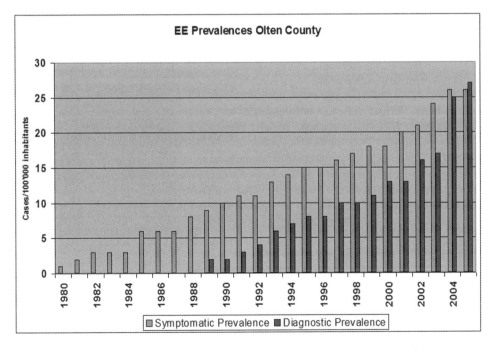

Figure 2. Symptomatic and diagnostic Prevalence of adult EE in Olten County between 1989 and 2005. (Cases per 100,000 population).

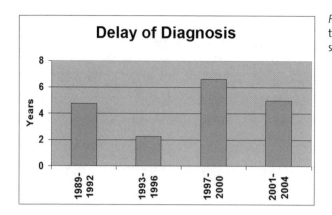

Figure 3. Diagnostic Delay (= time span between onset of symptoms and first diagnosis) between 1989 and 2005.

All patients presented here lived in Olten County, Switzerland, a well defined area having one single gastroenterology and pathology center, approximately 100,000 inhabitants, and having undergone no relevant demographic changes within recent decades. The diagnostic workup of patients presenting with the symptom "dysphagia" remained unchanged over the study period and consisted of EGD with biopsy-samples from the proximal and the distal esophagus (each at least 4) with histological examination and histometrical determination of the density of the eosinophilic infiltration.

Database inclusion criteria were (1) typical history, (2) consistent endoscopic abnormalities, and (3) peak infiltration of the esophageal epithelium with ≥ 24 eosinophils per high power field (400X) and epithelial proliferative changes. GERD was excluded clinically, endoscopically and with 24-h probe monitoring (optional).

Results

Throughout a 17-year observation period, an average annual incidence of 1.59/100,000 inhabitants was noted (range 0–6) with a marked increase in newly-diagnosed cases during the last years (Figure 1), leading to a current, cumulative prevalence of 27/100,000 inhabitants (Figure 2). Symptomatic prevalence (considered as onset of disease) and diagnostic prevalence (initial diagnosis of disease) showed a constant and parallel increase (Figure 2). No

patient had symptoms before 1980. The diagnostic delay remained unchanged throughout the study period (Figure 3).

Conclusions

Given the stability of demographic and recording conditions, the parallel increase of prevalence of symptoms and diagnosis and the non-improved diagnostic management, it is very likely that, (1) EE firstly appeared in the early eighties, (2) the constantly increased diagnosis reflects a real increase in EE and not just an enhanced awareness, (3) EE in adults occurs today at a considerable frequency that may soon reach that of classical IBD's, and (4) EE may be one of the leading causes of dysphagia.

References

1. Rothenberg ME, Mishra A, Collins MH, Putnam PE: Pathogenesis and clinical features of eosinophilic esophagitis (Editorial). J Allergy Clin Immunology 2001; 108:891–894.
2. Fox VL, Nurko S, Furuta GT: Eosinophilic esophagitis: it's not just kid's stuff. Gastrointest Endosc 2002; 56:260–270.
3. Straumann A, Bauer M, Fischer B, Blaser K, Simon HU: Idiopathic eosinophilic esophagitis is associated with a T(H)2-type allergic inflammatory response. J Allergy Clin Immunol 2001; 108:954–961.
4. Arora AS, Yamazaki K: Eosinophilic esophagitis: asthma of the esophagus? Clin Gastroenterol Hepatol 2004; 2:523–530.
5. Croese J, Fairley SK, Masson JW, Chong AK,

Whitaker DA, Kanowski PA, Walker NI: Clinical and endoscopic features of eosinophilic esophagitis in adults. Gastrointest Endosc 2003; 58:516–522.
6. Straumann A, Spichtin HP, Grize L, Bucher KA, Beglinger C, Simon HU: Natural history of primary eosinophilic esophagitis: a follow-up of 30 adult patients for up to 11.5 years. Gastroenterology 2003; 125:1660–1669.
7. Desai TK, Stecevic V, Chang C-H, Goldstein NS, Badiazdegan K, Furuta GT: Association of eosinophilic inflammation with esophageal food impaction in adults. Gastrointest Endosc 2005; 61:795–801.
8. Noel RJ, Putnam PE, Rothenberg ME: Eosinophilic esophagitis. N Engl J Med 2004; 351:940–941.

Alex Straumann

Department of Gastroenterology, Kantonsspital Olten, Roemerstrasse 7, CH-4600 Olten, Switzerland, Tel. +41 62 212-5577, Fax +41 62 212-5564, E-mail alex.straumann@hin.ch

Interleukin-4 Regulates the Expression of Thymus- and Activation-Regulated Chemokine (TARC)/CCL17

by a Signal Transducer and Activator of Transcription 6 (STAT6)-Dependent Mechanism

J. Horejs-Hoeck, G. Wirnsberger, D. Hebenstreit, G. Posselt, and A. Duschl

Department of Molecular Biology, University of Salzburg, Austria

Summary: *Background:* The recruitment of inflammatory cells, a hallmark of allergic reactions, is mediated via a number of chemokines and their receptors. The CC-chemokine TARC/CCL17 is considered to be a key mediator in the maintenance of allergic diseases, as it selectively binds the chemokine receptor CCR4, which is preferentially expressed on Th2 cells. In the present study, we have investigated the regulation of this Th2-related chemokine in primary human T-cells. *Methods:* We examined TARC/CCL17 mRNA and protein expression in human primary T-cells by quantitative real-time (RT)-PCR and ELISA techniques. Promoter studies were carried out in the STAT6-deficient cell line HEK 293. *Results:* In this study, we demonstrate that TARC/CCL17 is expressed by primary human T-cells cultured with IL-4 in a time-dependent way. Activation of the TARC/CCL17 promoter was only observed upon introduction of functional STAT6. Moreover, point mutations in either of the STAT6 binding sites identified in the TARC/CCL17 promoter led to a significant loss of cytokine responsiveness, whereas mutation of both STAT6 binding motifs resulted in complete abrogation of TARC/CCL17 promoter activity. *Conclusion:* The present study shows that human T-cells serve as a source of TARC/CCL17 when stimulated with IL-4. Moreover, we report that the transcription factor STAT6 is essentially involved in this mechanism. As TARC/CCL17 can be added to the list of STAT6-regulated genes, our study underlines the potential of this transcription factor as a therapeutic target in allergic disease.

Keywords: allergy, chemokines, TARC/CCL17, human T-cells, interleukin-4, STAT6

Introduction

Chemokines are regarded as key players in the pathogenesis of allergic inflammation. Their biological effects include the regulation of leukocyte trafficking, activation of cellular responses, release of inflammatory mediators, and promotion of Th2 responses [1]. Chemo- kines act through chemokine receptors, a family of G-protein coupled receptors. Among these, at least three receptors, CCR3, CCR4, and CCR8, are implicated in Th2-mediated inflammation, as they are preferentially expressed on Th2 cells [2]. TARC/CCL17, which, besides MDC/CCL22, represents one of the main CCR4 ligands, was shown to clearly enhance local dominance of Th2 cells during allergic responses [3, 4]. TARC/CCL17 is constitutively expressed in the thymus and, upon stimulation with various stimuli, also in several cell types including PBMCs, macrophages, dendritic cells, endothelial cells, and epithelial cells [3, 5–8]. Recent findings showed that TARC/CCL17 is also expressed in a Th2-biased cytokine environment. IL-4 as well as IL-13 induce TARC/CCL17 in airway smooth muscle cells, while IL-4, but not IL-13 was sufficient to stimulate TARC/CCL17 expression in the keratinocyte cell line HaCaT [9, 10].

Although several distinct signal transduction pathways are involved in IL-4 and IL-13 signaling, the transcription factor STAT6 arguably plays a key role in mediating the effects triggered by these cytokines. We have recently demonstrated that STAT6 is involved in the IL-4-induced regulation of the CC-chemokines Eotaxin-1/CCL11 and Eotaxin-3/CCL26 [11, 12] which are also known to be implicated in allergic inflammation.

In the present study, we describe IL-4-stimulated primary human T-cells as potent source of TARC/CCL17 expression. Moreover, we demonstrate that the stimulatory effect of IL-4 is mediated by the transcription factor STAT6.

Material and Methods

Peripheral blood was obtained from healthy adult donors and peripheral blood mononuclear cells (PBMCs) were separated by density-gradient centrifugation. Nonadherent lymphocytes were collected and T-cells were further purified using nylon wool chromatography (Polysciences, Eppelheim, Germany). Human primary T-cells were cultured in RPMI 1640, 10% FCS, 100 µg/ml streptomycin, 100U/ml penicillin and stimulated with increasing amounts of human IL-4 (R&D Systems, Minneapolis, MN). Detection of TARC/CCL17 protein in cell culture supernatants was performed using ELISA reagents specific for human TARC/CCL17 (R&D Systems, Minneapolis, MN). Total RNA was isolated using the TRIzol reagent

(Life Technologies, Gaithersburg, MD) according to the supplier's instructions. For real-time PCR analysis of TARC/ CCL17 mRNA a Rotorgene 2000 (Corbett Research, Sydney, Australia) was used.

TARC/CCL17 promoter studies were carried out in the human embryonic kidney cell line HEK 293, which endogenously expresses an inactive version of STAT6. HEK 293 cells were transiently transfected with a reporter gene expressing Luciferase under the control of wild-type or mutated promoter constructs featuring 239bp of the TARC/CCL17 promoter in the presence or absence of a STAT6 expression vector. To create the promoter mutants, two point mutations were introduced into the STAT6 consensus sequence. These substitutions were previously shown to efficiently abrogate STAT6 binding [11]. 24 h after transfection, cells were induced with 50 ng/ml of IL-4 or left unstimulated. IL-4 inducibility was measured after another 12 h by means of the Promega Luciferase Assay System (Promega, Mannheim, Germany).

Results

To analyse TARC/CCL17 mRNA and protein expression, T-cells from 5 different donors were cultured in the absence or presence of IL-4 for different times, ranging from 2 to 96 h.

We observed rapid induction of TARC/ CCL17 mRNA as well as protein expression, since mRNA levels were detectable after 2 h and protein levels after 24 h of IL-4 treatment. These findings indicated a possible role for the transcription factor STAT6.

Visual inspection of the proximal TARC/ CCL17 promoter region revealed the presence of two putative STAT6 binding sites, which are located in close proximity to the transcriptional start site of the chemokine. To carry out promoter gene assays, which allowed functional studies on the observed STAT6 binding sites, a 239bp TARC/CCL17 promoter fragment carrying both potential STAT6 binding motifs was cloned upstream of the LUC gene. HEK 293 cells were transiently transfected with wild-type or mutated reporter constructs in the absence or presence of a STAT6 expression vector. Our data clearly demonstrate that the promoter was inducible only upon introduction of functional STAT6. Moreover, point mutations in either of the STAT6 binding sites led to a significant loss of cytokine responsiveness, whereas mutation of both STAT6 binding sites resulted in complete abrogation of TARC/CCL17 promoter activity.

Discussion

In the present study, we show for the first time that the CC-chemokine TARC/CCL17 is expressed by primary human T-cells upon stimulation with IL-4. Rapid induction of TARC/ CCL17 mRNA expression (2 h) in response to IL-4 and the presence of two putative STAT6 binding motifs in the TARC/CCL17 promoter suggested a possible involvement of the transcription factor STAT6 in TARC/CCL17 regulation. STAT6 was already reported to be involved in the regulation of MDC/CCL22, the second main ligand of CCR4, upon stimulation with Th2 cytokines [13, 14]. Our data clearly demonstrate that TARC/CCL17 is also expressed by IL-4-stimulated T-cells in a STAT6-dependent way. Since both chemokines are stimulated in a Th2 environment and are further described to be major Th2 cell attractants, these findings suggest a regulatory feedback loop for T-cell recruitment and indicate increased expression of both CCR4 ligands during Th2-mediated responses.

Moreover, this study describes one more candidate for STAT6-regulated genes and emphasizes the potential of this transcription factor as a possible therapeutic target. In contrast to most other STAT molecules, STAT6 activation is unique to the signal transduction pathway employed by IL-4 and IL-13 [15]. The strictly limited modes of STAT6 activation and the important role it plays in allergic diseases make this transcription factor an excellent target for elucidation of the mechanistic basis of Th2-mediated immune disorders and for development of potent therapeutics.

Acknowledgments

This work was supported by the research program "Biomedicine and Health," University of Salzburg, Austria.

References

1. Gangur V, Oppenheim JJ: Are chemokines essential or secondary participants in allergic responses? Ann Allergy Asthma Immunol 2000; 84(6):569–579; quiz 579–581.
2. Rot A, von Andrian UH: Chemokines in innate and adaptive host defense: basic chemokinese grammar for immune cells. Annu Rev Immunol 2004; 22:891–928.
3. Imai T et al.: Selective recruitment of CCR4-bearing Th2 cells toward antigen-presenting cells by the CC chemokines thymus and activation-regulated chemokine and macrophage-derived chemokine. Int Immunol 1999; 11(1):81–88.
4. Imai T et al.: Macrophage-derived chemokine is a functional ligand for the CC chemokine receptor 4. J Biol Chem 1998; 273(3):1764–1768.
5. Imai T et al.: Molecular cloning of a novel T-cell-directed CC chemokine expressed in thymus by signal sequence trap using Epstein-Barr virus vector. J Biol Chem 1996; 271(35):21514–21521.
6. Nomura T et al.: Interleukin-13 induces thymus and activation-regulated chemokine (CCL17) in human peripheral blood mononuclear cells. Cytokine 2002; 20(2):49–55.
7. Sallusto F et al.: Distinct patterns and kinetics of chemokine production regulate dendritic cell function. Eur J Immunol, 1999. 29(5): 1617–25.
8. Sekiya T et al.: Inducible expression of a Th2-type CC chemokine thymus- and activation-regulated chemokine by human bronchial epithelial cells. J Immunol 2000; 165(4):2205–2213.
9. Faffe DS et al.: IL-13 and IL-4 promote TARC release in human airway smooth muscle cells: role of IL-4 receptor genotype. Am J Physiol Lung Cell Mol Physiol 2003; 285(4):907–914.
10. Kakinuma T et al.: IL-4, but not IL-13, modulates TARC (thymus and activation-regulated chemokine)/CCL17 and IP-10 (interferon-induced protein of 10kDA)/CXCL10 release by TNF-α and IFN-γ in HaCaT-cell line. Cytokine 2002; 20(1):1–6.
11. Hoeck J, Woisetschlager M: STAT6 mediates eotaxin-1 expression in IL-4 or TNF-α-induced fibroblasts. J Immunol 2001; 166(7):4507–4515.
12. Hoeck J, Woisetschlager M: Activation of eotaxin-3/CCl126 gene expression in human dermal

fibroblasts is mediated by STAT6. J Immunol 2001; 167(6):3216–3222.

13. Zhang S et al.: Cutting edge: differential expression of chemokines in Th1 and Th2 cells is dependent on Stat6 but not Stat4. J Immunol 2000; 165(1):10–14.

14. Bonecchi R et al.: Divergent effects of interleukin-4 and interferon-γ on macrophage-derived chemokine production: an amplification circuit of polarized T helper 2 responses. Blood 1998; 92(8):2668–2671.

15. Dent AL et al.: T helper type 2 inflammatory disease in the absence of interleukin 4 and transcription factor STAT6. Proc Natl Acad Sci USA 1998; 95(23):13823–13828.

Jutta Horejs-Hoeck

Department of Molecular Biology, University of Salzburg, Hellbrunner Str. 34, A-5020 Salzburg, Austria, Tel. +43 662 8044-5736, Fax +43 662 8044-5751, E-mail jutta.horejs_ hoeck@sbg.ac.at

The Functional Role of Hepatocyte Growth factor in Allergic Inflammation

W. Ito[1], A. Kanehiro[2], T. Chiba[1], H. Kato[1], M. Takeda[1], S. Ueki[1], N. Saito[1], H. Kayaba[1], and J. Chihara[1]

[1]*Department of Clinical and Laboratory Medicine, Akita University School of Medicine,*
[2]*Department of Internal Medicine, Okayama University Graduate School of Medicine and Dentistry, Akita, Japan*

Summary: *Background:* Hepatocyte growth factor (HGF) is recognized as a humoral mediator of epithelial-mesenchymal interactions in tissue regeneration. We demonstrate that HGF has significant regulatory effects in allergic diseases including bronchial asthma. *Methods:* We investigated the role of HGF in a murine model of allergen-induced airway inflammation and airway hyperresponsiveness. After ovalbumin (OVA) sensitization and airway challenge, airway function, lung inflammatory cells and Th2 cytokines levels in bronchoalveolar lavage fluid (BALF) were monitored. Next, we investigated the effect of HGF on human eosinophil chemotaxis. Human peripheral blood eosinophils were purified by the negative selection method using anti-CD16 immunomagnetic beads. Chemotaxis of eosinophils in human peripheral blood was conducted in Boyden chambers. *Results:* Administration of HGF during OVA challenge significantly prevented airway hyperresponsiveness, eosinophil numbers, and Th2 cytokines levels in BALF. Moreover, HGF inhibited eosinophil chemotaxis toward eotaxin. *Conclusions:* These data indicate that HGF plays an important role in the development of asthma, and treatment with HGF may be considered a new therapeutic strategy for allergic diseases.

Keywords: hepatocyte growth factor, eosinophil, chemotaxis

Bronchial asthma is a syndrome associated with allergen-induced chronic airway inflammation and airway hyperresponsiveness (AHR). Allergic airway inflammation is characterized by an influx of activated eosinophils and T lymphocytes, and numerous investigations have identified that Th2 cytokines play critical roles in orchestrating the allergic inflammatory response leading to AHR.

In contrast to cytokines/chemokines, the function of growth factors such as transforming growth factor-β (TGF-β), platelet-derived growth factor (PDGF), and nerve growth factor (NGF) in asthma have been less fully delineated and the results have not always been consistent. Some papers have reported that these growth factors contribute to airway inflammation, AHR, and airway remodeling [1–3].

Another growth factor, hepatocyte growth factor (HGF), which was originally identified and cloned as a potent mitogen for mature hepatocytes, is recognized as a multifunctional and essential cytokine, transducing signals for normal morphogenesis and regeneration. Further, there is now evidence that HGF plays an essential role in parenchymal repair and protection in various organs [4–6]. In some studies, administration of human recombinant HGF prevented the onset and progression of hepatic, renal, and lung fibrosis/cirrhosis [7–9]. In the present review, we will show that HGF has significant regulatory effects on allergic diseases including bronchial asthma.

In vivo, a murine model of asthma, OVA-sensitized and challenged BALB/c mice, showed increased airway responsiveness to

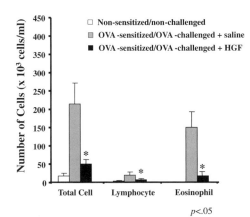

Figure 1. Treatment with hepatocyte growth factor prevents the development of inflammatory cell accumulation in bronchoalveolar fluid of asthmatic mice.

inhaled methacholine. Furthermore, eosinophils, lymphocytes and concentrations of Th2 cytokines (IL-4, IL-5) in BAL fluid increased compared to nonsensitized and nonchallenged mice. Administration of exogenous HGF significantly attenuated the increase of AHR, reduced the numbers of eosinophils and lymphocytes, and decreased the levels of Th2 cytokines in an asthmatic mouse model (see Figure 1). Furthermore, in sensitized and challenged HGF-treated mice, BALF IL-12, which is associated with the induction of IFN-γ production and has suppressive effects on eosinophilopoiesis in bone marrow, was significantly increased compared with vehicle-treated mice [10]. Consistent with our study, Okunishi and coworker have reported that the injection of HGF expression plasmid markedly suppressed the development of airway eosinophilia and AHR, and further, inhibited the production of IL-5 from CD4+ T-cells of Ag-sensitized mice

[11]. However, Okunishi has also found that HGF suppressed IL-12 production from DC activated by Ag-sensitized mice *in vitro* [11]. Regarding IL-12, the divergent results seen between these studies may be related to the different study style including *in vivo vs in vitro*. Moreover, treatment with HGF also suppressed the levels of some growth factors including TGF-β, which plays an important role in allergic airway remodeling [10, 11]. Consistent with our results, some studies have reported that HGF prevents the progression of diseases such as liver cirrhosis and lung fibrosis dependent on the suppression of TGF-β [7–9]. These results suggest that HGF also has a therapeutic benefit in reducing allergic inflammation in bronchial asthma.

Eosinophils play a pivotal role in the mechanism of allergic diseases including bronchial asthma. Moreover, the chemotaxis of eosinophils is one of the most important events in the pathogenesis of allergic inflammation. Th2 cytokines play an important role in the activation, survival, and chemotaxis of eosinophils; therefore, our *in vivo* studies suggested that HGF suppresses eosinophil accumulation in the airway through the inhibition of Th2 cytokine release. On the other hand, in our in vitro study, HGF tended to attenuate eotaxin-induced chemotaxis of human eosinophils in the absence of IL-4 or IL-5 (data not shown, manuscript in preparation). These results indicate that HGF negatively regulates allergic airway inflammation by eosinophils through not only the suppression of Th2 cytokines but also direct action against cell migration (see Figure 2).

In the future, further studies are necessary to elucidate the detailed mechanism of HGF

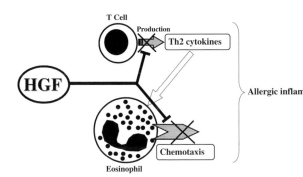

Figure 2. The model of the function of hepatocyte growth factor (HGF) in allergic inflammation. HGF may regulate allergic airway inflammation by eosinophils through not only the suppression of Th2 cytokines but also direct action against cell migration.

activity in allergic diseases; however, this result may provide new further insights into allergic reactions, and treatment with HGF may be considered a new therapeutic strategy for allergic diseases.

References

1. Minshall EM, Leung DYM, Martin RJ, Song YL, Cameron L, Ernst P, Hamid Q: Eosinophil-associated TGF-β_1 mRNA expression and airways fibrosis in bronchial asthma. Am J Respir Cell Mol Biol 1997; 17:326–333.
2. Yamashita N, Sekine K, Miyasaka T, Kawashima R, Nakajima Y, Nakano J, Yamamoto T, Horiuchi T, Hirai K, Ohta K: Platelet-derived growth factor is involved in the augmentation of airway responsiveness through remodeling of airways in the diesel exhaust particulate-treated mice. J Allergy Clin Immunol 2001; 107:135–142.
3. Fox AJ, Patel HJ, Barnes J, Belvisi MG: Release of nerve growth factor by human pulmonary epithelial cells: role in airway inflammatory diseases. Eur J Pharmacol 2001; 424:159–162.
4. Schmidt C, Bladt F, Goedecke S, Brinkmann V, Zschiesche W, Sharpe M, Gherardi E, Birchmeier C: Scatter factor/hepatocyte growth factor is essential for liver development. Nature 1995; 373:699–702.
5. Boros P, Miller CM: Hepatocyte growth factor: a multifunctional cytokine. Lancet 1995; 345:293–295.
6. Uehara Y, Minowa O, Mori C, Shiota K, Kuno J, Noda T, Kitamura N: Placental defect and embryonic lethality in mice lacking hepatocyte growth factor/scatter factor. Nature 1995; 373:702–705.
7. Ueki T, Kaneda Y, Tsutsui H, Nakanishi K, Sawa Y, Morishita R, Matsumoto K, Nakamura T, Takahashi H, Okamoto E, Fujimoto J: Hepatocyte growth factor gene therapy of liver cirrhosis in rats. Nat Med 1999; 5:226–230.
8. Mizuno S, Kurosawa T, Matsumoto K, Mizuno-Horikawa Y, Okamoto M, Nakamura T: Hepatocyte growth factor prevents renal fibrosis and dysfunction in a mouse model of chronic renal disease. J Clin Invest 1998; 101:1827–1834.
9. Yaekashiwa M, Nakayama S, Ohnuma K, Sakai T, Abe T, Satoh K, Matsumoto K, Nakamura T, Takahashi T, Nukiwa T: Simultaneous or delayed administration of hepatocyte growth factor equally represses the fibrotic changes in murine lung injury induced by bleomycin. Am J Respir Crit Care Med 1997; 156:1937–1944.
10. Ito W, Kanehiro A, Matsumoto K, Hirano A, Ono K, Maruyama H, Kataoka M, Nakamura T, Gelfand EW, Tanimoto M: Hepatocyte growth factor attenuates airway hyperresponsiveness, inflammation, and remodeling. Am J Respir Cell Mol Biol 2005; 32:268–280.
11. Okunishi K, Dohi M, Nakagome K, Tanaka R, Mizuno S, Matsumoto K, Miyazaki J, Nakamura T, Yamamoto K: A novel role of hepatocyte growth factor as an immune regulator through suppressing dendritic cell function. J Immunol 2005; 175:4745–4753.

Junichi Chihara

Department of Clinical and Laboratory Medicine, Akita University School of Medicine, 1–1-1, Hondo, Akita 010–8543, Japan, Tel. +81 18 884-6180, Fax +81 18 836-2624, E-mail chihara@hos.akita-u.ac.jp

Involvement of Periostin in Subepithelial Fibrosis of Bronchial Asthma Downstream of IL-4 and IL-13 Signals

K. Izuhara[1], G. Takayama[1], K. Arima[1], T. Kanaji[1], S. Kanaji[1], S. Ohta[1], H. Tanaka[2], and H. Nagai[2]

[1]Division of Medical Biochemistry, Department of Biomolecular Sciences, Saga Medical School, Saga, Japan, [2]Department of Pharmacology, Gifu Pharmaceutical University, Gifu, Japan

Summary: *Background:* Subepithelial fibrosis is a cardinal feature of bronchial asthma. Collagen I, III, and V; fibronectin; and tenascin-C are deposited in the lamina reticularis. Extensive evidence supports the pivotal role of IL-4 and IL-13 in subepithelial fibrosis, however, the precise mechanism remains unclear. We have previously identified the *POSTN* gene encoding periostin as an IL-4/IL-13-inducible gene in bronchial epithelial cells. Periostin is thought to be an adhesion molecule because it possesses four fasciclin I domains. Here, we explore the possibility that periostin is involved in subepithelial fibrosis in bronchial asthma. *Methods:* We have analyzed induction of periostin in lung fibroblasts by IL-4 or IL-13. We next analyzed expression of periostin in asthma patients and in OVA-sensitized and inhaled mice. Furthermore, we examined the binding ability of periostin to other extracellular matrix proteins. *Results:* Both IL-4-and IL-13-induced secretion of periostin in lung fibroblasts independently of TGF-β. Periostin co-localized with other extracellular matrix proteins involved in subepithelial fibrosis in both asthma patients and OVA-sensitized and inhalation challenged wild-type mice, but not in either IL-4 or IL-13 knockout mice. Periostin had an ability to bind to fibronectin, tenascin-C, collagen V, and periostin itself. *Conclusion:* Periostin secreted by lung fibroblasts in response to IL-4 and/or IL-13 is a novel component of subepithelial fibrosis in bronchial asthma. Periostin may contribute to this process by binding to other extracellular matrix proteins.

Keywords: bronchial asthma, interleukin-4, interleukin-13, periostin, TGF-β, subepithelial fibrosis, basement membrane, extracellular matrix protein, fibronectin, tenascin-C

Introduction

Subepithelial fibrosis is a cardinal feature of bronchial asthma. Extensive evidence supports its correlation with the clinical and functional severity of bronchial asthma. Subepithelial fibrosis is caused by the deposition of extracellular matrix proteins such as collagens I, III, and V; fibronectin; and tenascin-C [1, 2]. IL-4 and IL-13 are reported to have a critical role in subepithelial fibrosis [3–5]. It has been proposed that this IL-13-induced ECM deposition could be caused by TGF-β [6]. We have previously identified IL-4- or IL-13-inducible genes in human bronchial epithelial cells, in which the *POSTN* gene encoding periostin was included [7]. It has been assumed that periostin is an adhesion molecule, because periostin has the FAS1 domain, characteristic of a family of adhesion molecules [8]. We explore the possibility that periostin is involved in subepithelial fibrosis of bronchial asthma downstream of IL-4 or IL-13

Materials and Methods

MRC5, a normal embryonic lung fibroblast cell line or primary lung fibroblasts were stimulated with 10 ng/ml of human IL-4, 50 ng/ml of human IL-13, or 10 ng/ml of human TGF-β_1 for the indicated period. Western blotting was performed using anti-periostin antibody against the C-terminal portion of periostin. Bronchial tissues examined for immunostaining were autopsy specimens derived from seven asthma patients and eight nonasthma patients. For the generation of a model of more chronic asthma, mice were actively sensitized by intraperitoneal injections of 50 mg ovalbumin (OVA) with 1 mg alum on day 0 and 12. Starting on day 22, they were exposed to OVA or saline by inhalation for 30 min every day for three consecutive weeks. For the binding assay, we coated the plates with fibronectin; tenascin-C; collagen I, III, or V; or periostin and incubated the plates with biotinylated periostin and the signals of the bound periostin were developed.

Results

Induction of Periostin by IL-4 or IL-13 in Lung Fibroblasts

We first examined expression of periostin by IL-4 or IL-13 in a normal embryonic lung fibroblast cell line, MRC5, using RT-PCR. Upon stimulation of IL-4 or IL-13, expression of periostin became detectable at 3 h, and reached a peak after 24 h. In accordance with expression of periostin at the mRNA level, either IL-4 or IL-13 caused expression of periostin at the protein level in both cell lysates and supernatants of MRC5 cells and primary lung fibroblasts. TGF-β_1, a fibrogenic cytokine in the lung, induced only low amounts of

periostin compared to IL-4 or IL-13. Furthermore, anti-TGF-β Ab blocked only slightly the secretion of periostin induced by IL-13. These results demonstrated that expression of periostin by IL-4 or IL-13 in lung fibroblasts was independent of TGF-β.

Deposition of Periostin in Bronchial Tissues of Asthma Patients

The airway subepithelial region, observed by light microscopy to be homogeneous and hyaline, were obviously thickened in bronchial asthma patients, with periostin specifically localized, whereas deposition of periostin was not detected in bronchial tissues of nonasthma patients. Periostin co-localized with other ECM proteins such as collagens I, III, and V; fibronectin; and tenascin-C, deposited in the subepithelial region of asthmatic airways. These results demonstrate that periostin was a novel matrix protein involved in subepithelial fibrosis of bronchial asthma patients.

Deposition of Periostin in Bronchial Tissues of OVA-sensitized and Inhaled Mice

We generated a "chronic asthma model" using wild-type mice or IL-4 or IL-13 knockout mice and analyzed deposition of periostin. In parallel with subepithelial fibrosis, periostin was also deposited in the airway subepithelial regions in OVA-inhaled wild-type mice, but not in saline-exposed mice, and significantly decreased in IL-4 or IL-13 knockout mice. These results suggested that periostin was also involved in subepithelial fibrosis in this mouse model of bronchial asthma downstream of IL-4 and/or IL-13 signals.

Binding of Periostin with ECM Proteins in Heterophilic and Homophilic Manners

We analyzed the binding abilities of periostin to fibronectin, tenascin-C, and collagens, known components of subepithelial fibrosis of bronchial asthma. Periostin appeared to have the ability to bind to ECM proteins such as tenascin-C, fibronectin, collagen V (but not to collagens/and III), and to periostin itself, in both heterophilic and homophilic manners, which may explain how periostin would contribute to subepithelial fibrosis in bronchial asthma.

Author's Note

The content of this article was published in J Allergy Clin Immunol 2006; 118:98–104.

References

1. Roche WR, Beasley R, Williams JH, Holgate ST: Subepithelial fibrosis in the bronchi of asthmatics. Lancet 1989; 1:520–524.
2. Laitinen A, Altraja A, Kampe M, Linden M, Virtanen I, Laitinen LA: Tenascin is increased in airway basement membrane of asthmatics and decreased by an inhaled steroid. Am J Respir Crit Care Med 1997; 156:951–958.
3. Zhu Z, Homer RJ, Wang Z, Chen Q, Geba GP, Wang J, Zhang Y, Elias JA: Pulmonary expression of interleukin-13 causes inflammation, mucus hypersecretion, subepithelial fibrosis, physiologic abnormalities, and eotaxin production. J Clin Invest 1999; 103:779–788.
4. Kumar RK, Herbert C, Yang M, Koskinen AM, McKenzie AN, Foster PS: Role of interleukin-13 in eosinophil accumulation and airway remodeling in a mouse model of chronic asthma. Clin Exp Allergy 2002; 32:1104–1111.
5. Komai M, Tanaka H, Masuda T, Nagao K, Ishizaki M, Sawada M, Nagai H: Role of Th2 responses in the development of allergen-induced airway remodeling in a murine model of allergic asthma. Br J Pharmacol 2003; 138:912–920.
6. Lee CG, Homer RJ, Zhu Z, Lanone S, Wang X, Koteliansky V, Shipley JM, Gotwals P, Noble P, Chen Q, Senior RM, Elias JA: Interleukin-13 induces tissue fibrosis by selectively stimulating and activating transforming growth factor β_1. J Exp Med 2001; 194:809–821.
7. Yuyama N, Davies DE, Akaiwa M, Matsui K, Hamasaki Y, Suminami Y, Berger A, Richards I, Roberds SL, Yamashita T, Kishi F, Kato H, Arai K, Ohshima K, Tadano J, Hamasaki N, Miyatake S, Sugita Y, Holgate ST, Izuhara K: Analysis of novel disease-related genes in bronchial asthma. Cytokine 2002; 19:287–296.
8. Kawamoto T, Noshiro M, Shen M, Nakamasu K, Hashimoto K, Kawashima-Ohya Y, Gotoh O, Kato Y: Structural and phylogenetic analyses of RGD-CAP/βig-h3, a fasciclin-like adhesion protein expressed in chick chondrocytes. Biochim Biophys Acta 1998; 1395:288–292.

Dr. Kenji Izuhara

Department of Biomolecular Sciences, Saga Medical School, 5-1-1, Nabeshima, Saga, 849-8501 Japan, E-mail kizuhara@cc.saga-u.ac.jp

CD48 Is Critically Involved in Experimental Asthma

A. Munitz[1], I. Bachelet[1], R. Eliashar[2], M. Khoudon[3], F.D. Finkelman[3], M.E. Rothenberg[4], and F. Levi-Schaffer[1,5]

[1]*Department of Pharmacology, School of Pharmacy, Faculty of Medicine, The Hebrew University of Jerusalem, Jerusalem, Israel,* [2]*Department of Otolaryngology-Head and Neck Surgery, The Hebrew University School of Medicine, Hadassah Medical Center, Jerusalem, Israel,* [3]*Department of Medicine, University of Cincinnati College of Medicine, Cincinnati, OH, USA,* [4]*Division of Allergy and Immunology, Department of Pediatrics, Cincinnati Children's Hospital Medical Center, University of Cincinnati College of Medicine, Cincinnati, OH, USA,* [5]*The David R. Bloom Center for Pharmacology, The Hebrew University of Jerusalem, Jerusalem, Israel*

Summary: *Background:* Despite ongoing research, the molecular mechanisms underlying asthma pathogenesis are still elusive. CD48 is a glycosyl-phosphatidyl-inositol anchored protein involved in lymphocyte adhesion, activation and co-stimulation. While CD48 is widely expressed on hematopoietic cells and commonly studied in the context of NK and cytotoxic T-cell functions, its role in Th2-settings such as asthma has not been examined. *Objective:* To evaluate the expression and function of CD48 and its recognized ligands; CD2 and 2B4, in a murine model of allergic-eosinophilic airway inflammation. *Methods:* Allergic-eosinophilic airway inflammation was induced by OVA/Alum sensitization and intranasal inoculation of OVA or by repeated intranasal inoculation of *Aspergillus fumigatus* in wild type, STAT-6-deficient, and IL-4/IL-13-deficient mice. Gene profiling of whole-lung was performed, followed by northern blot and flow cytometric analysis. Anti-CD48, -CD2 and -2B4 antibodies were administered before OVA challenge and cytokine expression and histology were assessed. *Results:* Human eosinophils from atopic asthmatics display enhanced levels of CD48 expression and IL-3 upregulates CD48 expression both on human and murine eosinophils. Cross-linking of CD48 on human eosinophils triggers the release of eosinophil granule proteins but not cytokines. Microarray data analysis demonstrated upregulation of CD48 in the lungs of allergen-challenged mice. Allergen-induced CD48 expression was STAT-6-, IL-13- and IL-4-independent. Neutralization of CD48 but not 2B4 in allergen-challenged mice abrogated lung inflammation. Neutralization of CD2 inhibited the inflammatory response to a lesser extent *Conclusions:* Our results suggest that CD48 is an IL-3-induced activating receptor on eosinophils, likely involved in promoting allergic inflammation. As such, CD48 may provide a new potential target for the suppression of asthma.

Keywords: allergy, asthma, eosinophils, CD2-subfamily, CD48, IL-3

Eosinophil Activation

Eosinophils are thought to participate and function as effector cells in various disorders such as allergic inflammation (asthma, atopic rhinitis, atopic dermatitis etc.), neoplastic and myeloproliferative diseases, parasitic infections (schistosomiasis, trichinosis etc.), gastrointestinal eosinophil disorders, hypereosinophilic syndromes and many other inflammatory diseases [1, 2]. Their activation and consequent mediator release, both in allergic setting and in other diseases can be induced by a series of agonists. In fact, receptors for several proinflammatory mediators (i.e., C5a, PAF); cytokines (i.e., IL-5, GM-CSF, IL-3, IL-2, IFN-γ etc.), immunoglobulins (i.e., IgG, IgA) and chemokines (i.e., CCR3) are expressed on the eosinophil's surface [1, 2]. Notably, while much data has accumulated on pathways regulating eosinophil activation, most activation pathways that were examined and have been reported to regulate eosinophil activation are confined to "classical" activation pathways (e.g., cytokines, chemokines, proinflammatory components and adhesion molecules) and the presence of other activation molecules which might be disease specific is rather limited [1].

Thus, the need to identify new pathways that regulate eosinophil activation is indeed a warranted goal as it can expand our knowledge on this peculiar cell and provide us insight into important questions regarding this cell type. Two important queries are which cells interact with eosinophils and what are the molecules governing this interaction.

CD48

CD48 is a GPI anchored protein [3] that exists in both a membrane-associated and a soluble form [4]. It belongs to the CD2-subfamily and lacks a transmembrane domain, so how it transduces signals to the cell interior is an intriguing question [5]. A possible explanation is that GPI anchored proteins are preferentially restricted within distinct microdomains on the cell membrane known as glycosphingolipid-cholesterol rafts [6]. Indeed, cross-linking of CD48 on the surface of lymphocytes triggers their activation [7–9]. Furthermore, CD48 is upregulated in various diseases states [10, 11]. As such, we hypothesized that CD48 can deliver independent or co-stimulatory signals for eosinophil activation and hence may play a fundamental role in eosinophil related diseases such as asthma.

For this we characterized the expression and function of CD48 on murine and human eosinophils. Our studies revealed three major findings.

First, cross-linking of CD48 was sufficient to induce eosinophil degranulation but not cytokine release. Apparently, CD48 triggers piecemeal degranulation of eosinophils. Since CD48 is a GPI-linked protein it probably activates intracellular signaling cascades by reshuffling lipid rafts on the cell surface. Our study is the first to demonstrate activation of eosinophils through a GPI-linked receptor.

Second, is the finding that IL-3 specifically regulates CD48 expression on eosinophils.

This phenomenon was found to be conserved to both murine and human cells, suggesting that IL-3 is capable to induce signal transduction independent of the IL-3/IL-5/GM-CSF common β chain, and unforeseen roles for this cytokine in eosinophil biology. Interestingly, cross-linking of CD48 on human eosinophils triggers EPO release but no cytokine release even in the presence of IL-3. We speculate that under certain circumstances IL-3 can potentiate the responses elicited by CD48.

Third, CD48 was upregulated on tissue and blood eosinophils obtained from asthmatic donors. This finding may be especially important in the context of defining disease-specific pathways that may regulate eosinophil functions in asthma. Strengthening this observation is our findings that CD48 upregulated in the lungs of allergen challenged mice and is a component of the asthma genome signature described recently by Zimmerman et al [12].

Interestingly, key regulators of the asthmatic response such as STAT6, IL-4 and IL-13 that have been shown to regulate several genes from the asthma genome list [13], do not regulate CD48 expression. In order to establish a role for CD48 and its ligands (CD2 and 2B4) in asthma we neutralized these epitopes prior to allergen challenge in a murine asthma model. Strikingly, neutralization of CD48 was capable to abrogate eosinophilic inflammation, Th2 and proinflammatory cytokine expression, lung inflammation, mucus production and smooth muscle hyperplasia. These effects of anti-CD48 treatment are only partially dependent on interactions with CD2 expressed on lymphocytes, as anti-CD2 treatment induced a relatively modest effect.

Last, our in-vivo data suggests that 2B4 does not participate in murine asthmatic response. However, due to its limited expression on murine cells and its boundless expression on human leukocytes it may play a significant role in human asthma.

Conclusions

Our observations that CD48 is upregulated on human eosinophils from asthmatic donors (tissue and peripheral blood) together with its abundant expression on lung eosinophils in vivo and the relatively low effect of anti-CD2 treatment reinforce our hypothesis that CD48 is a critically involved in human asthma pathogenesis and is therefore a potential target for asthma therapy.

References

1. Bochner BS: Verdict in the case of therapies versus eosinophils: the jury is still out. J Allergy Clin Immunol 2004; 113:3.
2. Rothenberg ME, Hogan SP: The eosinophil. Annu Rev Immunol 2006; 24:147.
3. Korinek V, Stefanova I, Angelisova P, Hilgert I, Horejsi V: The human leucocyte antigen CD48 (MEM-102) is closely related to the activation marker Blast-1. Immunogenetics 1991; 33:108.
4. Smith GM, Biggs J, Norris B, Anderson-Stewart P, Ward R: Detection of a soluble form of the leukocyte surface antigen CD48 in plasma and its elevation in patients with lymphoid leukemias and arthritis. J Clin Immunol 1997; 17:502.
5. Hin JS, Abraham SN: Glycosylphosphatidylinositol-anchored receptor-mediated bacterial endocytosis. FEMS Microbiol Lett 2001; 197:131.
6. Horejsi V, Drbal K, Cebecauer M, Cerny J, Brdicka T, Angelisova P, Stockinger H: GPI-microdomains: a role in signaling via immunoreceptors. Immunol Today 1999; 20:356.
7. Maschek BJ, Zhang W, Rosoff PM, Reiser H: Modulation of the intracellular Ca^{2+} and inositol trisphosphate concentrations in murine T lymphocytes by the glycosylphosphatidylinositol-anchored protein sgp-60. J Immunol 1993; 150:3198.
8. Reiser H: sgp-60, a signal-transducing glycoprotein concerned with T-cell activation through the T-cell receptor/CD3 complex. J Immunol 1993; 145:2077.
9. Klyushnenkova EN, Li L, Armitage RJ: Choi CD48 delivers an accessory signal for CD40-mediated activation of human B-cells. Cell Immunol 1996; 174:90.
10. Thorley-Lawson DA, Schooley RT, Bhan AK, Nadler LM: Epstein-Barr virus superinduces a new human B-cell differentiation antigen (B-LAST 1) expressed on transformed lymphoblasts. Cell 1982; 30:415.
11. Yokoyama S, Staunton D, Fisher R, Amiot M, Fortin JJ, Thorley-Lawson DA: Expression of the Blast-1 activation/adhesion molecule and its identification as CD48. J Immunol 1991; 146:2192.
12. Zimmermann N, King NE, Laporte J et al.: Dissection of experimental asthma with DNA microarray analysis identifies arginase in asthma pathogenesis. J Clin Invest 2003; 111:1863.
13. Fulkerson PC, Zimmermann N, Hassman LM, Finkelman FD, Rothenberg ME: Pulmonary chemokine expression is coordinately regulated by STAT1, STAT6, and IFN-γ. J Immunol 2004; 173:7565.

Francesca Levi-Schaffer

Department of Pharmacology, School of Pharmacy, The Faculty of Medicine, The Hebrew University of Jerusalem, Jerusalem 91120, Israel, Tel. +972 2 6757512, Fax +972 2 6758144, E-mail fls@cc.huji.ac.il

Interaction of Allergic Rhinitis and Bacterial Sinusitis in a Mouse Model

R.M. Naclerio[1], V. Kirtsreesakul[1,3], T. Luxameechanporn[1], J.J. Klemens[1], K. Thompson[2], and Fuad Baroody[1]

[1]*Department of Surgery, Section of Otolaryngology-Head and Neck Surgery and* [2]*Department of Pathology, The University of Chicago, Chicago, IL, USA,* [3]*Department of Otolaryngology, Faculty of Medicine, Prince of Songkla University, Hat Yai, Songkla, Thailand*

Summary: We studied the interaction of allergic inflammation and allergy in mice. We showed that when mice were infected during an ongoing allergic reaction, they showed significantly higher bacterial recovery and phagocytic cell influx into the sinus mucosa compared to nonsensitized, OVA-challenged, and infected mice. The augmented infectious response persisted during long-term allergen challenge and was diminished when the allergen was removed. We demonstrated that C57BL/6 mice, with a Th1 tendency, can be made allergic. However, allergic and infected BALB/c mice, with a Th2 tendency, showed more allergic inflammation and a greater infectious response than C57BL/6 mice. Infected BALB/c mice without allergy, in contrast to C57BL/6 mice, had a significant number of bacteria at day 28. These results demonstrated that BALB/c mice were less able to clear infection than were C57BL/6 mice and emphasize the importance of the Th1 and Th2 genetic background, which played a role in the severity and course of infection. Our data suggests that the Th genetic background plays an important role in allergy induction, augmentation of infection, and infection control with the Th2 tendency leading to an exaggeration of all these responses. We hypothesize that the T-cells responding to allergens induce cytokines, e.g., IL4, which inhibit Th1 anti-inflammatory cell function [1]. This hypothesis might explain augmented bacterial and inflammatory reactions when allergy and bacterial infection interact.

Keywords: allergic rhinitis, Infection, Streptococcus pneumoniae, sinusitis, mice

Introduction

Man's nasal immune system is often obligated to respond to more than one foreign stimulus. We previously developed a mouse model of acute *Streptococcus pneumoniae* (*S. pneumoniae*) bacterial rhinosinusitis. In this model, an ongoing allergic reaction augmented the bacterial load in BALB/c mice 5 days after inoculation, and the infection was associated with an augmented inflammatory response [2]. In this study, we evaluated and compared the effect of long-term intranasal OVA challenge on the augmented infectious effect between sensitized and nonsensitized mice, and also the difference between BALB/c and C57BL/6 mice.

Materials and Methods

BALB/c and C57BL/6 mice, aged 6–8 weeks, were obtained from Jackson Laboratory. Mice were OVA-sensitized by IP injection (PBS IP injection for controls) on days 0 and 8, followed by IN challenge with OVA starting on day 9, and were then infected by IN inoculation with *S. pneumoniae* on day 10. We conducted 2 parallel studies. The distinction between the 2 studies was the length of OVA exposure, 5 vs. 28 days. At 5, 14, 21 and 28 days after infection, groups of mice were sedated with a respiratory-failure dose of pentobarbital sodium and nasal lavage with 200 ml of PBS was performed. The lavage fluid was cultured. After nasal lavage, mice were decapitated and sinus tissue was removed and processed for flow cytometry. Cells were stained with anti-CD11b FITC for CD11b$^+$ myeloid cells (mainly macrophages and neutrophils) and double stained with anti-GR1 PE & CCR3 FITC for GR1^{hi+} CCR3– neutrophils, and GR1$^{lo-int+}$ CCR3$^+$ eosinophils. Histamine challenges were done 2 days prior to the final endpoint.

Results

We compared the augmented infectious response between allergic, OVA-exposed and infected BALB/c mice and nonsensitized, OVA-exposed, and infected BALB/c mice. At 5 days after inoculation, allergic and infected BALB/c mice showed significantly more bacteria, macrophages, neutrophils, and eosinophils compared to the nonsensitized, OVA-exposed, and infected BALB/c mice. The number of bacteria and inflammatory cells remained statistically significantly elevated from 5 to 28 days after infection in the allergic group which received the prolonged OVA exposure (28 days). After short exposure to allergen (5 days) in a similar experiment, the number of bacteria and inflammatory cells decreased and became comparable to that in nonsensitized, OVA-challenged, and infected BALB/c mice at 21 and 28 days after infection. Long-term IN OVA challenge without prior sensitization slowly induced an allergic inflammation in BALB/c mice, with a significantly higher number of macrophages and eosinophils cells in sinuses at 28 days and these mice had increased nasal responsiveness to histamine at the third and fourth weeks after challenge compared to infected-only BALB/c mice.

Allergic-only C57BL/6 mice showed typical allergic inflammation, as indicated by an increased number of eosinophils cells in the sinuses and nasal responsiveness to histamine. The allergic and infected C57BL/6 mice had a significantly higher number of bacteria, macrophages and eosinophils, and more nasal responsiveness to histamine compared to nonsensitized, OVA-challenged, and infected C57BL/6 mice. Long-term (28 days) intranasal OVA challenge in nonsensitized and infected C57BL/6 did not increase the number of eosinophils or nasal responsiveness. They also cleared bacteria in sinuses at day 28.

Comparing these two mouse strains, allergic and infected BALB/c mice showed more bacteria, macrophages, eosinophils, and nasal responsiveness to histamine than did allergic and infected C57BL/6 mice. We also showed that nonsensitized and infected C57BL/6 mice were able to clear infection, in contrast to nonsensitized, PBS-challenged, and infected BALB/c mice, which showed a significant number of bacteria at 28 days after infection.

Discussion

We showed that the induction and severity of allergic inflammation and the augmented infectious response were affected by the duration of allergen stimulation and the Th1/Th2 genetic background of the mice. When mice were infected during an ongoing allergic reaction, they showed significantly higher bacterial recovery and phagocytic cell influx into the sinus mucosa compared to nonsensitized, OVA-challenged, and infected mice. The augmented infectious response persisted during long-term allergen challenge and was diminished when the allergen was removed. The experiments mimic epidemiologic data in man that show an increased incidence of rhinosinusitis during the allergy season [3], suggesting that control of allergic inflammation might be helpful in reducing infections.

We demonstrated that C57BL/6 mice, with a Th1 tendency, can be made allergic. The intraperitoneally exposed C57BL/6 mice had significantly more bacteria recovered and more phagocytic cells in sinuses compared to nonsensitized, OVA-exposed, and infected C57BL/6 mice. However, allergic and infected

BALB/c mice, with a Th2 tendency, showed more allergic inflammation and a greater infectious response than C57BL/6 mice.

Interestingly, 28 days after infection, nonsensitized, OVA-challenged, and infected BALB/c mice had a large number of bacteria in the sinuses, in contrast to nonsensitized, OVA-challenged, and infected C57BL/6 mice, which essentially resolved the infection. The earlier timepoints (up to 14 days) didn't show a significant difference. Infected BALB/c mice without allergy, in contrast to C57BL/6 mice, had a significant number of bacteria at our last time point. These results demonstrated that BALB/c mice were less able to clear infection than were C57BL/6 mice and emphasize the importance of the Th1 and Th2 genetic background, which played a role in the severity and course of infection.

Our data suggests that the Th genetic background plays an important role in allergy induction, augmentation of infection, and infection control with the Th2 tendency leading to an exaggeration of all these responses. We hypothesize that the T-cells responding to allergens induce cytokines, e.g., IL4, which inhibit Th1 anti-inflammatory cell function [1]. This hypothesis might explain augmented bacterial and inflammatory reactions when allergy and bacterial infection interact.

Acknowledgments

Funding from National Institutes of Health.

References

1. Ogasawara H, Asakura K, Saito H, Kataura A: Role of CD4-positive T-cells in the pathogenesis of allergy in the murine model. Int Arch Allergy Immunol 1999; 118:37–43.
2. Blair C, Nelson M, Thompson K, Boonlayangoor S, Haney L, Gabr U, Baroody FM, Naclerio RM: Allergic inflammation enhances bacterial sinusitis in mice. J Allergy Clin Immunol 2001; 108: 424–429.
3. Ferguson BJ, Johnson JT: Allergic rhinitis and rhinosinusitis. Is there a connection between allergy and infection? Postgrad Med 1999; 105:55–58.

Robert M. Naclerio

The University of Chicago, 5841 S. Maryland Ave., MC 1035, Chicago, IL 60637, E-mail rnacleri@surgery.bsd.uchicago.edu

Retinol Concentrations After Birth Are Inversely Associated with Atopic Manifestations in Children and Young Adults

M. Pesonen, M. Kallio, M. Siimes, and A. Ranki

Department of Dermatology, the Skin and Allergy Hospital and the Hospital for Children and Adolescents, Helsinki University Hospital, University of Helsinki, Finland

Summary: *Background:* Vitamin A is known to have immunomodulatory effects so that its deficiency results in impaired specific and innate immunity. Since gut immune response in early infancy is likely to regulate immune maturation and also atopic sensitization, and since vitamin A was recently shown to regulate the gut-homing of T-cells, we looked for an association of plasma retinol concentrations and the subsequent development of allergic symptoms in healthy infants. *Methods:* A cohort of 200 unselected, full-term newborns were followed-up from birth to age 20 years. The plasma retinol concentration was determined in cord blood, at ages of 2, 4 and 12 months, and at ages 5 and 11 years . They were repeatedly examined for the occurrence of allergic symptoms, skin prick test results (SPT), and serum IgE. *Results:* Subjects with atopic manifestations in childhood and adolescence had lower retinol concentrations in infancy and childhood than symptom-free subjects . The difference was most pronounced at age 2 months: the plasma retinol concentration correlated inversely with positive SPT at ages of 5 and 20 years, and with allergic symptoms at age 20 years. Furthermore, the retinol concentration at age 5 years was inversely associated with the prevalence of atopic dermatitis at that age. *Conclusion:* Retinol concentration in young infants is inversely associated with the subsequent development of allergic symptoms. We assume that the low concentration of retinol in the newborn infant may disturb $CD4^+$ T-cell homing to the gut and, subsequently, the development of normal Th1 type responses elicited by gut microflora.

Keywords: atopy, retinol, vitamin A

Introduction

The gut immune response, induced by microbial antigens, is assumed to play an important role in maturing the peripheral immune response. The majority of the body's T-cells reside in the gut. It was recently shown in mice that low levels of vitamin A (retinol) inhibit CD4-positive T-cell homing to the gut [1]. Under such circumstances, the T-cells rather home to the lung, and to the skin. Retinoic acid increased the expression of $\alpha4\beta7$ integrin and CCR9 on T lymphocytes, which provides them with tropism for the gut, and a Th1/T reg1 cytokine profile. Since an impaired gut immune response in early infancy may contribute to the development of atopic sensitization, we looked for an association of plasma retinol concentrations and the subsequent development of allergic symptoms in healthy infants.

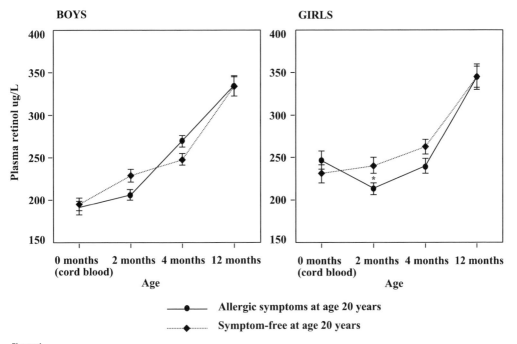

Figure 1.

Material and Methods

A cohort of 200 unselected, full-term new-borns were followed-up from birth to age 20 years [2]. All infants received vitamin A supplementation; therefore, a dietary deficiency of vitamin A was unlikely. The plasma retinol concentration was determined in cord blood (*n* = 97), at ages of 2, 4, and 12 months (*n* = 95), and at ages 5 (*n* = 155) and 11 years (*n* = 151) [3]. The subjects were re-examined at ages of 5, 11, and 20 years with assessment for allergic symptoms, skin prick testing (SPT), and measurement of sIgE. Statistical significances were tested with ANOVA and the two-tail un-paired Student's *t* test. Logistic regression analyses were performed to control for the effect of potential covariates (i.e., gender, duration of exclusive breast-feeding, a family history of allergy).

Results

Subjects with allergic symptoms or a positive SPT in childhood or adolescence had lower retinol concentrations in infancy and childhood

than symptom-free subjects (Figure 1). The difference was most pronounced at age 2 months. Retinol concentration at 2 months correlated inversely with positive SPT at ages 5 and 20 years (*p* = .03 and < .01, respectively). Furthermore, the retinol concentration at age 5 years was inversely associated with the prevalence of atopic dermatitis at that age (*p* = .03).

Discussion

The most important contact between the environmental antigens (allergens) and the immune system is likely to occur through the mucosal membranes of the gastrointestinal tract, the intestinal microflora being the major external driving force in the postnatal maturation of the immune system [4]. Thus, we can assume that if the newborn infant has a low concentration of retinol, as we have shown to be the case for those who later develop atopy, the CD4+ T-cell homing to the gut will be inhibited. Under such circumstances, the Th1 type responses, initiated by the intestinal microflora and other antigens, become weak and an environment favorable for the development of allergic sensitization may ensue. This may lead to the expression of the atopic phenotype and to the subsequent development of allergic symptoms.

References

1. Iwata M et al.: Retinoic acid imprints gut-homing specificity on T-cells. Immunity 2004; 21:527–538.
2. Pesonen M, Kallio MJT, Ranki A, Siimes MA: Prolonged exclusive breastfeeding is associated with increased atopic dermatitis: a prospective follow-up study of unselected healthy newborns from birth to age 20 years. Clin Exp Allergy 2006; 36:1011–1018.
3. Pesonen M, Kallio, MJT, Siimes MA, Ranki A: Retinol concentrations after birth are inversely associated with atopic manifestations in children and young adults. Clin Exp Allergy 2007; 37: 54–61.
4. Howie D, Spencer J, DeLord D, Pitzalis C, Wathen NC, Dogan A, Akbar A, MacDonald TT: Extra-thymic T-cell differentiation in the human intestine early in life. J Immunol 1998; 161:5862–5872.

Annamari Ranki

Skin and Allergy Hospital, P.O. Box 160, FIN-00029 HUS Helsinki, Finland, Tel. +358 9 47186301, Fax +358 9 471 86500, E-mail Annamari.Ranki@hus.fi

Evaluation of Chronic Rhinosinusitis and the Role of Nitric Oxide Measurements

G.K. Scadding

RNTNE Hospital, London, UK

Summary: Rhinosinusitis (including nasal polyps) is defined as: (1) inflammation of the nose and the paranasal sinuses characterized by two or more symptoms, one of which should be either nasal blockage/obstruction/congestion or nasal discharge (anterior/posterior nasal drip): (a) facial pain/pressure, (b) reduction or loss of smell; and either (2) endoscopic signs of (a) polyps and/or (b) mucopurulent discharge primarily from middle meatus and/or (c) oedema/mucosal obstruction primarily in middle meatus; and/or (3) CT changes: (a) mucosal changes within the ostiomeatal complex and/or sinuses. Therapy for this condition, which involves improvement of sinus ventilation and drainage either medically or surgically, has been poorly investigated to date, partly because defined outcome measures are lacking, nasendoscopes are not always available and repeated use of CT scans is inadvisable because of eye irradiation. Nasal NO measurements made either with the patient on topical nasal corticosteroids or while humming could prove useful in assessment of therapy, probably relate to ostiomeatal complex patency and may reduce the need for CT scans.

Keywords: nitric oxide, chronic rhinosinusitis, ostiomeatal complex

Introduction

The paranasal sinuses are air-filled bony cavities surrounding the nose. They communicate via sinus ostia with the nose. Fluid and gases pass in both directions via this ostiomeatal complex and proper ventilation is crucial for sinus integrity [1]. Blockage of the ostia by mucosal swelling due to viruses or allergic reaction is a major factor for the development of sinusitis [2, 3].

Upper and Lower Airways

Recent investigations have demonstrated the importance of the upper airway in asthma [4] with rhinitis/rhinosinusitis predisposing to asthma development [5], and rhinoviral upper respiratory tract infections causing most asthma exacerbations in both adults and children [6, 7]. There is a correlation between eosinophil numbers in the upper and lower airways [8], and rhinosinusitis is strongly associated with asthma, which is usually severe [9].

Our prospective randomized study of medical or surgical treatment for rhinosinusitis showed improvement in asthma control in both groups [10].

There is difficulty in defining chronic rhinosinusitis for 3 reasons:

1. Symptoms and signs such as facial pain and headache are not diagnostic, but can have a variety of other causes.
2. Viral colds lead to abnormalities on sinus CT scans which can persist for several

weeks, thus in unselected populations CT scans are abnormal in over 30% of adults and 45% of children [11, 12].

3. No correlation exists between CT changes and symptoms [13].

The EAACI definition of chronic rhinosinusitis [14] thus employs at least 2 modalities.

Chronic Rhinosinusitis (CRS) Definition

Rhinosinusitis (including nasal polyps) is defined as:

- Inflammation of the nose and the paranasal sinuses characterized by two or more symptoms, one of which should be either nasal blockage/obstruction/congestion or nasal discharge (anterior/posterior nasal drip):
  - facial pain/pressure,
  - reduction or loss of smell;

and either

- Endoscopic signs of:
  - polyps and/or;
  - mucopurulent discharge primarily from middle meatus and/or;
  - oedema/mucosal obstruction primarily in middle meatus,

and/or

- CT changes:
  - mucosal changes within the ostiomeatal complex and/or sinuses.

The disease can also be divided into mild and moderate/ severe based on visual analogue scores.

Treatment

Given the problems with assessment it is not surprising that the present state of knowledge regarding effective treatments for chronic rhinosinusitis is poor with few double blind prospective randomized controlled trials

Assessment of therapy for chronic rhinosinusitis has proved difficult since the response to treatment is based largely on subjective symptoms. In a patient who remains symptomatic it is necessary to assess whether there is continuing infection or inflammation present and whether the sinuses remain patent. Nasendoscopy while allowing a view of the nasal mucosa and turbinates may not always give visual access to the sinus orifices, even after decongestion of the nasal mucosa. Repeated CT scanning is not advisable because of the dose of irradiation given to the eyes.

As yet a simple objective measure has not been found although surrogate measures of the nasal airway (rhinomanometry, acoustic rhinometry, nasal inspiratory peakflow) or of mucosal function (saccharine clearance time, ciliary beat frequency, nasal cytology), have been employed [15].

Nitric Oxide

Prior to 1980, this colourless, odourless gas was considered only as part of noxious fumes [16, 17]. However it was identified as the endothelial derived relaxant molecule involved in arterial dilatation [18, 19] and subsequently as an important regulatory factor in multiple bodily processes such as blood flow, neurotransmission, renal function and in inflammation [20, 21]. In 1991 Gustaffson showed nitric oxide in the air exhaled from the bronchi [22], two years later Alving demonstrated that levels were raised in asthma [23]. Exhaled NO is now recognized as an important monitor of inflammation in the lower airways and is probably a useful guide to the most effective use of inhaled corticosteroids [24].

NO is derived from arginine by several nitric oxide synthases which are constitutive in endothelia, and the nervous system [25, 26], but inducible in macrophages in response to inflammation [27].

The upper respiratory tract produces far more nitric oxide in the lower as was demonstrated in tracheotomised patients [17, 28, 29]. In the upper respiratory tract the sinuses are the major source of nitric oxide which is continuously produced by a calcium independent nitric oxide synthase [30,31]. Nitric oxide is also formed in the nasal mucosa by an inducible form of nitric oxide synthase in response to inflammation [32–35].

Nitric Oxide in Chronic Rhinosinusitis

We have previously shown that nitric oxide levels are reduced in nasal polyposis [36], although polyp epithelium is a rich source of inducible nitric oxide synthase (iNOS) [37]. The degree of reduction of nitric oxide is inversely proportional to the quantity of polyp tissue [36]. More recently in a randomized prospective controlled study of medical versus surgical therapy in chronic rhinosinusitis we have observed that nitric oxide levels initially are proportional to the degree of change in the sinuses as assessed by CT scans using the Lund/MacKay score [38].

Therapy for chronic rhinosinusitis is aimed at improving sinus ventilation and drainage. In the Ragab study there was a rise in initially low nitric oxide levels in both surgically and medically treated patients. The percentage rise in nasal nitric oxide seen on both treatments correlated with changes in symptom scores ($p < .001$), saccharine clearance time ($p < .001$), endoscopic changes ($p < .001$), polyp grades ($p < .05$ at 6 months, $p < .01$ at 12 months) and surgical scores ($p < .01$). There was no significant correlation with age, sex, smoking or allergy [38]. These results were obtained while patients were being maintained on regular topical nasal corticosteroids which are known to reduce the elevated nasal nitric oxide seen in inflammatory rhinitis [39]. This suggests that they reflect emanation of sinus nitric oxide into the nose and thus relate to ostiomeatal complex potency. It would seem that measurements of nitric oxide under these circumstances accurately reflect what is happening in the sinuses and that such measures could be useful in assessing the response of chronic rhinosinu-

sitis to therapy. They should also reduce the use of repeated CT scans since normal elevated levels are unlikely if there is a significant degree of sinus obstruction.

Of particular interest is the close relationship of nitric oxide to saccharine clearance time with significant improvement shown in the latter post CRS therapy. It is known that in patients with primary ciliary dyskinesia inducible nitric oxide synthase is absent from the nasal mucosa and nasal nitric oxide levels are consequently very low usually less than 100 ppb [40].

An alternative approach has recently been suggested by Maniscalco [41] based on the observation that that the ventilation of the paranasal sinuses increases greatly when a person is humming. Measurements of nasal nitric oxide during humming may represent a test of sinus osteal function since in human studies in vivo and in a sinus/nasal model oscillating airflow generated during humming increases the nitric oxide measurements in nasally exhaled air. He explored the different factors determining the humming peak and found that sinus ostium size was the most important although humming frequency also influenced the sinus nitric oxide release [42]. In patients with severe nasal polyposis and completely blocked sinus ostium the humming peak in nitric oxide was abolished.

Summary

Chronic rhinosinusitis is common, has marked effects on quality of life and is frequently associated with severe or difficult asthma. Diagnostic criteria involving a complex of symptoms plus nasendoscopic signs or CT abnormalities have been suggested. Therapy has been poorly investigated to date, partly because defined outcome measures are lacking. Nasal NO measurements made either with the patient on topical nasal corticosteroids or while humming could prove useful in assessment of therapy and may reduce the need for CT scans.

References

1. Aust R, Flack B, Svanholm H: Studies of the gas exchange and pressure in the maxillary sinuses in normal and infected humans. Rhinology 1979; 17:245–251.
2. Aust R, Stierna P, Drettner B: Basic experimental studies of ostial patency and local metabolic environment of the maxillary sinus. Acta Otolaryngol Suppl 1994; 515:7–10.
3. Alho OP: Nasal airflow, mucociliary clearance and sinus functioning during viral colds: effects of allergic rhinitis and susceptibility to recurrent sinusitis. Am J Rhinol 2004; 18:349–355.
4. Bousquet J, Van Cauwenberge P, Khaltaev N et al.: Allergic rhinitis and its impact on asthma. J Allergy Clin Immunol 2001; 108:147–334.
5. Linneberg A, Henrik Nielsen N, Frolund L et al.: The link between allergic rhinitis and allergic asthma: a prospective population-based study. The Copenhagen Allergy Study. Allergy 2002; 57:969–971.
6. Heymann PW, Platts-Mills TA, Johnston SL: Role of viral infections, atopy and antiviral immunity in the etiology of wheezing exacerbations among children and young adults. Pediatr Infect Dis J 2005.
7. Wark PA, Gibson PG, Johnston SL: Exacerbations of asthma: addressing the triggers and treatments. Monaldi Arch Chest Dis 2001.
8. Gaga M, Lambrou P, Papageorgiou N, Koulouris NG, Kosmas E, Fragakis S, Sofios C, Rasidakis A, Jordanoglou J: Eosinophils are a feature of upper and lower airway pathology in nonatopic asthma, irrespective of the presence of rhinitis. Clin Exp Allergy 2000; 30:663–669.
9. ten Brinke A, Grootendorst DC, Schmidt JT, De Bruine FT, van Buchem MA, Sterk PJ, Rabe KF, Bel EH: Chronic sinusitis in severe asthma is related to sputum eosinophilia. J Allergy Clin Immunol 2002;109(4):621–626.
10. Ragab S, Lund VJ, Scadding GK: Evaluation of medical and surgical management of chronic rhinosinusitis: a prospective randomized controlled trial. Laryngoscope 2004; 114:923–930.
11. Gwaltney JM Jr, Phillips CD, Miller RD, Riker DK: Computed tomographic study of the common cold. N Engl J Med 1994; 330:25–30.
12. Gordts F, Clement PA, Destryker A, Desprechins B, Kaufman L: Prevalence of sinusitis signs on MRI in a non-ENT paediatric population. Rhinology 1997; 35(4):154–157.
13. Patel K, Chavda V, Violaris N Pahor AL: Incidental paranasal sinus inflammatory changes in a British population. J Laryngol Otol 1996; 110:649–645.
14. Fokkens W, Lund V, Mullol J et al.: EAACI position paper on rhinosinusitis and nasal polyps. Rhinology suppl 20, 2007; 1–136.
15. Parikh A, Scadding GK, Gray P, Belvisi MG, Mitchell JA: High levels of nitric oxide synthase activity are associated with nasal polyp tissue from aspirin-sensitive patients. Acta Otolaryngol 2002; 122:302–305.
16. Pryor WA, Dooley MM, Church DF: Mechanisms of cigarette smoke toxicity: the inactivation of human α-1 proteinase inhibitor by nitric oxide/isoprene mixtures in air. Chem Biol Interact 1985; 54:171–183.
17. Borland C, Higenbottam T: Nitric oxide yields of contemporary UK, US and French cigarettes. Int J Epidemiol 1987; 16:31–34.
18. Ignarro LJ, Buga GM, Wood KS, Byrns RE, Chaudhuri G: Endothelium-derived relaxing factor produced and released from the artery and vein is nitric oxide. Proc Natl Acad Sci USA 1987; 84:9265–9269.
19. Palmer RM, Ferrige AG, Moncada S: Nitric oxide release accounts for the biological activity of endothelium-derived relaxing factor. Nature 1987; 327:524–526.
20. Moncada S, Palmer RM, Higgs EA: Nitric oxide: physiology, pathophysiology and pharmacology. Pharmacol Rev 1991; 43:109–142.
21. Coleman JW: Nitric oxide in immunity and inflammation. Int Immunopharmacol 2001; 1:1397–1406.
22. Gustafsson, LE, Leone MAM, Persson MG, Wiklund NP, Moncada S: Endogenous nitric oxide is present in the exhaled air or rabbits, guinea pigs and humans. Biochem Biophys Res Commun 1991; 181:852–857.
23. Alving K, Weitzberg E, Lundberg JM: Increased amount of nitric oxide in exhaled air of asthmatics. Eur Respir J 1993; 6:1368–1370.
24. Kharitonov SA, Barnes PJ: Does exhaled nitric oxide reflect asthma control? Yes, it does! Am J Respir Crit Care Med 2001;164(5):727–728.
25. Nakane M, Schmidt HH, Pollock JS, Frosterman U, Murad F: Cloned human brain nitric oxide synthase is highly expressed in skeletal muscle. FEBS Lett 1993; 316:175–180.
26. Marsden PA, Heng HH, Scherer SW, Stewart RJ, Hall AV, Shi XM et al.: Structure and chromosomal localization of the human constitutive endothelial nitric oxide synthase gene. J Biol Chem 1993; 268:17478–17488.
27. Nathan C, Xie QW: Nitric oxide synthases: roles, tolls and controls. Cell 1994; 78:915–918.

28. Lundberg JO, Weitzberg E, Nordvall SL, Kuylenstierna R, Lundberg JM, Alving K: Primarily nasal origin of exhaled nitric oxide and absence in Kartagener's syndrome. Eur Respir J 1994; 7:1501–1504.

29. Lundberg JO, Weitzberg E: Nasal nitric oxide in man. Thorax 1999; 54:947–952.

30. Lundberg JO, Farkas-Szallasi T, Weitzberg E, Rinder J, Lidholm J, Anggaard A et al.: High nitric oxide production in human paranasal sinuses. Nat Med 1995; 1:370–373.

31. Lundberg JO, Weitzberg E, Rinder J, Rudehill A, Jansson O, Wiklund NP et al.: Calcium-independent and steroid-resistant nitric oxide synthase activity in human paranasal sinus mucosa. Eur Respir J 1996; 9:1344–1347.

32. Haight JS, Djupesland PG, Qjan W, Chatkin JM, Furlott H, Irish J et al.: Does nasal nitric oxide come from the sinuses? J Otolaryngol 1999; 28:197–204.

33. Kawamoto H, Takimuda M, Takeno S et al.: Localization of nitric oxide synthase in human nasal mucosa with nasal allergy. Acta Otolaryngol Suppl 1998; 539:65–70.

34. Kawamoto H, Takeno S, Yajin K: Increased expression of inducible nitric oxide synthase in nasal epithelial cells in patients with allergic rhinitis. Laryngoscope 1999; 109:2015–2020.

35. Gianessi F, Fattori B, Ursino F et al.: Ultrastructural and ultracytochemical study of the human nasal respiratory epithelium in vasomotor rhinitis. Acta Otolaryngol 2003; 123:943–949.

36. Colantonio L, Brouillette L, Parikh A, Scadding GK: Paradoxical low nasal nitric oxide in nasal polyposis. Clin Exp Allergy 2002; 32:698–701.

37. Parikh A, Scadding GK, Gray P, Belvisi MG, Mitchell JA: High Levels of nitric oxide synthase activity are associated with nasal polyp tissue from aspirin-sensitive asthmatics. Acta Otolaryngol 2002; 122:3.

38. Ragab S, Lund VJ, Saleh HA, Scadding GK: Nasal nitric oxide in objective evaluation of chronic rhinosinusitis therapy. Allergy 2006; 61(6):717–724.

39. Kharitonov SA, Rajakulasingam K, O'Connor B, Durham SR, Barnes PJ: Nasal nitric oxide is increased in patients with asthma and allergic rhinitis and may be modulated by nasal glucocorticoids. J Allergy Clin Immunol 1997; 99(1 Pt 1):58–64.

40. Wodehouse T, Kharitonov SA, Mackay IS, Barnes PJ, Wilson R, Cole PJ: Nasal nitric oxide measurements for the screening of primary ciliary dyskinesia. Eur Respir J 2003; 21(1):43–47.

41. Maniscalco M, Sofia M, Weitzberg E, de Laurentiis G, Stanziola A, Rossillo V, Lundberg JO: Humming-induced release of nasal nitric oxide for assessment of sinus obstruction in allergic rhinitis:pilot study. Eur J Clin Invest 2004; 34:555–560.

42. Maniscalco M, Sofia M, Weitzberg E, Carratu L, Lundberg JO: Nasal nitric oxide measurements before and after repeated humming maneuvers. Eur Respir J 2003; 22:323–329.

Glenis K. Scadding

Royal National Throat, Nose & Ear Hospital, Gray's Inn Rd., London WC1X 8DA, UK, E-mail g.scadding@ucl.ac.uk

Epigallocatechine-3-gallate Reduces Allergic Lung Inflammation in Guinea Pig Asthma-Like Reaction

Y. Suzuki[1], F. Fabrizi[3], L. Giannini[3], S. Nistri[3], P.F. Mannaioni[3], H. Suzuki[2], D. Bani[4], and E. Masini[3]

[1]Department of Pediatrics, University of Verona, [2]Department of Neuroscience and Vision, Section of Biochemistry, University of Verona, Verona, [3]Department of Preclinical and Clinical Pharmacology, University of Florence, [4]Department of Anatomy, Histology and Forensic Medicine, Section of Histology, University of Florence, all Italy

Summary: Asthma is a common inflammatory airway disease whose prevalence is ever-increasing, and whose major pathophysiological hallmarks are mast cell activation, increased endothelial expression of adhesion molecules and enhanced leukocyte recruitment. In this study we used an animal model of asthma-like reaction to test the possible therapeutic effect of the polyphenol epigallocatechin-3-gallate (EGCG), the major and most active catechin derivative from green tea. Ovalbumin-sensitized guinea pigs placed in a respiratory chamber were challenged with ovalbumin. In 10 of them EGCG (25 mg/kg b.wt.) was given i.p. 20 min before ovalbumin challenge. In all animals we analyzed the changes in respiratory activity, lung tissue histopathology, mast cell activation (by granule release), eosinophilic infiltration (by major eosinophilic protein, eMBP), bronchial inflammatory response (by PGD_2 and LTB_4 measurement in bronchoalveolar lavage fluid). Severe respiratory abnormalities appeared in the sensitized animals soon after the antigen challenge, accompanied by bronchoconstriction, alveolar inflation and a marked increase in the assayed parameters of inflammatory cell recruitment and release of proinflammatory molecules in bronchoalveolar fluid. Pretreatment with EGCG significantly reduced all the above parameters. These findings indicate that EGCG can counteract allergic asthma-like reactions in sensitized guinea pigs and suggest that it may be useful for the treatment of asthma in the future.

Keywords: epigallocatechine-3-gallate, allergic, inflammation, asthma-like reaction, cytokines

Introduction

Asthma, defined by airway inflammation and hyperresponsiveness, is a major medical problem but despite decades of research the therapy of this pathological condition has remained essentially unchanged for the past 30 years. A large number of studies indicate that mast cells play a central role in the anaphylactic reactions [1]. Mast cells, activated by binding to allergen, release inflammatory mediators such as histamine, prostaglandins, and leukotrienes that eventually lead to severe lung tissue injury [2]. Mast cells also regulate the levels of allergic inflammatory response in the airways by producing cytokines, such as IL-5 and IL-13, which are reported to be critical for leukocyte recruitment, especially eosinophils [3]. Eosinophils, upon activation, release large amounts of oxygen-derived free radicals, high-energy oxidants and leukotrienes that in turn contribute to exacerbate the pathophysiological features of asthma [4].

Green tea and black tea contain various flavonoids, generally known as catechins. Epigallocatechine-3-gallate (EGCG) is the major catechin present in green tea. Several experimental studies have reported beneficial effects of EGCG in inflammation [5]. These effects are likely due to its anti-oxidant properties [6], as well as to the inhibition of cytokine gene expression [7], reduction of neutrophil migration [8], and inhibition of mast cell activation [9].

In this study we evaluated the anti-inflammatory effect of EGCG in a well established *in vivo* model of allergic asthma-like reaction in sensitized guinea pigs.

Materials and Methods

Male albino guinea pigs (Harlan, Milan, Italy) were used. The experimental protocol was basically the same used previously for similar purposes [10]. It complied with the recommendations of the European Economic Community (86/609/CEE) for the care and use of laboratory animals and was approved by the animal care committee of the University of Florence (Florence, Italy).

Group 1

Ten guinea pigs were injected with phosphate-buffered saline (PBS) (5 ml/kg i.p., plus 5 ml/kg s.c.). Two weeks later, they were treated with an aerosol of ovalbumin (OVA) (5 mg/ml) (Fluka, Buchs, Switzerland) suspended in PBS. They are referred to as naïve controls.

Other guinea pigs were sensitized with OVA (100 mg/Kg i.p., plus 100 mg/Kg s.c.), dissolved in water to a concentration of 20 mg/ml. Two weeks later, they were challenged with an aerosol of OVA (5 mg/ml PBS) to verify that sensitization had occurred. The animals that developed a clear-cut airway hyperresponsiveness to the inhaled antigen are referred to as sensitized controls. After 4–8 days, the sensitized animals were randomly di-

vided in 4 further groups, 10 animals each, and treated as indicated below.

Group 2

No further treatment. These animals are referred to as sensitized, not challenged controls.

Group 3

Treatment with a s.c. injection of 1 ml PBS. Thirty min later, the animals underwent challenge with OVA aerosol and are referred to as sensitized OVA-challenged animals.

Group 4

Treatment with a s.c. injection of EGCG (Sigma, Milan, Italy: 25 mg/kg b.wt.), dissolved in 1 ml of PBS. Thirty min later, the animals underwent challenge with OVA aerosol and are referred to as EGCG-pretreated OVA challenged animals.

The guinea pigs of all the groups, except group 2, were placed, one by one, in a whole body respiratory chamber, as described previously [10]. The changes in inner pressure in the respiratory chamber induced by breathing were monitored with a pressure transducer (Battaglia-Rangoni, Comerio, Italy) connected with a multichannel polygraph (Battaglia-Rangoni) for the registration of the respiratory activity. Upon stabilization of the breathing pattern, the animals were challenged with an aerosol of OVA for 10 sec. The changes in the respiratory activity of the animals subjected to the different treatments were recorded for 10 min after the aerosol administration. At the end of the period of observation, the animals were extracted from the respiratory chamber and killed. Bronchoalveolar lavage (BAL) was carried out by insertion of a cannula into the trachea and instillation of 3 ml of PBS. Bronchi were washed 3 times before collection of bronchoalveolar fluid, which was then centrifuged at 1100 g for 30 min. The cell-free supernatant was collected, its volume measured and used to evaluate the release of prostaglandin D_2 (PGD_2), the major cyclooxygenase product generated by activated mast cells dur-

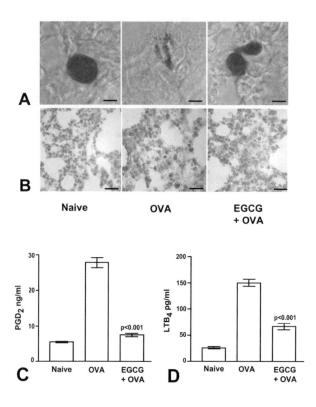

Figure 1. (A) Astra-Blue-stained mast cell granules from guinea pig lung of the different experimental groups. *Bar* 10 μm. (B) Immunohistochemical detection of eosinophilic major basic protein (eMBP) from guinea pig lung of the different experimental groups. *Bar* 50 μm. Pretreatment with EGCG prevents mast cell degranulation and lung eosinophils recruitment compared to the sensitized OVA challenged guinea pigs. (C) PGD_2 and (D) LTB_4 levels in BAL fluid of guinea pigs from the different experimental groups. Significance of differences (one-way ANOVA: each group n = 4) p < .001 *vs* sensitized OVA challenged guinea pigs. Pretreatment with EGCG reduces PGD_2 and LTB_4 levels in BAL fluid compared to the sensitized OVA challenged guinea pigs.

ing allergic response, and leukotriene B_4 (LTB_4), released by leukocytes and known to be involved in the recruitment of inflammatory cells in the tissue.

In all the animals, the thorax was then opened allowing for the gross appearance of lungs to be examined. Tissue specimens from the middle and the lower lobes of the right lung were excised and processed for histological and immunohistochemical analysis.

To reveal mast cell granules, histological sections, 5 μm thick, of Mota-fixed, paraffin-embedded lung tissue fragments were stained with Astra Blue (Fluka, Buchs, Switzerland). Immunohistochemistry for eosinophilic major basic protein (eMBP) was carried out to evaluate eosinophil infiltration in the tissue, as previously reported [10].

The pulmonary production of PGD_2 and LTB_4 in BAL fluid, were measured using a commercial enzyme-linked immunosorbent assay (ELISA) kit (Cayman Chemical, Ann Arbor, MI, USA), following the protocol provided by the manufacturer. Results are ex-

pressed as ng/ml and pg/ml of BAL fluid respectively.

Results and Discussion

In the sensitized OVA-challenged animals, severe respiratory abnormalities appeared soon after antigen challenge accompanied by bronchoconstriction and alveolar inflation (data not shown). In Astra-blue stained sections, mast cells showed a weakly stained cytoplasm, and frequent images of degranulating mast cells were detected (Figure 1A). The immunohistochemical analysis revealed a marked increase of eMBP-positive cells in the lung of sensitized OVA-challenged animals compared with the naïve controls (Figure 1B). Upon OVA challenge, the release of the proinflammatory mediators PGD_2 and LTB_4 in BAL fluid were significantly increased compared to naïve control guinea pigs (Figure 1C and 1D).

EGCG (25 mg/Kg b. wt.), given i.p. 30 min before OVA challenge, induced a clear-cut reduction of degranulated mast cells, whose cytoplasm appeared markedly stained for the presence of numerous secretion granules (Figure 1A), as well as of eosinophils infiltrating the lung tissue, as revealed by the decrease in eMBP-positive cells (Figure 1B).

The pretreatment of guinea pigs with EGCG before challenge with OVA significantly reduced the release of PGD_2 and LTB_4 in BAL fluid (Figure 1C and 1D).

Acute airway response to allergens chiefly depends on mast cells as well as eosinophils. Mast cell mediators may cause bronchoconstriction, smooth muscle cell proliferation, recruitment of other inflammatory cells, especially eosinophils, in the lung tissue, thereby sparkling a vicious circle that may exaggerate the pathophysiological aspects of asthma. The present study demonstrates that systemic pretreatment of OVA-sensitized guinea pigs with EGCG, the main polyphenol present in the green tea leaves, is able to reduce mast cell activation and release of PGD_2 by these cells, as well as eosinophil infiltration and production of LTB_4. This beneficial effect of EGCG can prevent severe lung tissue injury typical of asthmatic process, thus confirming the results obtained with this substance in other models of acute inflammation [11].

In summary, these findings provide evidence that EGCG can counteract allergic asthma-like reaction in sensitized guinea pigs and suggest its possible future use for the treatment of asthma.

Acknowledgment

This work was supported by a grant from the University of Florence and a grant from the Italian Ministry of Education, University and Research.

References

1. Boyce JA: The role of mast cells in asthma. Prostaglandins Leukot Essent Fatty Acids 2003; 69:195–205.
2. Schwartz LB, Austen KF: Structure and function of the chemical mediators of mast cells. Prog Allergy 1984; 34:271–321.
3. Hamelamann E, Gelfand EW: IL-5-induced airway eosinophilia – the key to asthma. Immunol Rev 200; 179:182–191.
4. Brightling CE, Pavord ID: Eosinophils in asthma and hyperresponsiveness. Am J Respir Crit Care Med 2004; 169:131–132.
5. Middleton E Jr, Kandaswami C, Theoharides TC: The effects of plant flavonoids on mammalian cells: implications for inflammation, heart disease, and cancer. Pharmacol Rev 2000; 52:673–751.
6. Nagai K, Jiang MH, Hada J, Nagata T, Yajima Y, Yamamoto S, Nishizaki T: Epigallocatechin gallate protects against NO stress-induced neuronal damage after ischemia by acting as an anti-oxidant. Brain Res 2002; 956:319–322.
7. Aneja R, Hake PW, Burroughs TJ, Denemberg AG, Wong HR, Zingarelli B: Epigallocatechin, a green tea polyphenol, attenuates myocardial ischemia reperfusion injury in rats. Mol Med 2004; 10:55–62.
8. Dona M, Dell'Aica I, Calabrese F, Benelli R, Morini M, Albini A, Garbisa S: Neutrophil restraint by green tea: inhibition of inflammation, associated angiogenesis, and pulmonary fibrosis. J Immunol 2003; 170:4335–4341.
9. Li GZ, Chai OH, Song CH: Inhibitory effects of epigallocatechin gallate on compound 48/80-induced mast cell activation and passive cutaneous anaphylaxis. Exp Mol Med 2005; 37:290–296.
10. Masini E, Bani D, Vannacci A, Pierpaoli S, Mannaioni PF, Comhair SAA, Xu W, Muscoli C, Erzurum SC, Salvemini D: Reduction of antigen-induced respiratory abnormalities and airway inflammation in sensitized guinea pigs by a superoxide dismutase mimetic. Free Radical Bio Med 2005; 39:520–531.
11. Townsend PA, Scarabelli TM, Pasini E, Menegazzi M, Suzuki H, Knight RA, Latchman DS, Stephanou A: Epigallocatechin-3 gallate inhibits STAT-1 activation and protects cardiac myocytes from ischemia/reperfusion-induced apoptosis. FASEB J 2004; 18:1621–1623.

Emanuela Masini

Department of Preclinical and Clinical Pharmacology, University of Florence, Viale Pieraccini 6, I-50139 Florence, Italy, Tel +39 55 427-1233, Fax +39 55 427-1280, E-mail emanuela.masini@unifi.it

Epidemiology of the Allergic Respiratory Syndrome in Residents of Urban US Public Housing Communities

A. Togias[1,2], Edward Horowitz[1], David Collins[1], Tasia Richards[1], Timothy Green[1], Kathleen Barnes[1], and Julian Poyser[1]

[1]Division of Allergy & Clinical Immunology and [2]Division of Respiratory and Critical Care Medicine, Johns Hopkins University School of Medicine, Baltimore, MD, USA

Summary: *Background:* Low-income urban communities in the US suffer from high asthma morbidity and mortality and efforts to understand the causes of this problem are needed. We report preliminary findings from a study conducted in Public Housing communities of Baltimore City. The goals are to determine a) the point prevalence of asthma, b) the point prevalence of nasal/sinus-related symptoms and their relationship to asthma and c) risk factors for asthma. *Methods:* The study is conducted in two phases, a door-to-door population survey using an upper and lower airway symptom questionnaire and a clinical evaluation for determination of allergic status, bronchial hyperresponsiveness or albuterol reversibility in a subgroup of the surveyed population. *Results:* In 600 participants, prevalence of "probable" and "possible asthma" by survey reaches 40%. With objective outcomes (clinical evaluation, $N = 101$) taken into account, the estimated point prevalence of asthma is 29.2%. Rhinitis/rhinosinusitis is present in 85.9% of asthmatics and the number of reported nasal/sinus symptoms is a predictor of asthma. Asthma is also predicted by the number of aeroallergen sensitivies with cockroach being the most common sensitizer. Sensitization to at least 2 allergens is present in 49% of nonasthmatic, nonrhinitic participants. *Conclusions:* Asthma is prevalent at epidemic proportions in these communities and is accompanied by very high rates of rhinitis/rhinosinusitis. The frequent presence of atopy in the absence of asthma or rhinitis indicates the existence of additional risk factors for this respiratory syndrome.

Keywords: asthma prevalence, rhinitis prevalence, rhinosinusitis prevalence, cockroach allergy, inner-city asthma, asthma diagnosis, rhinitis diagnosis, rhinosinusitis diagnosis

Introduction

The rationale for conducting this study derives from the fact that the residents of low income, urban communities have the highest asthma morbidity and mortality in the USA [1–3]. One of the factors contributing to this problem could be overall higher asthma prevalence, but the prevalence of this condition in African Americans, who constitute the majority of these communities, is only slightly higher than that of European Americans [4]. The point prevalence of asthma in the low-income, urban communities is not known.

Asthma and rhinitis/rhinosinusitis are strongly related and it has been proposed that they should be considered manifestations of the same syndrome in two parts of the respiratory tract [5]. The unusually high morbidity and mortality from asthma in the low-income, urban residents of the USA calls for examination of the relationships between upper and lower airway disease in this population in the context of assessing whether the clinical phenotype is similar to that of the general population.

Several studies have indicated that the severity of asthma in low-income, urban US populations is associated with allergy to cockroaches [6–8]. It is unknown, however, whether cockroach allergy is also a risk factor for asthma within a population that is almost uniformly exposed to these pests as a result of housing conditions.

Methods

Our study involves two phases: in the first phase, we are conducting a door-to-door survey in which we administer a respiratory questionnaire that queries the occurrence of specific upper and lower respiratory symptoms, within the previous 12 months, in the absence of a respiratory infection. In addition, the questionnaire records a previous physician diagnosis of asthma or rhinitis/sinus disease, as well as smoking history. An algorithm categorizes participants into groups utilizing the number of upper or lower respiratory symptoms they report in the survey questionnaire and the physician diagnosis of rhinitis/sinus disease or asthma. In the second phase of the study, a subgroup of first phase participants (≥ 6 years of age), selected to represent the clinical phenotype categories derived from the survey (no asthma, possible asthma, probable asthma) undergoes clinical evaluations, which include skin prick testing or serum specific IgE quantitation for 12 common aeroallergens, spirometry and methacholine bronchoprovocation or albuterol reversibility testing.

Both phases of the study have been approved by the Johns Hopkins University Institutional Review Board and written consent/assents are obtained from all participants.

Results

We currently have survey data (phase 1) from 600 individuals representing approximately 50% of the population of 2 public housing communities. The age of the participant population is 29.5 ± 21.8 (mean ± *SD*). African Americans represent 85.9%, 66.3% are female and 51.8% are younger than 18 years. In phase 2, 101 individuals have received clinical evaluation (age: 24.6 ± 15.9, African Americans: 93.1%, females: 65.4%, children: 52.5%).

Our algorithm places 22.5% of the surveyed population into the "probable asthma" category. Another 17.3% was categorized as "possible asthma." The clinical evaluation protocol confirmed that, out of the 51 participants with "no asthma" by survey, 84.3% had no objective evidence of lower airways disease, whereas airways hyperresponsiveness to methacholine or reversibility by albuterol was found in the remaining subjects (3 of those reported lower airway symptoms upon readministration of the survey questionnaire). Of the 26 individuals with "possible asthma" by survey, 65.4% were confirmed as asthmatics by the clinical evaluation; among the 24 participants with "probable asthma," 79% were confirmed, whereas another 12.5% had a COPD component. By extrapolating the clinical evaluation findings to the entire survey population, we report that the estimated point prevalence of asthma in the community is 29.2%. This prevalence is at least three times that of the reported prevalence of asthma in the US African American population [4].

Our survey diagnostic algorithm assigned the diagnosis of "probable rhinitis/rhinosinusitis" to those participants who reported the presence of at least 3 out of 5 nasal/sinus symptoms or those who reported at least 2 symptoms plus a diagnosis of "hay fever," "allergic rhinitis" or "sinus disease" by a physician. These criteria were fulfilled by 49.6% of the surveyed population. Of the 135 participants with "probable asthma" by survey, 116 (85.9%) had a "probable rhinitis" diagnosis. In contrast, among the 328 participants with "no asthma" by survey, 106 (32.3%) were classified as "probable rhinitis." A linear relationship was found between the number of reported nasal/sinus symptoms and the prevalence of "probable asthma" ($R^2 = 0.83$): among 134 participants who reported no nasal/sinus symptoms, the prevalence of "probable asthma" is 8%, whereas, among the 115 with 5 nasal/sinus symptoms, 41% have "probable asthma."

We have skin test or serum specific IgE data from 79 subjects who fall under the "no asthma/no rhinitis/rhinosinusitis" ($N = 21$), "asthma" ($N = 34$) and "no asthma/probable rhinitis/rhinosinusitis" ($N = 24$) final diagnoses. The number of aeroallergen sensitivities clearly differentiates the 3 groups with an average of 1.5, 5.3 and 2.9 sensitivities (out of 12 tested), respectively (ANOVA, $p = .0002$). The most common sensitization in the asthmatic group is against German cockroach (62%). Interestingly, German cockroach sensitization is also present in 34% of the "no asthma, no rhinitis/rhinosinusitis" subjects and does not differentiate these individuals from those with "no asthma/probable rhinitis/rhinosinusitis" (22%). Although, compared to the other two groups, the asthmatic participants appear to have higher prevalence of sensitization against every allergen tested, the indoor allergens that are, at this point of our investigation, statistically significant risk factors for asthma in comparison to rhinitis/rhinosinusitis alone are German and American cockroach, mouse and cat.

Discussion

Our data indicate that asthma should be considered an epidemic in the urban public housing communities of the US and should be treated as such. The associations of upper respiratory disease and of atopy with asthma are as strong as in other populations with the most important aeroallergens being those against which the residents of these communities are probably highly exposed to. However, the high prevalence of allergen sensitization in individuals with no upper or lower respiratory symptoms indicates that additional factors need to be considered in order to understand the reasons behind this major health problem.

Acknowledgment

The study was supported by US NIH grants R18-AI44840 and UO1-HL72455. Kathleen Barnes was supported in part by the Mary Beryl Patch Turnbull Scholar Program.

References

1. Wissow L, Gittelsohn A, Szklo M, Starfield B, Mussman M: Poverty, race, and hospitalization for childhood asthma. Am J Public Health 1988; 78:777–782.
2. Weiss K, Wagener D: Changing patterns of asthma mortality identifying target populations at high risk. J Am Med Assoc 1990; 264:683–1687.
3. Gupta R, Carrion-Carire V, Weiss K: The widening black/white gap in asthma hospitalizations and mortality. J Allergy Clin Immunol 2006; 117:351–358.
4. MMWR, Asthma prevalence and control characteristics by race/ethnicity – United States, 2002. MMWR 2004; 53:145–148.
5. Togias A: Rhinitis and asthma: evidence for respiratory system integration. J Allergy Clin Immunol 2003; 111:1171–1183.
6. Togias A, Horowitz E, Joyner D, Guydon L, Malveaux F: Evaluating the factors that relate to asthma severity in adolescents. Int Arch Allergy Immunol 1997; 113:87–95.
7. Rosenstreich D, Eggleston P, Kattan M, Baker D, Slavin R, Gergen P, Mitchell H, McNiff-Mortimer K, Lynn H, Ownby D, Malveaux F: The role of cockroach allergy and exposure to cockroach allergen in causing morbidity among inner-city children with asthma. N Engl J Med 1997; 336:1356–1363.
8. Gruchalla R, Pongracic J, Plaut M, Evans RI, Visness C, Walter M, Crain E, Kattan M, Morgan W, Steinbach S, Stout J, Malindzak G, Smart E, Mitchell H: Inner city asthma study: Relationship among sensitivity, allergen exposure, and asthma morbidity. J Allergy Clin Immunol 2005; 115:478–485.

Alkis Togias

DAIT/NIAID/NIH, 6610 Rockledge Drive, Bethesda, MD 20892, USA, Tel. +1 301 496-8973, Fax +1 301 402-0175, E-mail togiasa@niaid.nih.gov

Caspase Activation and Loss of Mitochondrial Membrane Potential Precedes Phosphatidylserine Exposure in CD45-Dependent Eosinophil Apoptosis

G.M. Walsh[1], M.G. Blaylock[1], and D.W. Sexton[2]

[1]*School of Medicine, Institute of Medical Sciences, University of Aberdeen, Foresterhill, UK*
[2]*BMRC, School of Medicine, Health Policy and Practice, University of East Anglia, Norwich, UK*

Summary: *Background:* Caspases are key molecules in the control of apoptosis but their contribution to eosinophil apoptosis is poorly understood. We examined the role of caspase-3, -8 and -9 in eosinophils ligated with CD45 mAb in parallel with externalization of phosphatidylserine and changes in mitochondrial transmembrane potential ($\Delta\Psi_m$). *Methods:* Purified human eosinophils were cultured for 2, 4 and 8 h with CD45RA, CD45RB, CD45RO, isotype-matched control mAb or dexamethasone (10^{-6} M). Caspase activity was analyzed using fluorochrome inhibitor of caspases technology in parallel with phosphatidylserine externalization measured by Annexin V binding. Both parameters and changes in $\Delta\Psi_m$ were analyzed using flow cytometry. *Results:* Eosinophils treated with CD45RA or CD45RB mAb did not exhibit significant increases in phosphatidylserine exposure at up to 8 h postligation. CD45RB mAb ligation induced caspase-3 activation at 4 and 8 h posttreatment. Significant ($p < .05$) caspase-8 activation followed CD45RB treatment at 2, 4 and 8 h while CD45RA failed to elicit a significant response. Caspase-9 activation was evident at all time points studied following CD45RB ligation while CD45RA activated caspase-9 at 8 h. CD45RO or dexamethasone treatment failed to activate caspases above constitutive levels at these early time-points although significant apoptosis was observed in dexamethasone-treated eosinophils after 24 h of treatment. CD45RB-dependent caspase activation was associated with changes in $\Delta\Psi_m$ at 8 h posttreatment. *Conclusions:* These observations suggest that different caspase pathways are involved in the very early apoptosis-inducing events following eosinophil CD45-dependent receptor-ligation and may aid development of more targeted and effective asthma therapy.

Keywords: eosinophils, apoptosis, CD45, caspases, mitochondria, cell surface molecules

Introduction

Much of the inflammation that underlies asthma pathogenesis is thought to be a consequence of the inappropriate accumulation of eosinophils in the tissues of the lung and the subsequent release of their potent proinflammatory arsenal of granule-derived basic proteins, mediators, cytokines and chemokines [1]. Apoptosis or programmed cell death is a central and essential process in the resolution of inflammation. Furthering our understanding of the processes controlling apoptosis and phagocytic clearance of eosinophils in the asthmatic lung is therefore an important and growing area of research [2, 3]. Caspases, aspartate-specific cysteine proteases, regulate the execution phase of apoptosis [4]. Two main pathways, the intrinsic and the extrinsic, have been defined for caspase activation in cells undergoing apoptosis. Previous studies on the role of caspases in human eosinophil apoptosis have reported conflicting findings. For example, caspase-3 and -8 involvement in glucocorticoid-induced [5] or Fas-induced eosinophil apoptosis [6, 7] have been reported while, in contrast, others have reported that dexamethasone-induced apoptosis failed to induce specific caspase-3 or -8 activity in eosinophils compared with spontaneous apoptosis [8]. However, the majority of these studies relied on apoptosis and caspase detection at relatively late periods ($\geq$ 18 h). Our previous findings demonstrated that mAb-dependent ligation of the transmembrane protein tyrosine phosphatase CD45 is a potent and rapid inducer of apoptosis in human eosinophils [9]. We therefore investigated the differential and early activation of caspases-3, -9, and -8 using the novel FLICA (fluorochrome inhibitor of caspases) technique and flow cytometry together with examination of changes in phosphatidylserine (PS) exposure and mitochondrial transmembrane potential ($\Delta\Psi_m$) in human peripheral blood eosinophils following mAb-dependent membrane receptor ligation of CD45 and CD45 isoforms.

Materials and Methods

Purified human eosinophils were incubated for varying time points in 96-well flexible flat-bottomed plates alone or with experimental antibodies or isotype-matched controls as described [9]. All isotype control and experimental mAb were used at a final concentration of 10 µg/ml. Eosinophils were assessed for concurrent apoptosis and viability as determined by annexin V-FITC binding to exposed phos-

phatidylserine and propidium iodide (PI) uptake as previously described [9]. Assay of caspase activity and mitochondrial membrane potential ($\Delta\Psi_m$) were both performed using established protocols [10].

Results

Eosinophils treated with CD45RA or CD45RB mAb did not exhibit significant increases in phosphatidylserine exposure at up to 8 h postligation. The same cells exhibited significant ($p < .05$) caspase-3 activation at 4 and 8 h posttreatment with CD45RB mAb. Significant ($p < .05$) caspase-8 activation followed CD45RB treatment at 2, 4, and 8 h, while CD45RA failed to elicit a significant response. Caspase-9 activation was evident at all time points studied following CD45RB ligation while CD45RA activated caspase-9 at 8 h. CD45RO ligation or dexamethasone treatment failed to activate caspases above constitutive levels at these early time-points although significant apoptosis was observed in dexamethasone-treated eosinophils after 24 h of treatment. CD45RB-dependent caspase activation was associated with changes in $\Delta\Psi m$ at 4 h posttreatment; the same loss of $\Delta\Psi m$ was not seen with CD45RA.

Discussion

These observations suggest that different caspase pathways are involved in the apoptosis-inducing events following eosinophil CD45-dependent receptor-ligation and these precede membrane phosphatidylserine exposure. We clearly demonstrated that both the extrinsic (caspase 8) and intrinsic (caspase 9) pathways are activated in a time dependent fashion following CD45 receptor ligation and that there was significant mitochondrial involvement in CD45RB induced eosinophil apoptosis. This is an interesting observation as there is evidence that the priority of mitochondrial function in eosinophils is to initiate apoptosis, even though they do not provide significant respiration [11]. Both caspase and mitochondrial involvement were observed at very early time-points and preceded phosphatidlyserine exposure following CD45-dependent receptor-ligation. In contrast, dexamethasone did not activate caspases at these early time-points. These findings emphasize the early nature of the intracellular events controlling mAb-dependent apoptosis induction in human eosinophils and may aid development of more targeted and effective asthma therapy.

Acknowledgment

This work was supported by the Scottish Hospitals Research Trust and Tenovus Scotland.

References

1. Walsh GM: Advances in the immunobiology of eosinophils and their role in disease. Crit Rev Clin Lab Sci 1999; 36:453–496.
2. Walsh GM: Eosinophil apoptosis: mechanisms and clinical relevance in asthmatic and allergic inflammation. Brit J Haematol 2000; 111:61–67.
3. Walsh GM, Sexton DW, Blaylock MG: Eosinophils, bronchial epithelial cells and steroids – new insights into the resolution of inflammation in asthma. J Endocrinology 2003; 178:37–43.
4. Riedl SJ, Shi, Y: Molecular mechanisms of caspase regulation during apoptosis. Nat Rev Mol Cell Biol 2004; 5:897–907.
5. Létuvé S, Druilhe A, Grandsaigne M, Aubier M, Pretolan M: Critical role of mitochondria, but not caspases, during glucocorticosteriod-induced human eosinophil apoptosis. Am J Respir Cell Mol Biol 2002; 26:565–571.
6. Letuve S, Druilhe A, Grandsaigne M, Aubier M, Pretolani M: Involvement of caspases and mitochondria in Fas ligation-induced eosinophil apoptosis: modulation by interleukin-5 and interferon-γ. J Leuk Biol 2001; 70:167–175.
7. Zangirilli J, Robertson N, Shetty A: Effect of IL-5, glucocorticoid, and Fas ligation on Bcl-2 homologue expression and caspase activation in circulating human eosinophils. Clin Exp Immunol 2000; 120:12–21.
8. Zhang JP, Wong CK, Lam WK: Role of caspases in dexamethasone-induced apoptosis and activation of c-Jun NH2-terminal kinase and p38 mitogen-activated protein kinase in human eosinophils. Clin Exp Immunol 2000; 122:20–27.
9. Blaylock MG, Sexton DW, Walsh GM: Ligation of CD45 and the isoforms CD45RA and CD45RB accelerates the rate of constitutive apoptosis in human eosinophils. J Allergy Clin Immunol 1999; 104:1244–1250.
10. Al-Rabia MW, Blaylock MG, Sexton DW, Walsh GM: Membrane receptor-mediated apoptosis and caspase activation in the differentiated EoL-1 eosinophilic cell line. J Leukoc Biol 2004; 75:1045–1055.
11. Peachman KK, Lyles DS, Bass DA: Mitochondria in eosinophils: functional role in apoptosis but not respiration. PNAS 2001; 98:1717–1722.

Garry M. Walsh

School of Medicine, IMS Building, University of Aberdeen, Foresterhill, Aberdeen AB25 2ZD, UK, Tel. +44 1224-552786, Fax +44 1224-555766, E-mail g.m.walsh@abdn.ac.uk

Impact of IL-13 on Epidermal Inflammation in Atopic Dermatitis

M. Wittmann, R. Purwar, and T. Werfel

Department of Dermatology and Allergology, Hannover Medical School, Germany

Summary: *Background:* Skin inflammation in atopic dermatitis (AD) is characterized by lymphocytic infiltration. Recent studies have described that IL-13 acts on epithelial cells via inducing chemokines. In this study we investigated the role of IL-13 stimulated human primary keratinocytes (HPKs) in recruitment of lymphocytes and further delineated the mechanism of enrichment of these cells. *Methods:* Responsiveness of HPK to IL-13 was determined by ELISA based detection of secreted chemokines and active matrix metalloproteinase 9 (MMP-9). We performed migration assays with CD4+ T-cells. *Results:* We observed preferential migration of CCR4+ CD4+ T-cells toward IL-13 stimulated HPKs. Interestingly, CCR4+ CD4+ T-cells from AD patients showed a higher chemotactic response than those from healthy individuals. We observed a marked increase in the expression of CCL-22/MDC in IL-13 stimulated HPKs as compared to unstimulated cells. In addition we found that IL-13 stimulated HPKs secreted biologically active MMP-9 which could degrade collagen type IV of the basement membrane. *Conclusions:* Taken together our data suggest that IL-13 stimulated HPKs participate in enriching Th2-cells in lesional skin of acute AD and facilitate their infiltration into the epidermal compartment by degrading the basement membrane.

Keywords: keratinocytes, atopic dermatitis, IL-13/IL-4, matrix metalloproteinases, human, chemokines

Introduction

IL-13 has been shown to be a crucial mediator of Th-2 dominant immune responses [1]. It has been described that, in AD skin lesions, there is a higher number of IL-13 positive cells in the acute phase as compared to the chronic phase [2]. CD4+ T-cells and mast cells are major sources of IL-13 in acute lesions and in peripheral blood of AD [3]. IL-13 does not exert direct effects on T-cells, which lack a functional IL-13 receptor (IL-13R). In murine models of asthma IL-13 has been shown to modulate the expression of chemokine, matrix metalloproteinases and TGF-β_1 and therefore facilitates cell migration and induces tissue fibrosis [4, 5]. Tissue remodeling is also a pathophysiological feature of chronic eczematous skin diseases. The aim of this study was to investi-

gate the influence of IL-13 stimulated human primary keratinocytes (HPKs) on attraction of effector subsets of CD4+ T-cells and the modulation of matrix metalloproteinases (MMP), which play an important role in tissue remodeling.

Material and Methods

CD4+ T-cells from healthy individuals or AD patients were purified using negative selection (Miltenyi Biotech, Bergisch Gladbach, Germany). Primary cultures of normal human keratinocytes were prepared as described previously [6]. For flow cytometric analysis labeled mAb were used. For migration assays CD4+ T-cells were added to the top chamber of 5-μm pore size polycarbonate transwell culture insert containing either un-stimulated or IL-13 stimulated HPKs in the bottom chamber. The numbers of migrated cells were counted by Truecount tubes (BD Biosciences, Heidelberg, Germany). Concentrations of CCL-22 (DuoSet ELISA, R&D Systems, Wiesbaden, Germany) and MMP-9 (Biotrak MMP-9 activity assay, Amersham Biosciences Europe GmbH, Germany) were determined in the cell free supernatants.

Results

IL-13 Stimulated HPKs Preferentially Attract CCR4+ CD4+ T-Cells

In a transwell chemotaxis assay, we observed after 3 h a significant increase in absolute number of migrated CD4$^+$ T-cells in response to IL-13 stimulated HPKs as compared to negative controls. A significant enrichment of CCR4$^+$ CD4$^+$ T-cells but not CXCR3$^+$CD4$^+$ T-cells was observed by IL-13 stimulated HPKs as compared to un-stimulated cells.

IL-13 Stimulated HPKs Attract More CCR4+ CD4+ T-Cells from AD Patients than Healthy Individuals

Interestingly, chemotaxis indices of CCR4$^+$ CD4$^+$ T-cells from AD (chemotaxis index 1.64 ± 0.15, p = .01) were significantly higher than those from healthy individuals (chemotaxis index 1.34 ± 0.11, p = .02).

IL-13 Induces CCL22/MDC but No CCL17/TARC. CCL22/MDC Is Responsible for CCR4+ CD4+ T-Cells Migration

To confirm that the observed effect on migration of Th2-cells was due to chemokine production by HPKs, we studied the ability of HPKs to synthesize chemokines. We showed that CCL22/MDC mRNA was upregulated 2–8 fold by IL-13 stimulation. However, CCL17/TARC was not detected in IL-13 stim-

ulated HPKs. HPKs produced pg/ml quantities of CCL22/MDC (mean 73.54 ± 17.26, range 24.5–157 pg/ml, p = .0004) upon stimulation with IL-13 (50 ng/ml). Blocking of CCL-22/MDC in IL-13 stimulated HPKs by a neutralizing antibody resulted in 70–90% inhibition in migration of CCR4$^+$ CD4$^+$ T-cells.

IL-13 Induces MMP-9 in Epidermal KCs

We investigated the bioactivity of MMP-9 in cell free supernatants of HPK by a BioTrak Activity Assay (Amersham Biosciences, Munich, Germany). IL-13 induced a functionally active form of MMP-9 in HPK. To compare *in vitro* data with *ex vivo* findings, we used 3 mm punch biopsies from healthy individuals and cultured them in a HPK growth medium with or without IL-13 (50 ng/ml). Biopsies were stained for MMP-9 which was very prominent in the basal epidermal layer in IL-13 stimulated biopsies as compared to un-stimulated ones.

Coexpression of MMP-9 and IL-13 in Eczema Patients

IL-13 and MMP-9 mRNA expression were analyzed by qRT-PCR in biopsies from lesional eczematous skin. As expected, we observed higher expression of IL-13 in acute eczema as compared to chronic eczematous skin lesions. We also found a higher expression of MMP-9 in acutely inflamed skin which point to a coexpression of IL-13 and MMP-9.

Discussion

During inflammation, the migration of inflammatory cells is tightly regulated by the coordinated expression of proteinases, cytokines and chemokines. Our study demonstrates that IL-13 stimulated HPKs express CCL22/MDC that preferentially attract CCR4$^+$ CD4$^+$ T-cells. Our results point to the fact that the higher rate of migration of CCR4$^+$ CD4$^+$ T-cells in AD patients may not be only due to a higher frequency of CCR4$^+$ cells in AD patients than those of healthy individuals [7] but also because of higher migratory capacity of CCR4+ cells from AD than healthy individuals. There are evidences suggesting that MMPs play a role in tissue remodeling and migration of cells within tissues. In this study, we have demonstrated that IL-13 increases the production of MMP-9 by human HPK. IL-13 activated HPKs preferentially enrich Th2-cells by means of CCL22/MDC. Secretion of MMP-9, which can degrade basement membrane components, may contribute to the infiltration of inflammatory cells into the epidermis in atopic dermatitis.

Acknowledgment

This study was supported by DFG grant SFB 566, A6.

References

1. Wynn TA: IL-13 effector functions. Annu Rev Immunol 2003; 21:425.
2. Hamid Q, Naseer T, Minshall EM, Song YL, Boguniewicz M, Leung DY: In vivo expression of IL-12 and IL-13 in atopic dermatitis. J Allergy Clin Immunol 1996; 98:225.
3. Obara W, Kawa Y, Ra C, Nishioka K, Soma Y, Mizoguchi M: T-cells and mast cells as a major source of interleukin-13 in atopic dermatitis. Dermatology 2002; 205:11.
4. Lee CG, Homer RJ, Zhu Z, Lanone S, Wang X, Koteliansky V, Shipley JM, Gotwals P, Noble P, Chen Q, Senior RM, Elias JA: Interleukin-13 induces tissue fibrosis by selectively stimulating and activating transforming growth factor β(1). J Exp Med 2001; 194:809.
5. Zhu Z, Homer RJ, Wang Z, Chen Q, Geba GP, Wang J, Zhang Y, Elias JA: Pulmonary expression of interleukin-13 causes inflammation, mucus hypersecretion, subepithelial fibrosis, physiologic abnormalities, and eotaxin production. J Clin Invest 1999; 103:779.
6. Wittmann M, Purwar R, Hartmann C, Gutzmer R, Werfel T: Human keratinocytes respond to interleukin-18: implication for the course of chronic inflammatory skin diseases. J Invest Dermatol 2005; 124:1225.
7. Nakatani T, Kaburagi Y, Shimada Y, Inaoki M, Takehara K, Mukaida N, Sato S: CCR4 memory CD4+ T lymphocytes are increased in peripheral blood and lesional skin from patients with atopic dermatitis. J Allergy Clin Immunol 2001; 107:353.

Miriam Wittmann

Hannover Medical School, Department of Dermatology and Allergology, Ricklinger Str. 5, D-30449 Hannover, Tel. +49 511 9246-278, Fax +49 511 9246-440, E-mail wittmann.miriam@mh-hannover.de

PPARγ- and Toll-Like Receptor-2 Agonists

Might Have Therapeutical Value in Respiratory Syncytial Virus (RSV)-Induced Airway Disease: PPARγ Agonists May Act in a PPARγ-Independent Manner

R. Arnold and W. König

Institute of Medical Microbiology, Otto-von-Guericke University, Magdeburg, Germany

Summary: Background: Respiratory syncytial virus (RSV) is worldwide the major causative agent of severe lower respiratory tract disease in infants. Despite 50 years of intense research there exist neither an active vaccine nor a promising antiviral and antiinflammatory therapy. Recently, we showed that peroxisome proliferator-activated receptor-γ (PPARγ) ligands diminish the inflammatory response of the infected human lung epithelial cells and significantly inhibit the replication of RSV. However, it is still not known whether these agonists act thereby in a PPARγ-dependent or – independent manner. Furthermore, it is important to know whether they still play a protective role when applied subsequently to RSV-infection. *Methods:* By means of FACS analysis we determined the expression of ICAM-1 and the viral F protein on RSV-infected human lung epithelial cells (A549) which were cultured in the presence or absence of the following PPARγ agonists: troglitazone, 15d-PGJ$_2$, and Fmoc-Leu, respectively. *Results:* We observed a markedly reduced cell surface expression of ICAM-1 on RSV-infected A549 cells when PPARγ agonists were added as late as 20 h postinfection. The PPARγ agonist-mediated inhibition of the viral F protein expression on RSV-infected A549 cells was not counter-regulated by the specific PPARγ antagonist GW-9662. *Conclusions:* Our data suggest that PPARγ agonists have still a protective effect in the course of RSV-infection when added at later times of infection. They may act thereby primarily via PPARγ-independent mechanisms.

Keywords: ICAM-1, viral F protein, inflammation, RSV, PPARγ, A549, TLR-2

Respiratory syncytial virus (RSV) is worldwide the leading cause for severe lower respiratory tract infection (LRTI) in infants requiring hospitalization [1]. Evidence accumulated that RSV-induced LRTI leads to bronchiolitis, pneumonia, airway hyperresponsiveness (AHR) and apparently asthma. Persistent lung function abnormalities were even observed 20 years following RSV infection [2]. Evidence accumulated that the lung endothelial cells in addition to lung epithelial cells are also permissive for productive RSV infection and that they contribute to the induced inflammatory response [3]. The viral lytic replication process, the fulminant cytopathic effect primarily mediated by the viral fusion protein (F protein), and the RSV-induced intense inflammatory lung response are considered to be responsible for the detrimental outcome of RSV infection. Peroxisome proliferator-activated receptors (PPARs) are ligand-activated transcription factors which form a subfamily of the nuclear receptor gene family consisting of three isotypes: PPARα, PPARβ and PPARγ [4]. Quite recently, we reported that the addition of specific peroxisome-proliferator activated receptor-γ (PPARγ) agonists (15d-PGJ$_2$, Fmoc-Leu, ciglitazone, and troglitazone) to RSV-infected human lung epithelial cells (A549) led to a significantly reduced cell surface expression of ICAM-1 [5]. Furthermore, the release of immunomodulatory (IL-6, GM-CSF) and proinflammatory cytokines (IL-1α, TNF-α) as well as of chemokines (IL-8, RANTES) was markedly reduced [6]. Most intriguingly, the replication of RSV was simultaneously inhibited [7]. As a consequence, the addition of PPARγ agonists might protect the RSV-infected lung by the counterregulation of the RSV-induced inflammatory host response as well as the inhibition of the viral lifecycle. In addition, we observed an RSV-dependent upregulation of toll-like receptor (TLR)-2 on A549 cells. Ligation of TLR-2 reduced the RSV-induced expression of ICAM-1 and release of GM-CSF suggesting an antiinflammatory potential. Our data suggest that specific stimulation of PPARγ and TLR-2 in RSV-infected human lung epithelial cells might have beneficial effects in the control of RSV-induced lung disease.

However, important questions remain to be answered. Do the PPARγ agonists still supply their protective potential when added to already infected cells? And do the agonists activate primarily PPARγ-dependent or PPARγ-independent signaling pathways?

To address these questions we performed *in vitro* experiments analyzing the ICAM-1 and F protein expression on RSV-infected A549 cells. Cell monolayers of the human pulmonary type II epithelial cell line A549 (ATCC) were treated with troglitazone, Fmoc-Leu (Merck Biosciences), 15-deoxy-Δ^{12,14}-prostaglandin J$_2$ (15d-PGJ$_2$) (Biomol), and solvent DMSO (Sigma), respectively, prior to and after RSV-infection (Long strain (ATCC), multiplicity of infection = 3). To determine whether PPARγ-dependent pathways are activated by the given PPARγ agonists, the cells were additionally preincubated with the PPARγ antagonist GW-9662 (Cayman Chemicals) for 30 min. Subsequently, PPARγ agonists were added for another 30 min before RSV infection proceeded for 2 h. Thereafter, cells were washed and compounds added again in the

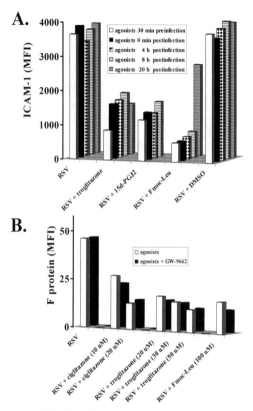

Figure 1. (A) Effect of PPARγ agonists on the RSV-induced ICAM-1 cell surface expression on A549 cells. The agonists troglitazone (50 μM), 15d-PGJ$_2$ (20 μM), Fmoc-Leu (200 μM), and the vehicle control DMSO (0.2%) were added to the RSV-infected cells at the given times. All cells were cultured for 48 h postinfection. The constitutive ICAM-1 expression was 391 ± 42 MFI. (B) Viral F protein expression on RSV-infected A549 cells. Cells were preincubated with ciglitazone, troglitazone, Fmoc-Leu, and medium, respectively, or in combination with the PPARγ antagonist GW-9662 (20 μM). Following infection the cells were incubated for 48 h in the presence of freshly added agonists and GW-9662, respectively.

same time order. After 48 h of incubation (DMEM, 2% FCS, streptomycin (100 μg/ml), penicillin (100 IU/ml)) the cells were stained with PE-labeled mouse anti-human ICAM-1 mAb (BD Biosciences) or with the mouse anti-RSV F protein mAb (Biotrend) plus a Cy3-labeled detecting goat anti-mouse IgG (H + L) (Dianova).

As can be seen from Figure 1A, the RSV-induced upregulation of ICAM-1 on A549 cells was significantly reduced when the PPARγ agonists under study, i.e., troglitazone,

15d-PGJ$_2$, and Fmoc-Leu, respectively, were added prior to infection (–30 min). Moreover, the ICAM-1 expression was potently suppressed when agonists were added directly after RSV-infection (0 min) suggesting that the agonists neither kill the virus nor interfere with the primary adhesion and fusion process. Most intriguingly, the agonists still inhibited the RSV-induced ICAM-1 expression when applied as late as 20 h postinfection. For control, RSV-infected cells were also incubated with DMSO alone, the solvent for the PPARγ agonists (0.2%). As shown, DMSO had no impact on the RSV-induced ICAM-1 expression.

The results presented in Figure 1B show that the PPARγ antagonist GW-9662 did not counter-regulate the ciglitazone-, troglitazone-, and Fmoc-Leu-mediated suppression of the viral F protein. Therefore, one may suggest that the observed antiviral and antiinflammatory activities of the PPARγ agonists may be performed by PPARγ-independent mechanisms. However, the PPARγ agonist mediated inhibition of the RSV-induced binding activity of NF-κB and AP-1 seems to be intimately involved [6]. Future studies have to address this point in more detail.

In summary, our presented *in vitro* data supply evidence that PPARγ agonists inhibit the RSV-induced upregulation of ICAM-1 even when applied 1 day after RSV-infection. Since the addition of the PPARγ antagonist GW-9662 was without any influence on viral protein synthesis PPARγ-independent signaling pathways seem to be activated by PPARγ agonists in the RSV-infected human lung epithelial cell.

References

1. Hall CB: Respiratory syncytial virus and parainfluenza virus. N Engl J Med 2001; 344:1917–1928.
2. Korppi, M, Piippo-Savolainen E, Korhonen K, Remes S: Respiratory morbidity 20 years after RSV infection in infancy. Pediatr Pulmonol 2004; 38:155–160.
3. Arnold, R, König W: Respiratory syncytial virus infection of human lung endothelial cells enhances selectively ICAM-1 expression. J Immunol 2005; 174:7359–7367.
4. Clark RB: The role of PPARs in inflammation and immunity. J Leukoc Biol 2002; 71:388–400.
5. Arnold, R, König W: Peroxisome proliferator-activated receptor-γ ligands have anti-inflammatory and antiviral activity in the course of respiratory syncytial virus infection. In H. Löwenstein et al. (Eds.), From genes to phenotypes. The basis of future allergy management. Proceedings of the 25th Symposium of the Collegium Internationale Allergologicum. Allergy Clin Immunol Int: J World Allergy Org 2005; Suppl. 2:97–99. Hogrefe & Huber.
6. Arnold R, König W: Peroxisome proliferator-activated receptor-γ agonists inhibit the release of proinflammatory cytokines from RSV-infected epithelial cells. Virology 2006; 346:427–439.
7. Arnold R, König W: Peroxisome proliferator-activated receptor-γ agonists inhibit the replication of respiratory syncytial virus in human lung epithelial cells. Virology 2006; 50:335–346.

Wolfgang König

Otto-von-Guericke University, Institute of Medical Microbiology, Leipzigerstr. 44, D-39120 Magdeburg, Germany, Tel. +49 391 671-3393, Fax +49 391 671-3384, E-mail wolfgang.koenig@medizin.uni-magdeburg.de

Author Index

Keyword Index